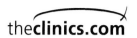

UROLOGIC CLINICS
OF NORTH AMERICA

Minimally Invasive
Genitourinary Procedures

GUEST EDITOR
Howard N. Winfield, MD

August 2008 • Volume 35 • Number 3

SAUNDERS

An Imprint of Elsevier, Inc.
PHILADELPHIA   LONDON   TORONTO   MONTREAL   SYDNEY   TOKYO

W.B. SAUNDERS COMPANY
A Division of Elsevier Inc.

1600 John F. Kennedy Boulevard • Suite 1800 • Philadelphia, Pennsylvania 19103-2899

http://www.theclinics.com

UROLOGIC CLINICS OF NORTH AMERICA   Volume 35, Number 3
August 2008   ISSN 0094-0143
Editor: Kerry Holland   ISBN-13: 978-1-4160-6366-7
                                                              ISBN-10: 1-4160-6366-8

Urologic Clinics of North America (ISSN 0094-0143) is published quarterly by Elsevier Inc., 360 Park Avenue South, New York, NY 10010-1710. Months of issue are February, May, August, and November. Business and Editorial Offices: 1600 John F. Kennedy Blvd., Suite 1800, Philadelphia, PA 19103-2899. Customer Service Office: 6277 Sea Harbor Drive, Orlando, FL 32887-4800. Periodicals postage paid at New York, NY and additional mailing offices. Subscription prices are $249.00 per year (US individuals), $394.00 per year (US institutions), $285.00 per year (Canadian individuals), $472.00 per year (Canadian institutions), $333.00 per year (foreign individuals), and $472.00 per year (foreign institutions). Foreign air speed delivery is included in all *Clinics* subscription prices. All prices are subject to change without notice. **POSTMASTER:** Send address changes to *Urologic Clinics of North America*, Elsevier Periodicals Customer Service, 6277 Sea Harbor Drive, Orlando, FL 32887-4800. **Customer Service: 1-800-654-2452 (US). From outside the United States, call 1-407-563-6020. Fax: 1-407-363-9661. E-mail: JournalsCustomerService-usa@elsevier.com.**

Reprints. For copies of 100 or more, of articles in this publication, please contact the Commercial Reprints Department, Elsevier Inc., 360 Park Avenue South, New York, New York 10010-1710. Tel.: (212) 633-3813, Fax: (212) 462-1935, e-mail: reprints@elsevier.com.

Urologic Clinics of North America is covered in MEDLINE/PubMed (*Index Medicus*), *Excerpta Medica*, *Current Contents/Clinical Medicine*, *Science Citation Index*, and *ISI/BIOMED.*

Printed in the United States of America.

GUEST EDITOR

HOWARD N. WINFIELD, MD, Professor of Urology; and Director, Urologic Laparoscopic Surgery & Endourology, University of Iowa Hospitals & Clinics, Iowa City, Iowa

CONTRIBUTORS

SERO ANDONIAN, MD, Endourology Fellow, Smith Institute for Urology, North Shore-Long Island Jewish Health System, New Hyde Park, New York

ANDRE BERGER, MD, Research Fellow, Department of Urology, Center for Laparoscopic and Robotic Surgery, Glickman Urological and Kidney Institute, Cleveland Clinic, Cleveland, Ohio

GEOFFREY N. BOX, MD, Endourology Fellow, Department of Urology, University of California, Irvine Medical Center, Orange, California

BENJAMIN K. CANALES, MD, MPH, Assistant Professor of Urology, University of Florida, Gainesville, Florida

DAVID CANES, MD, Clinical Fellow, Department of Urology, Center for Laparoscopic and Robotic Surgery, Glickman Urological and Kidney Institute, Cleveland Clinic, Cleveland, Ohio

RALPH V. CLAYMAN, MD, Professor and Chair, Department of Urology, University of California, Irvine Medical Center, Orange, California

JEAN J.M.C.H. DE LA ROSETTE, MD, PhD, Department of Urology, Academic Medical Center, University of Amsterdam, Meibergdreef, Amsterdam, The Netherlands

JOHN D. DENSTEDT, MD, Chair/Chief, Department of Surgery, University of Western Ontario, London, Ontario, Canada

MIHIR M. DESAI, MD, Associate Professor and Director, Stevan B. Streem Center for Endourology; and Department of Urology, Center for Laparoscopic and Robotic Surgery, Glickman Urological and Kidney Institute, Cleveland Clinic, Cleveland, Ohio

STEVEN G. DOCIMO, MD, Professor of Urology and Vice Chairman, Department of Urology, University of Pittsburgh Medical Center; and Director of Urology, Division of Pediatric Urology, Children's Hospital of Pittsburgh of UPMC, Pittsburgh, Pennsylvania

DAVID A. DUCHENE, MD, Assistant Professor of Urology; and Director of Minimally Invasive Urological Surgery and Stone Disease, University of Kansas Medical Center, Kansas City, Kansas

AMR F. FERGANY, MD, Staff, Center for Laparoscopy and Robotics, and Comprehensive Center for Urologic Oncology, Glickman Urological and Kidney Institute, Cleveland Clinic; and Associate Professor of Surgery, Cleveland Clinic Lerner School of Medicine at Case Western University, Cleveland, Ohio

JOHN M. FITZPATRICK, MCh, FRCSI, FC Urol (SA), FRCSGlas, FRCS, Department of Surgery, Mater Misericordiae Hospital, University College, Dublin, Ireland

MATTHEW T. GETTMAN, MD, Associate Professor, Department of Urology, Mayo Clinic, Rochester, Minnesota

INDERBIR S. GILL, MD, Chairman, Department of Urology, Glickman Urological and Kidney Institute, Cleveland Clinic; and Professor of Surgery, Cleveland Clinic Lerner School of Medicine at Case Western University, Cleveland, Ohio

MARK L. GONZALGO, MD, PhD, Department of Urology, James Buchanan Brady Urological Institute, The Johns Hopkins Medical Institutions, Baltimore, Maryland

STAVROS GRAVAS, MD, PhD, Department of Urology, University Hospital of Larissa, Larissa, Greece

MATTHEW H. HAYN, MD, Resident Physician, Department of Urology, University of Pittsburgh Medical Center, Pittsburgh, Pennsylvania

GÜNTER JANETSCHEK, MD, Professor of Urology, Department of Urology, Elisabethinen Hospital, Linz, Austria

KATHLEEN C. KOBASHI, MD, Head, Section of Urology and Renal Transplantation, Virginia Mason Medical Center, Seattle, Washington

JAIME LANDMAN, MD, Associate Professor and Director of Minimally Invasive Urology, Columbia University Medical Center, New York, New York

BENJAMIN R. LEE, MD, Associate Professor of Urology, Smith Institute for Urology, North Shore-Long Island Jewish Health System, New Hyde Park, New York

DANIEL S. LEHMAN, MD, Fellow, Department of Urology, Minimally Invasive Urology/Oncology, Columbia University Medical Center, New York, New York

RAYMOND J. LEVEILLEE, MD, FRCS-G, Clinical Professor of Urology, Radiology and Biomedical Engineering, Department of Urology, University of Miami Miller School of Medicine, Miami, Florida

ELSPETH M. McDOUGALL, MD, FRCSC, Professor of Urology, Director, Surgical Education Center, and Associate Dean of Clinical Sciences, University of California, Irvine; and Department of Urology, University of California, Irvine Medical Center, Orange, California

MANOJ MONGA, MD, Professor, Department of Urologic Surgery, University of Minnesota, Minneapolis, Minnesota

STEPHEN Y. NAKADA, MD, Chairman and Professor of Urology, Department of Urology, Clinical Science Center, University of Wisconsin, Madison, Wisconsin

MICHAEL C. OST, MD, Assistant Professor of Urology, Department of Urology, University of Pittsburgh Medical Center, Pittsburgh, Pennsylvania

VIPUL R. PATEL, MD, Global Robotics Institute, Florida Hospital, Orlando, Florida

NILESH PATIL, MD, Global Robotics Institute, Florida Hospital, Orlando, Florida

MARC C. SMALDONE, MD, Resident Physician, Department of Urology, University of Pittsburgh Medical Center, Pittsburgh, Pennsylvania

SAMUEL P. STERRETT, DO, Endourology Fellow, Department of Urology, Clinical Science Center, University of Wisconsin, Madison, Wisconsin

LI-MING SU, MD, Department of Urology, James Buchanan Brady Urological Institute, The Johns Hopkins Medical Institutions, Baltimore, Maryland

ROBERT M. SWEET, MD, Assistant Professor of Urologic Surgery and General Surgery; and Director, Simulation Perioperative Resource for Training and Learning, University of Minnesota, Minneapolis, Minnesota

ELIZABETH B. TAKACS, MD, Clinical Assistant Professor, Department of Urology, University of Iowa, Iowa City, Iowa

TOSHIRO TERASHI, MD, Professor and Chairman, Department of Urology, Tokai University School of Medicine, Bohseidai, Isehara, Japan

DAVID S. WANG, MD, Assistant Professor, Department of Urology, Boston University School of Medicine, Boston, Massachusetts

GEOFFREY R. WIGNALL, MD, Fellow, Department of Surgery/Urology, University of Western Ontario, London, Ontario, Canada

STEVE K. WILLIAMS, MD, Endourology Fellow, Radiology and Biomedical Engineering, Department of Urology, University of Miami Miller School of Medicine, Miami, Florida

HOWARD N. WINFIELD, MD, Professor of Urology; and Director, Urologic Laparoscopic Surgery & Endourology, University of Iowa Hospitals & Clinics, Iowa City, Iowa

MARSHALL S. WINGO, MD, Endourology Fellow, Radiology and Biomedical Engineering, Department of Urology, University of Miami Miller School of Medicine, Miami, Florida

CONTENTS

procedures. This article attempts to provide an overview of the current status of LRC, with technical details, modifications, and results of various techniques as reported by the authors' group and other groups.

Minimally Invasive Treatment of Stress Urinary Incontinence and Vaginal Prolapse

Elizabeth B. Takacs and Kathleen C. Kobashi

Multimedia Components available within this article at www.urologic.theclinics.com

Stress urinary incontinence and pelvic organ prolapse are prevalent conditions that can have detrimental effects on a woman's quality of life. Surgically, this has often been approached by means of a transvaginal route. With recent advances in laparoscopic and robotic instrumentation and operating systems, there is increasing interest in minimally invasive techniques for correction of pelvic organ prolapse. In this article, the authors briefly describe the laparoscopic and robotic approaches in terms of surgical techniques, operative anatomy, and results published in the literature.

Minimally Invasive Treatment of Vesicoureteral Reflux

Matthew H. Hayn, Marc C. Smaldone, Michael C. Ost, and Steven G. Docimo

Vesicoureteral reflux (VUR) is a common problem in childhood, affecting approximately 1% to 2% of the pediatric population. Mild cases of VUR are likely to resolve spontaneously, but high-grade VUR may require surgical correction. Pediatric urologists are familiar with open antireflux operations, which can be accomplished with minimal operative morbidity. Minimally invasive endoscopic and laparoscopic techniques that now exist may serve to reduce morbidity further. This article reviews the endoscopic materials, techniques, and outcomes in the treatment of VUR in addition to the techniques and outcomes of laparoscopic and robotic ureteroneocystotomy.

Minimally Invasive Surgical Approaches and Management of Prostate Cancer

Mark L. Gonzalgo, Nilesh Patil, Li-Ming Su, and Vipul R. Patel

Multimedia Components available within this article at www.urologic.theclinics.com

For clinically localized prostate cancer, radical prostatectomy remains the "gold standard" treatment. New forms of minimally invasive therapies are sought out by patients, however, because of the potential morbidity associated with open surgery. With quality-of-life aspects influencing patient decision making, minimally invasive therapeutic modalities have generated great interest among patients. Laparoscopic radical prostatectomy, robotic-assisted laparoscopic prostatectomy, brachytherapy, cryotherapy, and high-intensity focused ultrasound are all considered to be minimally invasive treatment options for the management of clinically localized prostate cancer.

Minimally Invasive Treatment of Lower Urinary Tract Obstruction

Jean J.M.C.H. de la Rosette, Stavros Gravas, and John M. Fitzpatrick

During the past decade, increasing numbers of minimally invasive treatments for managing male lower urinary tract symptoms caused by urinary tract obstruction have been positioned. On one hand, transurethral needle ablation and transurethral microwave thermotherapy bridge the gap between medical management and surgery, while on the other hand, outcomes of holmium laser enucleation of the prostate and Greenlight laser equal outcomes following transurethral resection of the prostate (TURP). With the introduction of the bipolar technology, however, TURP has reinforced its position.

Simulation and Computer-Animated Devices: The New Minimally Invasive Skills Training Paradigm

Robert M. Sweet and Elspeth M. McDougall

Multimedia Components available within this article at www.urologic.theclinics.com

Complex surgical technologies, restricted resident work hours, and limited case volumes in surgical practice have created new challenges to surgical education. At the same time, maintenance of established skills and development of new skills are becoming increasingly important for surgeons, especially skills related to technically challenging minimally invasive surgical therapies. In addition, minimally invasive therapies are highly dependent on uniquely specialized teams of health care workers. For all of these reasons, simulation is gaining attention in surgical education for the development and refinement of minimally invasive surgical skills and technique. This article summarizes developments and challenges related to simulation in surgical education, especially as it relates to minimally invasive surgical therapies in the field of urology.

GOAL STATEMENT

The goal of *Urologic Clinics of North America* is to keep practicing urologists and urology residents up to date with current clinical practice in urology by providing timely articles reviewing the state of the art in patient care.

ACCREDITATION

The *Urologic Clinics of North America* is planned and implemented in accordance with the Essential Areas and Policies of the Accreditation Council for Continuing Medical Education (ACCME) through the joint sponsorship of the University of Virginia School of Medicine and Elsevier. The University of Virginia School of Medicine is accredited by the ACCME to provide continuing medical education for physicians.

The University of Virginia School of Medicine designates this educational activity for a maximum of *15 AMA PRA Category 1 Credits™*. Physicians should only claim credit commensurate with the extent of their participation in the activity.

The American Medical Association has determined that physicians not licensed in the US who participate in this CME activity are eligible for *15 AMA PRA Category 1 Credits™*.

Credit can be earned by reading the text material, taking the CME examination online at http://www.theclinics.com/home/cme, and completing the evaluation. After taking the test, you will be required to review any and all incorrect answers. Following completion of the test and evaluation, your credit will be awarded and you may print your certificate.

FACULTY DISCLOSURE/CONFLICT OF INTEREST

The University of Virginia School of Medicine, as an ACCME accredited provider, endorses and strives to comply with the Accreditation Council for Continuing Medical Education (ACCME) Standards of Commercial Support, Commonwealth of Virginia statutes, University of Virginia policies and procedures, and associated federal and private regulations and guidelines on the need for disclosure and monitoring of proprietary and financial interests that may affect the scientific integrity and balance of content delivered in continuing medical education activities under our auspices.

The University of Virginia School of Medicine requires that all CME activities accredited through this institution be developed independently and be scientifically rigorous, balanced and objective in the presentation/discussion of its content, theories and practices.

All authors/editors participating in an accredited CME activity are expected to disclose to the readers relevant financial relationships with commercial entities occurring within the past 12 months (such as grants or research support, employee, consultant, stock holder, member of speakers bureau, etc.). The University of Virginia School of Medicine will employ appropriate mechanisms to resolve potential conflicts of interest to maintain the standards of fair and balanced education to the reader. Questions about specific strategies can be directed to the Office of Continuing Medical Education, University of Virginia School of Medicine, Charlottesville, Virginia.

The authors/editors listed below have identified no professional or financial affiliations for themselves or their spouse/partner:
Sero Andonian, MD; Andre Berger, MD; Geoffrey N. Box, MD; David Canes, MD; Steven G. Docimo, MD; David A. Duchene, MD; Amr F. Fergany, MD; John M. Fitzpatrick, MCh, FRCSI, FC Urol (SA), FRCSGlas, FRCS; Matthew T. Gettman, MD; Mark L. Gonzalgo, MD, PhD; Stavros Gravas, MD, PhD; Matthew H. Hayn, MD; Kerry K. Holland (Acquisitions Editor); Günter Janetschek, MD; Benjamin R. Lee, MD; Daniel S. Lehman, MD; Michael C. Ost, MD; Vipul R. Patel, MD; Nilesh N. Patil, MD; Marc C. Smaldone, MD; Samuel P. Sterrett, DO; Li-Ming Su, MD; Toshiro Terachi, MD; David S. Wang, MD; Geoffrey R. Wignall, MD; Steve K. Williams, MD; Howard N. Winfield, MD; and, Marshall S. Wingo, MD.

The authors/editors listed below identified the following professional or financial affiliations for themselves or their spouse/partner:
Benjamin K. Canales, MD, MPH owns stock in ForTec Litho, LLC.
Ralph V. Clayman, MD has received funding from Cook Urology, Boston Scientific, Vascular Technology, Inc., and Omeros, is a consultant for Cook Urology, Karl Storz, Inc., Omeros, and Galil, Inc., owns stock in Applied Urology, is a patent holder for Boston Scientific and Applied Urology, and received royalties from Cook Urology, Boston Scientific, Greenwald, Inc., and OSI.
Jean J.M.C.H. de la Rosette, MD, PhD is a consultant for Galil Medical, BSC, and AMS.
John D. Denstedt, MD is a consultant for Boston Scientific and serves on the Advisory Committee for Cook Urology and Olympus.
Mihir M. Desai, MD owns stock in Hansen Medical.
Inderbir S. Gill, MD owns stock in Hansen Medical.
Kathleen C. Kobashi, MD is a consultant and serves on the Advisory Committee for Coloplast, and has received researching funding and serves on the Speaker's bureau for Novartis and Astellas.
Jaime Landman, MD has received funding, is a consultant and serves on the Advisory Committee for Galil Medical.
Raymond J. Leveillee, MD, FRCS-G is a surgical proctor for Covidien and Intuitive Surgical, and has received funding from Lumasense and Angiodynamics.
Elspeth M. McDougall, MD, FRCSC is employed by Astellas Pharma, US, and is an industry funded research/investigator for Karl Storz, Simbionix, Ethicon, and Endocare.
Manoj Monga, MD has received funding from Sanofi-Aventis and Stryker Endoscopy, serves on the Speakers Bureau for Boehringer-Ingelheim, and is a patent holder for Cook Urological.
Stephen Y. Nakada, MD is a consultant for Cook Urologic.
Robert M. Sweet, MD is a consultant and has received research funding for Medical Education Technologies, Inc., owns stock in Red Llama Technologies, Inc., and has received research funding from Gyrus ACMI.
Elizabeth B. Takacs, MD has received funding from Pfizer and Astellas and serves on the Speaker's bureau for Pfizer.

Disclosure of Discussion of non-FDA approved uses for pharmaceutical products and/or medical devices:
The University of Virginia School of Medicine, as an ACCME provider, requires that all faculty presenters identify and disclose any "off label" uses for pharmaceutical and medical device products. The University of Virginia School of Medicine recommends that each physician fully review all the available data on new products or procedures prior to instituting them with patients.

TO ENROLL

To enroll in the Urologic Clinics of North America Continuing Medical Education program, call customer service at 1-800-654-2452 or visit us online at www.theclinics.com/home/cme. The CME program is available to subscribers for an additional fee of $195.00.

FORTHCOMING ISSUES

RECENT ISSUES

ELSEVIER
SAUNDERS

Urol Clin N Am 35 (2008) xiii

**UROLOGIC
CLINICS
of North America**

Preface

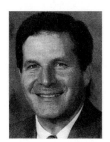

Howard N. Winfield, MD
Guest Editor

Urologists have always been the leading forces among other surgical disciplines in the use of the minimally invasive approach to surgery. In the late 1970s and early 1980s, the term "endourology," used for management of urolithiasis, was established. Although many believed this to be the end of urology as it had been known for previous decades, it became quickly apparent that the minimally invasive approach to all urologic organs was not a transient fad. The frontiers of minimally invasive surgery (MIS) have been pushed further with the advent of laparoscopic—and recently robotic—urologic surgery. There is no organ of the genitourinary system that has not been impacted by MIS.

In the summer of 2006, the late Dr. Martin Resnick invited me to be the guest editor for an edition of the *Urologic Clinics*, devoted solely to minimally invasive procedures. I was delighted to undertake this task and believe we have compiled a remarkable group of articles authored by world leaders in MIS. Up-to-date information on techniques and results of laparoscopic and robotic procedures of the adrenal gland, kidney, prostate, and bladder are discussed. Excellent reviews of the state-of-the-art MIS for upper tract urolithiasis, stress urinary incontinence/vaginal prolapse, and lower urinary tract obstruction are presented by distinguished authors. Finally, a comprehensive review of thermal ablative therapy and the application of simulation or computer-animated devices for teaching are discussed by world authorities.

It is hoped that the reader will gain significant understanding of these constantly evolving topics and will be confident in the knowledge that urology continues at the forefront of MIS. It is with regret that Marty is not here to see this final product, but I am certain that he would give his warm smile in acknowledgement towards this issue dedicated to MIS.

Howard N. Winfield, MD
Professor of Urology
Director, Urologic Laparoscopic Surgery &
Endourology
Department of Urology
University of Iowa Hospitals and Clinics
200 Hawkins Drive
Iowa City, IA 52242, USA

E-mail address: howard-winfield@uiowa.edu

0094-0143/08/$ - see front matter © 2008 Elsevier Inc. All rights reserved.
doi:10.1016/j.ucl.2008.05.013

ELSEVIER
SAUNDERS

Urol Clin N Am 35 (2008) 351–363

UROLOGIC
CLINICS
of North America

Laparoscopic Adrenalectomy

David S. Wang, MD[a],*, Toshiro Terashi, MD[b]

[a]Department of Urology, Boston University School of Medicine, 720 Harrison Avenue, Suite 606, Boston, MA 02118, USA
[b]Department of Urology, Tokai University School of Medicine, Bohseidai, Isehara 259-1193, Japan

Since originally reported by Gagner and colleagues [1] in 1992, laparoscopic adrenalectomy has become an established procedure that has replaced the open approach in virtually all cases. Numerous studies [2–9] have demonstrated the advantages of the laparoscopic approach, including decreased blood loss, less patient morbidity, shorter hospitalization, faster recovery, and cost-effectiveness [10]. The indications for laparoscopic adrenalectomy have increased, whereas the absolute contraindications have decreased. As such, laparoscopic adrenalectomy has become a standard of care and the technique of choice for most benign adrenal lesions.

This article discusses the diagnosis and evaluation, indications, surgical technique, and results of laparoscopic adrenalectomy for benign and malignant conditions.

Diagnosis

In the past, most adrenal lesions were diagnosed secondary to clinical manifestations resulting from hormonally active adrenal tumors. Because of widespread use of ultrasound, CT scans, and MRI, however, most adrenal lesions are diagnosed incidentally. Figs. 1 and 2 demonstrate examples of adrenal lesions diagnosed on CT and MRI. The differential diagnosis of an incidental adrenal mass includes benign nonfunctioning adenoma, hormonally active cortical tumor, myelolipoma, pheochromocytoma, adrenocortical carcinoma, and metastatic lesion.

* Corresponding author.
E-mail address: davids.wang@bmc.org (D.S. Wang).

Endocrinologic evaluation

Hormonal evaluation is required in all patients who have adrenal lesions, regardless of size, to determine whether there is functional activity present. This evaluation is particularly important in patients who are undergoing adrenal surgery because of postoperative considerations regarding blood pressure control, electrolyte status, volume status, and other anesthesia considerations. Box 1 lists standard laboratory tests used for evaluating patients who have adrenal lesions. In general, most hormonally active adrenal tumors should be removed. On occasion, medical management of aldosteronomas may be achieved with spironolactone, particularly when patients are poor surgical candidates [11].

Cushing's syndrome

Cushing's syndrome refers to the clinical condition that results from excess circulating glucocorticoids. There are several nonadrenal causes of Cushing's syndrome, but the urologist most commonly encounters a patient who has an adrenal cortical tumor as the cause of Cushing's syndrome. Features of Cushing's syndrome are well recognized, including hypertension, truncal obesity, moon facies, easy bruising, and mood disorders. Diagnosis is made by collecting a 24-hour urinary cortisol measurement [12]. The low-dose dexamethasone suppression test can be used to diagnose Cushing's syndrome further if the urinary cortisol measurement is equivocal. An abdominal CT scan and MRI are used to identify adrenal adenomas or bilateral adrenal hyperplasia. Adrenal adenomas causing Cushing's syndrome are amenable to laparoscopic adrenalectomy. Other than optimizing the patient's general medical

0094-0143/08/$ - see front matter © 2008 Elsevier Inc. All rights reserved.
doi:10.1016/j.ucl.2008.05.009

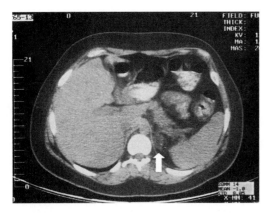

Fig. 1. CT scan of the abdomen demonstrates left adrenal lesion (*arrow*).

condition, there are no specific additional recommendations that are required in patients who have Cushing's syndrome before undergoing laparoscopic adrenalectomy.

Aldosteronoma

Primary hyperaldosteronism (Conn's syndrome) is the clinical syndrome that arises when elevated aldosterone levels result in increased total body sodium content and a decrease in potassium. It is a rare cause of hypertension, with other symptoms, including paresthesias, muscle weakness, and, on occasion, visual disturbances [11,13]. Adrenal aldosteronomas as small as 1 cm can be sufficient to cause the symptoms. Typical laboratory findings include hypokalemia, hypernatremia, elevated plasma and urine aldosterone levels, an elevated serum aldosterone-to-renin

ratio, and suppressed plasma renin activity [11,13]. Adrenal vein sampling is rarely required.

Once the diagnosis is confirmed, medical control of hypertension and correction of hypokalemia should be instituted several weeks before adrenalectomy. Spironolactone, a competitive antagonist of the aldosterone receptor, is the most effective medication for management of hyperaldosteronism. Alternative medications include potassium-sparing diuretics, calcium channel blockers, and converting enzyme inhibitors. Unless they are poor candidates for surgery, adrenalectomy is recommended in all patients, with hypertension being improved or cured in more than 90% of patients after surgery [13].

Pheochromocytoma

Pheochromocytomas are tumors that release adrenal catecholamines, which can result in hypertension, tachycardia, and a host of clinical manifestations. Laboratory diagnosis is made by identifying elevated levels of catecholamines in the

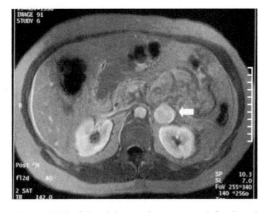

Fig. 2. MRI of the abdomen demonstrates left adrenal lesion (*arrow*).

blood and urine. Radiographic diagnosis is made with CT or MRI, with MRI demonstrating a bright image on a T2-weighted study. Additionally, MIBG nuclear medicine scanning can help to confirm and localize pheochromocytomas [14].

Because of the unique manifestations of catecholamine excess, successful laparoscopic adrenalectomy for pheochromocytoma requires collaboration with the surgeon, endocrinologist, and anesthesiologist. Although pheochromocytoma was once considered a relative contraindication to laparoscopic surgery, laparoscopic adrenalectomy for pheochromocytomas has now been performed successfully and reported in several series [15–17]. Preoperative medical preparation includes optimal control of blood pressure with alpha-blockade or calcium channel antagonists [14]. Beta-blockers may be used to control reflex tachycardia after initiation of the alpha-blockade. During surgery, aggressive fluid expansion is necessary to increase circulating plasma volume and prevent postoperative hypotension. Close monitoring during surgery includes careful attention to blood pressure, central venous pressure, and urinary output.

Indications for laparoscopic adrenalectomy

The indications for laparoscopic adrenalectomy have expanded as more surgeons have become proficient with the technique and the advantages of this approach have become apparent. In many centers, laparoscopic adrenalectomy has become the surgical procedure of choice for the management of functional tumors less than 6 cm in size. The current indications for performing laparoscopic adrenalectomy are listed in Box 2.

Box 2. Indications for laparoscopic adrenalectomy

Hormonally active adrenal tumor
  Aldosteronoma
  Pheochromocytoma
  Cortisol-producing adrenal tumor
Nonfunctioning adrenal lesion greater
  than 5 cm in size
Nonfunctioning adrenal lesion with
  progressive growth
Solitary adrenal metastasis with
  negative metastatic survey

In general, most hormonally active tumors should be removed unless patients are poor candidates for surgery. Conversely, hormonally inactive tumors are managed according to size. Tumors less than 3 cm in size are almost always benign adenomas and generally require no further treatment unless clinical signs of hormonal activity develop [18]. Most adrenocortical carcinomas are larger than 6 cm in size [19]. Because CT is thought to underestimate the size of such lesions by as much as 1 cm [20], surgery is recommended for lesions greater than 5 cm in size. Hormonally inactive lesions between 3 and 6 cm in size can be followed with serial imaging.

There are few absolute contraindications to laparoscopic adrenalectomy. In cases of suspected primary adrenal carcinoma, particularly with extension into surrounding organs, open surgery should be performed. Given the aggressive nature of the disease, the open approach allows for en bloc resection and potential removal of surrounding organs [21,22]. Other absolute contraindications to laparoscopic adrenalectomy include uncorrectable coagulopathy, severe cardiopulmonary disease, and uncontrolled pheochromocytoma.

Relative contraindications to laparoscopic adrenalectomy include extensive previous surgery and pregnancy. Caution should be used when doing laparoscopic adrenalectomy on lesions greater than 12 cm because of the increased risk for hemorrhage and injury to surrounding viscera. With increasing experience in performing laparoscopic adrenalectomy, relative contraindications have decreased.

Occasionally, the urologist encounters a patient who is suspected of having a solitary metastatic lesion to the adrenal gland. If the lesion is less than 6 cm in size and not obviously adherent to surrounding viscera, a laparoscopic approach is possible [23].

Surgical technique

Preoperative patient preparation and evaluation

Careful preoperative control and management of hormonally active tumors is necessary before performing laparoscopic adrenalectomy. Collaboration with an endocrinologist and anesthesiologist experienced with adrenal disorders is helpful. The urologist should have an understanding of the physiology of adrenal disorders to manage patients appropriately in the peri- and postoperative periods with regard to fluid management, electrolyte abnormalities, and blood pressure control. Hormonally functional tumors must be adequately evaluated, and appropriate preoperative interventions must be initiated in concert with an endocrinologist.

Before surgery, all patients should receive a mechanical bowel preparation. Clear liquids should be started the day before surgery. A broad-spectrum antibiotic should be administered on call to the operating room. Standard precautions for deep venous thrombosis prophylaxis, such as stockings and pneumatic compression devices, should be used.

Approach

There are several laparoscopic approaches to the adrenal gland. Commonly used approaches to the adrenal gland include the transperitoneal approach and the posterior and lateral retroperitoneal approaches. A transthoracic approach has been described for patients who have undergone extensive previous transperitoneal and retroperitoneal surgery [24]. Surgeon preference and experience seem to be the most important factors in determining the approach. Although each approach has purported advantages and disadvantages, there is no evidence that one is superior [25–27].

Transperitoneal approach for right adrenalectomy

The patient is positioned on a beanbag with the right side elevated at 45° to 70° with the table slightly flexed at the level of the umbilicus. Fig. 3 shows the general modified flank position used for laparoscopic adrenalectomy. Next, the patient should be secured with tape to allow the table to be tilted side to side to facilitate exposure. A catheter is placed to drain the bladder, and an orogastric tube is placed to decompress the stomach.

After pneumoperitoneum is achieved, four subcostal ports are placed below the costal margin (Fig. 4). Mobilization and retraction of the liver are necessary to expose the right adrenal gland. It is generally not necessary to mobilize the ascending colon and hepatic flexure fully. Incision of the posterior peritoneum and extension through the triangular ligaments of the liver allow for upward and medial retraction of the liver (Fig. 5).

Full mobilization of the duodenum is often not necessary, because the inferior vena cava (IVC) is often identified once there is adequate liver mobilization. Further dissection of the IVC allows for visualization of the right adrenal vein. Extreme caution should be used when dissecting out the right adrenal vein because it is short and sometimes broad. Hemorrhage resulting from avulsion or injury to the right adrenal vein is extremely difficult to control because of its direct drainage into the IVC. The adrenal vein should be carefully divided between standard clips (Fig. 6).

Ultrasonic laparoscopic coagulation instruments or bipolar cautery can be used to mobilize the adrenal gland further once the main vascular pedicle has been divided. After the right adrenal vein is divided, further dissection is continued toward the diaphragm, where the inferior phrenic

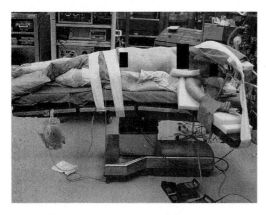

Fig. 3. Patient positioning for right transperitoneal adrenalectomy.

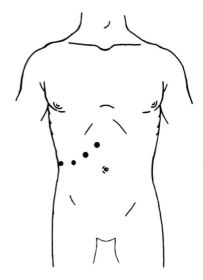

Fig. 4. Port placement for right transperitoneal adrenalectomy.

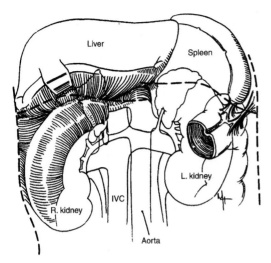

Fig. 5. T-shaped incision through the posterior perito-neum for left and right adrenalectomies. (*Right*) Incision from the second part of the duodenum to triangular lig-aments at the liver edge and then lateral to the hepatic flexure. (*Left*) Incision is developed across phrenocolic and splenocolic ligaments and at the inferior border of the spleen. IVC, inferior vena cava; L., left; R., right.

vessels can be divided. Next, the inferior pedicle of the adrenal gland is released, separating the adrenal gland from the upper pole of the kidney (Fig. 7). Gerota's fascia is next incised at the junc-tion of the upper pole of the kidney and the right adrenal gland. Finally, the lateral attachments of the adrenal gland, which are generally relatively avascular, are divided.

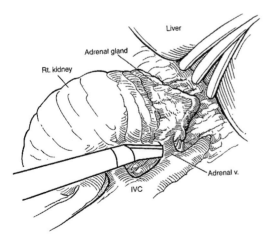

Fig. 6. The short right adrenal vein is carefully dissected out and then divided. Rt., right, v., vein. (*From* Bishoff JT, Kavoussi RL. Atlas of laparoscopic retroperitoneal sur-gery. Philadelpha: WB Saunders, 2000; with permission.)

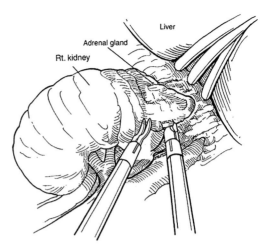

Fig. 7. With the right adrenal vein divided, the inferior surface of the right adrenal gland is dissected off of the right kidney. Rt., right. (*From* Bishoff JT, Kavoussi RL. Atlas of laparoscopic retroperitoneal surgery. Philadelpha: WB Saunders, 2000; with permission.)

Once the adrenal gland is completely sepa-rated, it should be placed in a specimen retrieval bag and removed en bloc. Hemostasis is con-firmed, and the ports are closed as necessary and removed under direct vision. A drain is not routinely used.

Transperitoneal approach for left adrenalectomy

The patient is positioned with the left side elevated 45° to 70° with the table slightly flexed at the level of the umbilicus. Three or four trocars are placed in a mirror image as for a right adrenalectomy (Fig. 8). Key anatomic landmarks to identify when performing a transperitoneal left laparoscopic adrenalectomy include the splenic flexure of the colon, spleen, tail of the pancreas, and left kidney. Mobilization of the splenic flexure of the colon is necessary to provide adequate ex-posure to the left adrenal gland.

The splenic flexure of the colon is mobilized, and the splenocolic and lienorenal ligaments are divided. This allows the splenic flexure of the co-lon and the spleen to fall away from the adrenal gland (see Fig. 5). On occasion, some surgeons prefer to incise the peritoneum lateral to the de-scending colon and the spleen up to the dia-phragm; in such case, the splenocolic ligament does not need to be divided. If necessary, the tail of the pancreas can be separated away from Ger-ota's fascia to allow the pancreas to fall away with the spleen to provide more exposure. Caution should be taken to avoid injury to the tail of the

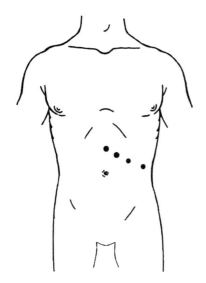

Fig. 8. Port placement for left transperitoneal adrenalectomy.

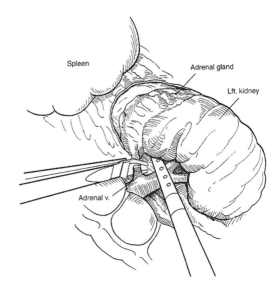

Fig. 9. The left adrenal vein is dissected out along the superior aspect of the left renal vein and then divided. Lft., left; v., vein. (*From* Bishoff JT, Kavoussi RL. Atlas of laparoscopic retroperitoneal surgery. Philadelpha: WB Saunders, 2000; with permission.)

pancreas, which often lies in close proximity to the left adrenal gland and the left kidney.

Next, Gerota's fascia is incised between the upper pole of the left kidney and the adrenal gland. Dissection along the medial aspect of the kidney is continued until the left renal vein is identified. Careful dissection along the superior aspect of the left renal vein should lead to the identification of the takeoff of the left adrenal vein. The left adrenal vein is then isolated, clipped, and divided (Fig. 9).

With the left adrenal vein divided, the remaining mobilization of the adrenal gland can proceed. The superior aspect of the adrenal gland is then mobilized, taking care to divide the phrenic vessels supplying the gland. It is important not to mistake the tail of the pancreas for the left adrenal gland; dissection should proceed along the superior aspect of the kidney to ensure that the correct plane is established (Fig. 10). The medial gland is mobilized off of the aorta, and, generally, the vasculature supplying the adrenal gland can be divided using ultrasonic shears or bipolar. Finally, the lateral attachments of the adrenal gland are divided to free the gland fully from all surrounding tissues. The specimen is then placed into a retrieval bag and removed intact, and standard closure is performed.

Retroperitoneal technique

The retroperitoneal approach to the adrenal gland is useful in the patient with a prior history

of extensive abdominal surgery. The patient is placed into the full flank position, with three or four ports typically used. Patient positioning and port placement are as shown in Fig. 11. Access

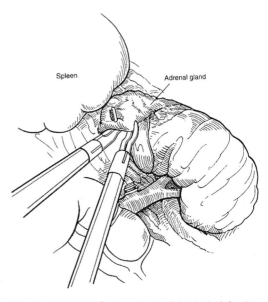

Fig. 10. With the left adrenal vein divided, the left adrenal gland is dissected off of the superior surface of the left kidney. (*From* Bishoff JT, Kavoussi RL. Atlas of laparoscopic retroperitoneal surgery. Philadelpha: WB Saunders, 2000; with permission.)

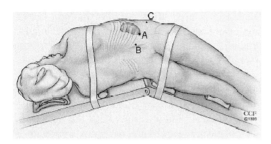

Fig. 11. Patient positioning and trocar placement for retroperitoneal adrenalectomy. A, camera port; B, C, working ports. (*Courtesy of* the Cleveland Clinic Foundation, Cleveland, OH; with permission.)

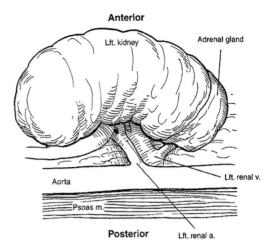

Fig. 12. Retroperitoneal approach to the left adrenal gland. The psoas muscle is identified, and dissection is performed superior to the upper pole of the kidney. a., artery; Lft., left; m., muscle; v., vein. (*From* Bishoff JT, Kavoussi RL. Atlas of laparoscopic retroperitoneal surgery. Philadelpha: WB Saunders, 2000; with permission.)

into the retroperitoneum requires the creation of a working space using a dilating balloon.

A Hasson technique is used to place the first port. First, a 2-cm incision is made below the tip of the twelfth rib, and S-type retractors are used to split the muscles until the lumbodorsal fascia is identified. Once the lumbodorsal fascia is incised, access into the retroperitoneal space is confirmed by inserting one finger in and palpating the twelfth rib, the iliac crest, and the psoas muscle. The balloon is then inflated to establish a working space, and carbon dioxide insufflation is attached to the trocar to generate pneumoretroperitoneum at a pressure of 15 mm Hg. Once the primary port is inserted, the working ports are placed. The second port is placed posterior to the primary port, below the angle formed by the twelfth rib and the paraspinous muscles. The third port is placed approximately 3 to 4 cm medial to the primary port in the anterior axillary line. An optional fourth port is placed in the anterior axillary line 5 to 7 cm inferior to the third port and may be used to assist with retraction throughout the duration of the case.

Once pneumoretroperitoneum is established, identification of key landmarks helps to establish the orientation. The psoas muscle is usually easily seen and establishes longitudinal orientation. By retracting the kidney upward and anteriorly, subsequent medial dissection eventually reveals the great vessels running parallel to the psoas muscle. The renal artery can be identified by identifying pulsations, although full mobilization of the renal hilar vessels is generally not necessary during adrenalectomy.

Left adrenalectomy

When performing a left retroperitoneal adrenalectomy, dissection should start on the psoas

muscle to the upper pole of the left kidney (Fig. 12). Dissection on the left side should be conducted along the psoas muscle to the upper pole of the kidney. Identification of the left renal hilum allows for identification of the left adrenal vein. The adrenal vein can be found along the inferomedial border of the adrenal gland. If difficulty is encountered in identifying the left adrenal vein, the adrenal vein can be found by first locating the left renal vessels and noting the junction of the left adrenal vein with the left renal vein. Unlike transperitoneal laparoscopy, the dissection and identification of the left adrenal vein must be done from a posterior approach. The left adrenal vein is then divided between clips, and the remainder of the adrenal gland can be detached. Next, the lateral and inferior surfaces of the adrenal gland are carefully dissected away from the kidney. Finally, the superior attachments of the kidney, including the inferior phrenic vessels, are divided using the ultrasonic shears.

After the adrenal gland is free, it is placed into a specimen retrieval bag and removed in standard fashion. The trocars and wounds are then closed in standard fashion.

Right adrenalectomy

The right adrenalectomy proceeds using the same principles of retroperitoneal laparoscopy.

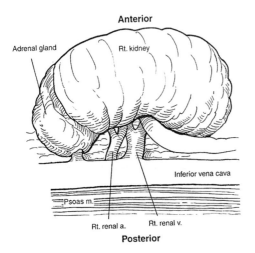

Anterior

Adrenal gland   Rt. kidney

Inferior vena cava

Psoas m.

Rt. renal a.   Rt. renal v.

Posterior

Fig. 13. Retroperitoneal approach to the right adrenal gland. The psoas muscle is identified, and the dissection moves superior to the upper pole of the right kidney. The vena cava is identified and dissected out to help localize the right adrenal vein. a., artery; m., muscle; Rt., right; v., vein. (*From* Bishoff JT, Kavoussi RL. Atlas of laparoscopic retroperitoneal surgery. Philadelpha: WB Saunders, 2000; with permission.)

The dissection proceeds along the psoas muscle in a superior direction (Fig. 13). The kidney may be retracted anteriorly to help facilitate exposure to the right adrenal gland. Of note, the right adrenal gland is situated more medial to the kidney than the left adrenal gland; as such, the upper pole of the kidney may interfere with exposure of the adrenal gland. The IVC is identified medial to the psoas. Along the posterolateral aspect of the IVC, the main adrenal vein is identified. Again, extreme caution must be exercised when manipulating the main right adrenal vein to prevent inadvertent avulsion or injury. The adrenal vein is then clipped and divided.

Once the adrenal vein is divided, the inferior and medial borders of the adrenal gland are dissected free from the right renal vein and the IVC. Small adrenal vessels can then be effectively ligated using the ultrasonic shears. The inferior phrenic vessels are then divided to release the adrenal gland, and the specimen is removed in the usual fashion.

Posterior retroperitoneal approach

The posterior retroperitoneal approach to the adrenal gland has been described [28]. With this technique, the operation is performed with the patient in the prone position. A three- to four-port

technique is used after standard balloon dilatation. Gerota's fascia is incised along the medial crus of the diaphragm. The medial surface of the adrenal gland, including the adrenal vessels, is exposed first before mobilization of the entire gland. Once the main vascular supply of the adrenal gland is divided, the remainder of the gland is dissected free. Although results with this technique are promising, experience with this approach is limited.

Transthoracic technique

Gill and colleagues [24] have reported the technique of thorascopic transdiaphragmatic adrenalectomy. This technique has potential for use in the unusual case in which the patient has undergone transperitoneal and retroperitoneal surgery. After double-lumen endotracheal intubation, the patient is placed in the prone position. A four-port transthoracic technique is used. To gain exposure to the adrenal gland, the diaphragm is incised under ultrasonographic guidance and the retroperitoneum is entered. The adrenal gland is then identified and dissected free. Once the adrenal gland is removed, the diaphragm is repaired. A chest tube is kept in place at the conclusion of the procedure.

Laparoscopic partial adrenalectomy

Laparoscopic partial adrenalectomy has been reported [29], with the goal of retaining functioning adrenal tissue to obviate the need for hormone replacement therapy, particularly in patients with a solitary adrenal gland. This procedure has limited applicability in highly selected and well-informed patients, however. Currently, this is not an accepted treatment modality in most adrenal disorders.

Robotic adrenalectomy

Robotic surgery has become prevalent in urology, particularly with regard to radical prostatectomy. Several groups have reported robotic-assisted laparoscopic adrenalectomy [30,31]. Robotic technology allows surgeons with limited laparoscopic experience to perform adrenalectomy. The advantages of this approach are unclear, however, and the added cost is a significant disadvantage.

Postoperative care

Patients generally have a rapid recovery. The orogastric tube is removed at the end of the case, and the Foley catheter is removed as soon as the patient is ambulatory. Postoperative pain is controlled with parenteral narcotics in the first 24 hours and with ketorolac or oral narcotics thereafter. Supplemental corticosteroids and appropriate antihypertensive medications are administered as needed depending on the type of tumor removed. Postoperative care can be coordinated in concert with an endocrinologist if necessary. Discharge is usually within 24 to 48 hours from surgery, and full recovery requires 10 to 14 days.

Complications

The most significant intraoperative complication is hemorrhage. On the right side, the adrenal vein drains directly into the vena cava. Severe hemorrhage during isolation of the right adrenal vein can necessitate conversion to the open procedure. On the left side, avulsion of the left adrenal vein can similarly result in severe hemorrhage. Extreme caution during dissection of the adrenal vein is required.

Other intraoperative complications from laparoscopic adrenalectomy are similar to those for any laparoscopic procedure and can include injuries to the colon, small bowel, liver, gallbladder, spleen, pancreas, and diaphragm [32]. Conversion to an open case should be done if hemorrhage is uncontrollable or intraoperative injury cannot be repaired through a laparoscopic approach.

Results

Worldwide experience with laparoscopic adrenal surgery has increased since its original introduction in 1992. Several centers have now reported large series in the literature documenting the decreased blood loss, shortened hospital stay, and faster return to normal activity. Selected series in the literature are summarized in Table 1.

Several large studies have been published. Shen and colleagues [34] reported on 456 laparoscopic adrenalectomies, with a conversion rate of 5.5%. Lezoche and colleagues [35] reported that a total of 216 laparoscopic adrenalectomies were performed through the anterior transperitoneal, lateral transperitoneal, and posterior retroperitoneal approaches. The study was a combined experience of surgeons in Italy and The Netherlands. The average operating time of all approaches was 100 minutes with a conversion rate of only 1.9%.

Shen and colleagues [34] reported 800 retroperitoneal adrenalectomies with a low complication rate of 1.5%. The largest published series of laparoscopic adrenalectomies is from Japan, reporting on nearly 5000 cases [36]. The overall complication rate was 2.89%.

The approach to laparoscopic adrenalectomy, whether transperitoneal or retroperitoneal, seems to depend largely on the surgeon. Several studies have demonstrated no advantage of one approach over another [25–27].

Comparison studies have been made between laparoscopic and open adrenalectomy [2–9]. In general, the operative times for laparoscopic surgery are longer than for the open technique, particularly early on in the learning curve. The operative times decrease as surgeon experience increases, however. It is clear that the morbidity after laparoscopic adrenalectomy is less than that for the open approach, and the laparoscopic approach seems to be cost-effective [10].

Laparoscopic adrenalectomy for malignant tumors

More recently, laparoscopic adrenalectomy has been performed for potentially malignant tumors. Henry and colleagues [50] performed laparoscopic adrenalectomies on 19 patients who had potentially malignant tumors, all of which were greater than 6 cm in size. The median operating time was 150 minutes, and conversion was necessary in 2 patients because of intraoperative evidence of invasive carcinoma. Six of the 19 patients had an adrenocortical carcinoma on pathologic diagnosis. One of these patients presented with liver metastasis 6 months after surgery and died. The other 5 patients are alive with a follow-up ranging from 8 to 83 months. These investigators concluded that laparoscopic adrenalectomy can be performed in select patients in experienced hands; however, conversion to open adrenalectomy should be performed if there is evidence of local invasion observed during surgery.

In addition, laparoscopic adrenalectomy has been safely performed in patients who have solitary adrenal metastases. Heniford and colleagues [23] performed laparoscopic adrenalectomy in 11 patients, 10 of whom had the adrenalectomy performed for metastatic disease. One patient required conversion to an open approach because of local invasion of the tumor into the lateral wall of the vena cava, which was removed with the specimen. Ten of the 11 patients were alive with a mean follow-up of 8.3 months.

Table 1
Selected laparoscopic adrenalectomy series

Authors	No. cases	Age (years)	Approach	OR time (minutes)	EBL (cm^3)	Hospital stay (days)	Conversion rate	Complications
Zhang et al [33]	800	—	Retroperitoneal	45	25	—	?	1.5% minor complications, no major complications
Shen et al [34]	456	—	Not specified	—	—	—	25/456	Not reported
Lezoche et al [35]	214	52.8	Transperitoneal	80 R 109 L	—	2.5	?	6 patients with intraoperative complications, 1 death from colonic perforation and sepsis
Japan series [36]	4909	—	3941 transperitoneal 822 retroperitoneal 146 other	—	—	—	3.24%	4.73% intraoperative 2.89% postoperative
MacGillivray et al [37]	60	—	Transperitoneal	183	63	2	0/60	—
Valeri et al [38]	91	—	Transperitoneal	92–148	—	3.5	2/91	2 postoperative hemorrhages, 1 port site bleed, 1 UTI, 1 death from myocardial infarction
Kebebew et al [39]	176	—	Transperitoneal	168	—	1.7	0/176	5.1%
Salomon et al [40]	115	49.3	115 retroperitoneal	118	77	4	1/118	3.5% intraoperative 12.1% postoperative
Guazzoni et al [41]	161	39.4	Transperitoneal	160	—	2.8	4/161	5.5%
Suzuki [42]	118	51.7	78 transperitoneal 40 retroperitoneal	171	96.3	—	6/118	2 paralytic ileus 4 shoulder tip pain

Study								
Soulie et al [43]	52	46.9	52 retroperitoneal	135	80	5	1/52	5.7% intraoperative 11.5% postoperative
Mancini et al [44]	172	—	Transperitoneal	132	—	5.8	12/172	8.7% 2 deaths
Shichman et al [45]	50	54	Transperitoneal	219	142	3	0/50	10%
Winfield et al [3]	21	52.2	Transperitoneal	219	183	2.7	0/21	1 subcutaneous bleed 2 pneumothorax 1 pulmonary edema
Yoshimura et al [4]	28	42	11 transperitonea 17 retroperitoneall	375	370	2.7	0/28	4 blood transfusions 4 subcutaneous emphysema 2 postoperative bleeds
Chee et al [46]	14	46.2	8 transperitoneal 6 retroperitoneal	135	Min	3	0/14	1 pneumonia
Gagner et al [47]	100	46	Transperitoneal	123	70	3	3/100	12%, 3 DVTs, 2 pulmonary emboli
Terachi et al [48]	100	—	Transperitoneal	240	77	—	3/100	—
Rutherford et al [49]	67	54	Transperitoneal	124	—	5.1	0/67	3 DVTs, 2 pulmonary emboli 1 port site hernia, 1 postoperative bleed

Abbreviations: DVT, deep vein thrombosis; L, left; OR, operation; R, right.

These data suggest that the laparoscopic approach to some malignant neoplasms originating from or metastasizing to the adrenal gland is reasonable, but the conversion to an open procedure should be performed if local invasion is present.

Summary

Laparoscopic adrenalectomy has become an accepted method for removing benign lesions of the adrenal gland. There is no question that the advantages of the laparoscopic approach include shorter hospitalization and convalescence. There are few contraindications to the laparoscopic approach, and the transperitoneal and retroperitoneal techniques yield excellent results. Virtually all benign lesions and select malignant lesions can be removed laparoscopically.

Laparoscopic adrenalectomy has been shown to be a safe and effective approach to many forms of adrenal pathologic conditions. It should be considered the standard of care in the management of benign lesions of the adrenal gland that require surgical removal.

References

[1] Gagner M, Lacroix A, Bolte E. Laparoscopic adrenalectomy in Cushing's syndrome and pheochromocytoma. N Engl J Med 1992;327:1033.

[2] Schell SR, Talamimi MA, Udelsman R. Laparoscopic adrenalectomy for nonmalignant disease: improved safety, morbidity, and cost-effectiveness. Surg Endosc 1999;13:30.

[3] Winfield HN, Hamilton BD, Bravo EL, et al. Laparoscopic adrenalectomy: the preferred choice? A comparison to open adrenalectomy. J Urol 1998; 160:235.

[4] Yoshimura K, Yoshioka T, Miyake O, et al. Comparison of clinical outcomes of laparoscopic and conventional open adrenalectomy. J Endourol 1998;12:555.

[5] Vargas HI, Kavoussi LR, Bartlett DL, et al. Laparoscopic adrenalectomy: a new standard of care. Urology 1997;49:673.

[6] Bolli M, Oertli D, Staub J, et al. Laparoscopic adrenalectomy: the new standard? Swiss Med Wkly 2002; 132:12.

[7] Hazzan D, Shiloni E, Golijanin D, et al. Laparoscopic vs open adrenalectomy for benign adrenal neoplasm. Surg Endosc 2001;15:1356.

[8] MacGillivray DC, Schichman SJ, Ferrer FA, et al. A comparison of open vs laparoscopic adrenalectomy. Surg Endosc 1996;10:987.

[9] Miccoli P, Raffaelli M, Berti P, et al. Adrenal surgery before and after the introduction of laparoscopic adrenalectomy. Br J Surg 2002;89:779.

[10] Ortega J, Sala C, Garcia S, et al. Cost-effectiveness of laparoscopic vs open adrenalectomy: small savings in an expensive process. J Laparoendosc Adv Surg Tech A 2002;12:1.

[11] Blumenfeld JD, Vaughan ED Jr. Diagnosis and treatment of primary aldosteronism. World J Urol 1999;17:15.

[12] Goldfarb DA. Contemporary evaluation and management of Cushing's syndrome. World J Urol 1999;17:22.

[13] Blumenfeld JD, Sealey JE, Schlussel Y, et al. Diagnosis and treatment of primary aldosteronism. Ann Intern Med 1994;121:877.

[14] Walther MM, Keiser HR, Linehan WM. Pheochromocytoma: evaluation, diagnosis, and treatment. World J Urol 1999;17:35.

[15] Edwin B, Kazaryan AM, Mala T, et al. Laparoscopic and open surgery for pheochromocytoma. BMC Surg 2001;1:2.

[16] Salomon L, Rabii R, Soulie M, et al. Experience with retroperitoneal laparoscopic adrenalectomy for pheochromocytoma. J Urol 2001;165:1871.

[17] Gotoh M, Ono Y, Hattori R, et al. Laparoscopic adrenalectomy for pheochromocytoma: morbidity compared with adrenalectomy for tumors of other pathology. J Endourol 2002;16:245.

[18] Murai M, Baba S, Nakashima J, et al. Management of incidentally discovered adrenal masses. World J Urol 1999;17:9.

[19] Belldegrun A, Hussain S, Seltzer S, et al. Incidentally discovered mass of the adrenal gland. Surg Gynecol Obstet 1986;163:203.

[20] Cerfolio RJ, Vaughan ED Jr, Brennan TG Jr, et al. Accuracy of computed tomography in predicting adrenal tumor size. Surg Gynecol Obstet 1993;176:307.

[21] Schulick RD, Brenna MF. Adrenocortical carcinoma. World J Urol 1999;17:26.

[22] Schulick RD, Brennan MF. Long-term survival after complete resection and repeat resection in patients with adrenocortical carcinoma. Ann Surg Oncol 1999;6:719.

[23] Heniford BT, Arca MJ, Walsh RM, et al. Laparoscopic adrenalectomy for cancer. Semin Surg Oncol 1999;16:293.

[24] Gill IS, Meraney AM, Thomas JC, et al. Thoracoscopic transdiaphragmatic adrenalectomy: the initial experience. J Urol 2001;165:1875.

[25] Lezoche E, Guerrieri M, Feliciotti F, et al. Anterior, lateral, and posterior retroperitoneal approaches in endoscopic adrenalectomy. Surg Endosc 2002;16:96.

[26] Suzuki K, Kageyama S, Hirano Y, et al. Comparison of 3 surgical approaches to laparoscopic adrenalectomy: a nonrandomized, background matched analysis. J Urol 2001;166:437.

[27] Rubinstein M, Gill IS, Aron M, et al. Prospective, randomized comparison of transperitoneal versus retroperitoneal laparoscopic adrenalectomy. J Urol 2005;174(2):442.

[28] Baba S, Ito K, Yanaihara H, et al. Retroperitoneo-scopic adrenalectomy by a lumbodorsal approach: clinical experience with solo surgery. World J Urol 1999;17:54.

[29] Nambirajan T, Janetschek G. Laparoscopic partial adrenalectomy. Minim Invasive Ther Allied Technol 2005;14(2):71.

[30] Wu JC, Wu HS, Lin MS, et al. Comparison of robot-assisted laparoscopic adrenalectomy with traditional laparoscopic adrenalectomy—1 year follow-up. Surg Endosc 2008;22(2):463.

[31] Winter JM, Talamini MA, Stanfield CL, et al. Thirty robotic adrenalectomies: a single institution's experience. Surg Endosc 2006;20(1):119.

[32] Henry JF, Defechereux T, Raffaelli M, et al. Compli-cations of laparoscopic adrenalectomy: results of 169 consecutive procedures. World J Surg 2000;24: 1342.

[33] Zhang X, Fu B, Lang B, et al. Technique of anatom-ical retroperitoneoscopic adrenalectomy with report of 800 cases. J Urol 2007;177(4):1254.

[34] Shen ZJ, Chen SW, Wang S, et al. Predictive factors for open conversion of laparoscopic adrenalectomy: a 13-year review of 456 cases. J Endourol 2007; 21(11):1333.

[35] Lezoche E, Guerrieri M, Crosta F, et al. Periopera-tive results of 214 laparoscopic adrenalectomies by anterior transperitoneal approach. Surg Endosc 2008;22(2):522.

[36] The Academic Committee of Japanese Society of Endoscopic Surgeons. Eighth nation wide survey. J Jpn Soc Endosc Surg 2006;5:527.

[37] MacGillivray DC, Whalen GF, Malchoff CD, et al. Laparoscopic resection of large adrenal tumors. Ann Surg Oncol 2002;9:480.

[38] Valeria A, Borrelli A, Presenti L, et al. The influence of new technologies on laparoscopic adrenalectomy. Surg Endosc 2002;16:1274.

[39] Kebebew E, Siperstein AE, Duh QY. Laparoscopic adrenalectomy: the optimal surgical approach. J Laparoendosc Adv Surg Tech A 2001;11:409.

[40] Salomon L, Soulie M, Mouly P, et al. Experience with retroperitoneal laparoscopic adrenalectomy in 115 procedures. J Urol 2001;166:38.

[41] Guazzoni G, Cestari A, Montorsi F, et al. Eight-year experience with transperitoneal laparoscopic adre-nal surgery. J Urol 2001;166:820.

[42] Suzuki K. Laparoscopic adrenalectomy: retroper-itoneal approach. Urol Clin North Am 2001;28: 85.

[43] Soulie M, Mouly P, Caron P, et al. Retroperitoneal laparoscopic adrenalectomy: clinical experience in 52 procedures. Urology 2000;56:921.

[44] Mancini F, Mutter D, Peix JL, et al. Experience with adrenalectomy in 1997. Apropos of 247 cases: a mul-ticenter prospective study of the French-speaking Association of Endocrine Surgery. Chirurgie 1999; 124:368.

[45] Shichman SJ, Herndon CD, Sosa RE, et al. Lateral transperitoneal laparoscopic adrenalectomy. World J Urol 1999;17:48.

[46] Chee C, Ravinthiran T, Cheng C. Laparoscopic ad-renalectomy: experience with transabdominal and retroperitoneal approaches. Urology 1998;51:29.

[47] Gagner M, Pomp A, Heniford BT, et al. Laparoscopic adrenalectomy: lessons learned from 100 consecutive procedures. Ann Surg 1997;226:238.

[48] Terachi T, Matsuda T, Terai A, et al. Transperito-neal laparoscopic adrenalectomy: experience in 100 patients. J Endourol 1997;11:361.

[49] Rutherford JC, Stowasser M, Tunny TJ, et al. Laparoscopic adrenalectomy. World J Surg 1996; 20:758.

[50] Henry JF, Sebag F, Iacobone M, et al. Results of laparoscopic adrenalectomy for large and poten-tially malignant tumors. World J Surg 2002;26:1043.

ELSEVIER
SAUNDERS

UROLOGIC
CLINICS
of North America

Urol Clin N Am 35 (2008) 365–383

Minimally Invasive Management of Upper Tract Malignancies: Renal Cell and Transitional Cell Carcinoma

Geoffrey N. Box, MD[a], Daniel S. Lehman, MD[b],
Jaime Landman, MD[b], Ralph V. Clayman, MD[a],*

[a]Department of Urology, University of California Irvine Medical Center,
333 City Boulevard West, Suite 2100, Orange, CA 92868, USA
[b]Department of Urology, Minimally Invasive Urology/Oncology,
Columbia University Medical Center, 161 Fort Washington Avenue,
Room 1111, New York, NY 10032, USA

Renal cell carcinoma

The incidence of renal tumors continues to increase with the more widespread use of abdominal imaging. With this increasing incidence, more tumors are detected that are potentially amenable to less invasive treatment. At the same time, technologic advances have created new minimally invasive options for the treatment of smaller lesions [1]. Since the performance of the first laparoscopic nephrectomy in 1990 [2], there has been an ever-growing incorporation of laparoscopic techniques into clinical practice; in fact, laparoscopic nephrectomy has become a standard treatment of renal tumors that are not candidates for nephron-sparing surgery. Currently, tumors that are amenable to a nephron-sparing approach may be treated with one of several options. Laparoscopic partial nephrectomy (LPN) has established its intermediate oncologic equivalency to the open method [3–5], although this technique has not experienced the same incorporation into clinical practice as laparoscopic radical nephrectomy (LRN), likely, in large part, because of the technical complexity of the procedure and the potentially higher complication rates. When treating the small renal mass, other alternatives have become available, specifically needle ablative

techniques. The clinical evidence is building in favor of cryoablation and radiofrequency ablation for the treatment of small renal tumors. Other experimental techniques that could further reduce the invasiveness of treatment, such as noninvasive high-intensity focused ultrasound (HIFU) and the gamma knife, have also been explored; however, to date, clinical results have been few and disappointing [6,7].

This article focuses primarily on the laparoscopic approaches to radical and partial nephrectomy for management of renal cell carcinoma (RCC). An in-depth discussion of treatment options for transitional cell carcinoma (TCC) is also covered.

Small renal tumors

Most solid renal tumors with a diameter of 4 cm or less are amenable to treatment with nephron-sparing surgery; the oncologic outcomes are excellent and equivalent to radical nephrectomy [8–10]. Tumors 3 cm or less are thought to be best suited for needle ablative treatment. The natural history and cancer potential of these small masses is an important consideration, given the fact they are often found in elderly patients who have significant comorbidities. One study looked at tumors 4 cm or less and reviewed the histopathologic results of 287 tumor excisions, attempting to characterize the aggressiveness of smaller renal

* Corresponding author.
E-mail address: rclayman@uci.edu (R.V. Clayman).

masses [11]. In this series, 19.5% of the masses were found to be benign. Among the patients who had RCC, high grade and high stage seemed to be correlated with tumor size; to wit, Fuhrman grade 3/4 or pT3a lesions were found in 4.2% and 4.2% (≤ 2 cm), 5% and 14.9% (2.1–3 cm), and 25.5% and 35.7% (3.1–4.0 cm), respectively. Distant metastases were seen in 2.4% of tumors 3 cm or less and in 8.4% of tumors 3.1 to 4.0 cm. This underscores the fact that tumor aggressiveness seems to increase dramatically in tumors larger than 3 cm, calling into question the reliability of the current T1a system, which includes tumors up to 4 cm in size. Indeed, not only aggressiveness but the likelihood of cancer seems to be related to the size of the mass. Regarding the latter, when looking at tumor sizes from less than 1 cm to greater than 7 cm, with each 1-cm increase in tumor size, the odds of cancer increase by 17% [12].

An ongoing concern with the treatment of the small renal mass is that upward of 20% to 25% of lesions 4 cm or less are benign [12,13]. This high incidence of benign lesions makes the natural history of untreated renal masses an area of interest. In a meta-analysis of untreated renal lesions, the mean growth rate was 2.8 mm/y and only 1% of the patients developed metastasis during the surveillance period [14]. Important questions, such as cancer-specific death in untreated lesions and how to differentiate benign from malignant growth patterns, remain unanswered. Indeed, surveillance rather than immediate ablative therapy has been proposed as one treatment strategy. To this end, the work of Kouba and colleagues [15] is most enlightening. In this study of 43 patients who had 46 solid or cystic (Bosniak IV) masses with a mean size of 2.9 cm who were followed for an average of 3 years, there was a median growth rate of 6 mm/y. Only 28% came to surgery (ie, growth rate of 9 mm/y), among whom 87% had cancerous lesions. During the same period, 10% of the patients died from unrelated causes, having had no renal surgery. Over the 3-year period, no patient developed metastatic disease, and among those coming to surgery, all still had a nephron-sparing procedure.

Laparoscopic partial nephrectomy

Winfield and colleagues [16] performed the first LPN in 1991 for benign disease, with McDougall and colleagues [17] subsequently extending the application to renal tumors in 1993. The traditional open approach to nephron-sparing surgery has established oncologic and functional outcomes with 10-year follow-up [8,9]. Several groups have published their results with the laparoscopic technique (Table 1) [3,4,18–25]. Lane and Gill [4] recently published the results on 58 patients who had undergone an LPN with at least 5 years of follow-up (median of 5.7 years; range: 5–6.9 years). The mean tumor size was 2.9 cm, and the 5-year overall and cancer-specific survival (CSS) rates were 86% and 100%, respectively, which is comparable to the published open series. There was one positive surgical margin (1.7%) and an overall complication rate of 21%. On average, the creatinine increased from 0.9 mg/dL before surgery to 1.0 mg/dL after surgery. No patient with a normal preoperative creatinine level developed postoperative chronic renal insufficiency, as defined by a serum creatinine level greater than 2 mg/dL. Thirty-seven patients (66%) had RCC on the final histopathologic analysis, and in this group of patients, there were no distant recurrences and a single local recurrence (1.7%). Allaf and colleagues [24] reported the oncologic outcomes of 48 patients who had pathologically proved RCC with a mean follow-up of 38 months. The mean tumor size was 2.4 cm, with 42 patients having pT1 tumors and 6 patients having pT3a tumors. All patients had a negative intraoperative frozen margin; however, one of these was determined to be positive on the final pathologic examination (2.1%). This patient remained disease-free with greater than 3 years of follow-up. Two patients (4.2%) developed a local recurrence at 18 and 46 months after surgery. Jeschke and colleagues [3] reported on their series of 51 patients undergoing LPN with a mean follow-up of 34 months (range: 3–78 months). The mean tumor size was 2 cm (range: 1–5 cm), with 35 patients having pT1 tumors and 3 having pT3a tumors; 38 patients (76%) were confirmed to have pathologic RCC. Surgical margins were negative in all cases. One patient (2.6%) developed a local recurrence 12 months after the initial surgery, and no distant recurrences were seen. The overall complication rate was 10%.

Three large series comparing laparoscopic with open partial nephrectomy (OPN) are summarized in Table 2 [5,26,27]. A direct comparative analysis of 100 consecutive LPNs to a contemporary cohort of 100 consecutive OPNs was reported by Gill and colleagues [28]. The LPN group had smaller tumors (2.8 versus 3.3 cm), a shorter operative time (3 versus 3.9 hours), less blood loss

Table 1
Summary of clinical series of laparoscopic partial nephrectomy

Authors	Institution	No. patients [tumors] (N)	Mean tumor size [cm] (range)	Mean warm ischemia time (minutes)	Mean EBL (mL)	Malignancy rate (%)	Positive surgical margin (%)	Length of follow-up/months (range)	Recurrence		Complications			Survival		
									Local	Distant	Intraoperative	Postoperative	Overall	Recurrence-free (%)	Cancer-specific (%)	Overall (%)
Lane et al [4]	Cleveland Clinic	56	2.9 (1.3–7.0)	—	—	66%	1 (1.7%)	68 (60–83)	1	0	6%	13%	18%	97%	100%	86%
Moinzadeh et al [18]	Cleveland Clinic	100	2.9	27	219	68%	2 (2%)	43 (24–62)	0	—	—	—	—	100%	100%	86%
Weld et al [19]	Washington University	60	2.5 (0.7–5.1)	26.9 (10–44)	226	60%	0 (0%)	25	0	0	—	—	30%	100%	—	—
Wille et al [20]	Humboldt University	44	2.8 (1–5)	21 (7–41)	—	82%	0	15 (6–37)	0	0	0%	—	—	100%	—	—
Link et al [21]	Johns Hopkins	217	2.6 (1–10)	27.8 (5–60)	385	66%	7 (3.5%)	24 (7–54)	2	0	—	10.6%	—	—	—	—
Ramani et al [22]	Cleveland Clinic	200	2.9 (1–10)	28.7 (15–58)	247	—	—	—	—	—	5.5%	27.5% (15.5% delayed)	33%	—	—	—
Abukora et al [23]	Elisabethinen Austria	78	2.4 (0.5–3.5)	33.8 (17–56)	212	83%	1 (1.2%)	16 (3–38)	0	0	9%	19%	28%	100%	—	—
Allaf et al [24]	Johns Hopkins	48	2.4 (1.0–4.0)	—	—	100%	1 (2.1%)	38 (22–84)	2	0	—	—	—	96%	100%	—
Seifman et al [25]	University of Michigan	40	2.3	—	300	73%	1 (2.5%)	24	0	0	—	—	38%	100%	—	—
Jeschke et al [3]	University of Innsbruck	51	2.0	—	282	76%	0 (0%)	34 (3–78)	0	0	2%	8%	10%	100%	100%	—

Data from Canes D. Long-term oncological outcomes of laparoscopic partial nephrectomy. Curr Opin Urol 2008;18:145–9.

Table 2
Summary of comparative clinical series of laparoscopic versus open partial nephrectomy

Authors	Institution	Surgery	Patients [tumors] (N)	Mean tumor size [cm] (range)	Mean warm ischemia time (minutes)	Mean EBL (mL)	OR time (minutes)	LOS (days)	Malignancy rate (%)	Positive surgical margin (%)	Length of follow-up [months] (range)	Recurrence Local	Recurrence Distant	Intra operative complications	Bleeding/ Urine leak	All post operative	Survival Recurrence-free (%)	Survival Cancer-specific (%)	Survival Overall (%)
Gill et al [26]	3 centers[a]	LPN	771	2.7 (0.5–7.0)	30 (4–68)	300	201	3.3	72%	22 (2.9%)	14 (0–84)	1.4%[b]	0.9%[b]	1.8%	4.2% 3.1%	25%	—	99%[b]	—
		OPN	1028	3.5 (0.6–7.0)	20 (4–52)	376	266	5.8	83%	13 (1.3%)	34 (0–91)	1.5%[b]	2.1%[b]	1.0%	1.6% 2.3%	19%	—	99%[b]	—
Permpongkosol et al [5]	Johns Hopkins	LPN	85	2.4 (0.5–5.3)	29.5	437	225	3.3	100%	2 (2.4%)	40 (18–96)	2 (2.3%)	1 (1.2%)	3.5%	—	7%	91%[c]	—	94%[c]
		OPN	58	2.9 (1–5)	48	428	276	5.4	100%	1 (1.7%)	49 (18–106)	1 (1.7%)	1	3.5%	—	22%	97%[c]	—	96%[c]
Gill et al [27]	Cleveland Clinic	LPN	100	2.8	28	125	180	2.0	70%	3	—	—	—	5%	3% 3%	16%	—	—	—
		OPN	100	3.3	18	250	231	5.0	85%	0	—	—	—	0%	0% 1%	13%	—	—	—

[a] Cleveland Clinic, Johns Hopkins, and Mayo Clinic.
[b] Three-year Kaplan-Meier estimates.
[c] Five-year Kaplan-Meier estimates.

(125 versus 250 mL), and a longer warm ischemia time (28 versus 18 minutes) when compared with the OPN group. The overall complication rate was similar, with 19% of patients in the LPN group and 13% in the OPN group experiencing complications. Five percent of the LPN group had intraoperative complications versus none in the OPN group, however. Additionally, the LPN group had more renal or urologic complications (11% versus 2%). This study confirmed that laparoscopic nephron-sparing surgery is an effective therapeutic approach, albeit a technically demanding and more morbid procedure than OPN even in highly experienced hands. Advantages of LPN included decreased narcotic use (20- versus 252-mg morphine equivalents), shorter hospital stay (2 versus 5 days), and a more rapid convalescence (4 versus 6 weeks). Permpongkosol and colleagues [5] reported the outcomes of 85 LPNs compared with 58 OPNs with pathologically proven RCC and mean follow-ups of 40 and 49 months, respectively. The 5-year recurrence-free and overall survival rates were 91% versus 97% and 94% versus 96% for LPN and OPN, respectively, demonstrating equivalent intermediate oncologic outcomes. The largest comparative study reported the outcomes of 771 LPNs compared with 1028 OPNs from three tertiary care centers [26]. The OPN group had larger tumors (3.5 versus 2.7 cm) and represented a higher risk group based on performance status, impaired renal function, and solitary tumor status. LPN was associated with a shorter operative time (201 versus 266 minutes) decreased blood loss (300 versus 376 mL), and a shorter hospital stay (3.3 versus 5.7 days) but had a longer warm ischemia time (30 versus 20 minutes) and more postoperative complications (25% versus 19%). Renal functional outcomes (98% versus 99%) and 3-year CSS (99% versus 99%) were similar with both approaches.

With regard to the morbidity of LPN, Ramani and colleagues [22] looked at the complications seen in 200 consecutive LPNs. A total of 66 patients (33%) experienced at least one complication. Hemorrhage was the most common complication and was seen in 19 patients (9.5%), occurring during surgery in 7 (3.5%), after surgery in 4 (2%), and delayed (after discharge) in 8 (4%) at a mean of 16 postoperative days. A urine leak was seen in 9 patients (4.5%) and was typically managed with a double-J stent. Again, this series came from the Cleveland Clinic, which has the largest experience with LPN, stressing that even

in the most experienced hands, the morbidity of LPN is a significant consideration.

Technique

Approach

LPNs have been successfully performed by means of transperitoneal and retroperitoneal approaches. The choice is typically based on surgeon preference, tumor location, and patient factors, although the transperitoneal approach provides a larger working space with more familiar anatomy, which may facilitate tumor excision and renorrhaphy. In general, for lesions that are directed posteriorly, a retroperitoneal approach is chosen, especially if no entry into the collecting system is anticipated because of the mass being largely exophytic (ie, less than 10 mm extension into the kidney).

Intraoperative ultrasound

The use of intraoperative laparoscopic ultrasound has become common to define the borders of the tumor and to assist in planning the plane of incision for removal. Additionally, the entire kidney may be surveyed to rule out other lesions.

Vascular control

Vascular clamping provides a bloodless field for more precise tumor excision. Vascular occlusion can be achieved with internalized bulldog vascular clamps or with an exteriorized handheld Satinsky clamp. When using bulldog clamps, one is typically placed on the artery and another on the vein, although clamping of the artery alone is also an option, because the renal venous blood flow is decreased by upward of 90% with a pneumoperitoneum pressure of 15 mm Hg [29].

The bulldog clamps seem to provide the most reliable occlusive force when placed entirely across the vessel to the end of the clamp [30]. Additionally, over time, some bulldogs fatigue and no longer provide supraphysiologic occlusion forces, which could explain some of the variability noted among bulldog clamps and recommendations of some surgeons to check for cessation of arterial inflow to the kidney with a laparoscopic ultrasound Doppler probe or to place at least two bulldog clamps on the artery (J. Landman, personal communication).

The Satinsky clamps are typically placed across the entire hilum without isolating the artery and vein individually. In the authors' experience, vascular control is not required for all tumors, and it is their policy to use vascular control only for tumors that are 10 mm or deeper from the kidney surface and are likely to entail closure of the collecting system; with this approach, warm ischemia time is avoided during the excision of most exophytic masses [31].

Warm ischemia

The acceptable duration of warm ischemia that can be tolerated without causing reversible nephron loss has not been firmly established, although minimizing warm ischemia time is generally agreed to be important. Typically, warm ischemia times 30 minutes or less are desirable, but some have shown that warm ischemia time up to 40 to 45 minutes may be well tolerated [32]. Of note, in the porcine model, warm ischemia times of 90 minutes are tolerated with complete return of function in 2 weeks [33]. All this depends more on the patient than on the absolute warm ischemia time, because the elderly patient, the hypertensive patient who has arteriosclerosis, patients with preexisting renal insufficiency, or the diabetic patient seems to be more prone to damage from warm ischemia even of short duration. This has led some surgeons to release the vascular clamps before completing the renorrhaphy, thereby producing warm ischemia times of 15 minutes or less [34].

Adjuncts

Bleeding is the most common complication after LPN, and several hemostatic agents exist to help achieve hemostasis. These include thrombin-impregnated gelatin matrix, fibrin sealants, and oxidized cellulose. Looking at risk factors for complications after LPN, thrombin-impregnated gelatin matrix has been shown to decrease the risk for postoperative bleeding complications [35].

Current technique: with warm ischemia

Using a transperitoneal approach, the kidney is mobilized and the renal hilum is isolated en bloc. The capsule of the kidney is exposed within Gerota's fascia to the edge of the tumor, leaving the peritumoral fat in place. Intraoperative ultrasound is used to confirm the size and depth of the tumor, and the argon beam monopolar cautery is then used to score the renal capsule around the tumor along the planned site of excision. All sutures (6-inch length of 2-0 Vicryl on SH needle and 10-inch length of 0 Vicryl on CT-1 needle) and bolsters needed for repair are placed into the abdominal cavity before applying the vascular clamp to minimize warm ischemia time. The handheld Satinsky clamp is applied across the renal hilum, the tumor is excised, and reconstruction is performed using a specific series of techniques in an attempt to minimize bleeding [36]. In this regard, at the authors' institution, tumor excision is performed using an energy-based device; either a bipolar or ultrasonic based sealing device. The argon beam monopolar cautery is then applied to the tumor base, followed by suture repair of the collecting system and exposed vessels. A absorbable polydioxanone suture anchor is used to secure the suture at either end, as previously described [37]. A layer of thrombin-impregnated gelatin matrix is applied, followed by oxidized cellulose bolsters; then, a series of simple sutures is used to close the parenchymal defect, again utilizing absorbable polydioxanone suture anchors. Finally, fibrin glue or thrombin-impregnated gelatin matrix is applied on the surface of the repair. Using this technique, no early or delayed postoperative bleeding complications have occurred over a 2-year period [36].

Current technique: without warm ischemia

In patients who have a 3-cm or smaller tumor that is nonhilar and does not extend into the renal parenchyma by more than 10 mm, the lesion can be excised without any warm ischemia. A spiral CT angiogram is performed with three-dimensional reconstruction to measure the depth of the tumor accurately and assess its proximity to the collecting system. This approach requires the use of a bipolar or ultrasonic sealing device to excise the lesion. Although questions have been raised concerning the integrity of the margin, in fact, neither the bipolar nor the ultrasonic modality precludes an accurate assessment of the margin status according to an extensive study recently completed at the authors' institution [38]. The approach to the tumor is based on its location, with retroperitoneoscopy being performed for posteriorly directed tumors and transperitoneal laparoscopy being performed for anteriorly directed tumors. The hilum can be dissected at the surgeon's discretion; however, this is not routinely done in the authors' operating room. Once the peritumoral fat is removed and the lesion is clearly seen for a complete 360° circumference, the planned site of incision is marked with monopolar electrocautery and the argon beam cautery. The renal capsule is then incised completely around the tumor. The pneumoperitoneum pressure is then elevated to 20 to 25 mm Hg, the anesthesiologist is notified, and a timer is set for 10 minutes. Using the bipolar or ultrasonic sealing device, the activated blade is passed to its full depth at the inferior point of the tumor; this is done so that one is always working away from any bleeding that may occur. Once the jaws of the device are closed and activated (ie, bipolar based sealing device) or activated and closed (ie, ultrasonic based sealing device), the dissection continues to the right and left side and upward. Throughout the process, the assistant can use the argon beam to stop any bleeding that occurs; the surgeon uses the suction unit in the nondominant hand continually to expose the next adjacent area to be incised. As the tumor is rolled upward and out of its parenchymal bed, the argon beam is used to continue to aid hemostasis on the parenchymal surface. In this manner, the tumor is mobilized and excised. As soon as the tumor is free, the parenchymal bed is treated with argon beam cautery, followed by fibrin glue, a layer of oxidized cellulose, and another layer of fibrin glue; a couple of minutes are allowed to pass to enable the fibrin glue to set up. Usually, this entire process should take less than 10 minutes. The pneumoperitoneum is then lowered to 5 mm Hg to check for any bleeding. In none of our cases have we found it necessary to place a bolster or to suture the edges of the capsule or parenchyma. A 5-mm round drain is placed at the end of the procedure.

Laparoscopic radical nephrectomy

Since Clayman and colleagues [2] performed the first laparoscopic nephrectomy (LRN) in June of 1990 at Washington University, this technique has become internationally accepted. In fact, many urologists consider this the standard of care for those patients who have T1, T2, or T3a tumors amenable to treatment by means of the laparoscopic approach but are not candidates for nephron-sparing surgery. The decreased morbidity of LRN has been well documented with reductions in postoperative pain, hospital stay, and convalescence. Several studies with maturing follow-up data have been published, establishing the oncologic equivalency to the open procedure (Table 3) [39–44]. Portis and colleagues [44] reported a multicenter series of 64 patients treated with LRN compared with a group of 69 patients treated with open radical nephrectomy (ORN). With a median follow-up of 54 months (range: 0–94 months), no difference was seen between the two approaches, with a 5-year recurrence-free survival, 5-year CSS, and overall survival rates of 92%, 98%, and 81%, respectively, in the laparoscopic group. Permpongkosol and

colleagues [42] reported on a series of 67 patients who had an LRN with a median follow-up of 73 months (range: 12–164 months) that was compared with 54 patients who had renal cancer and had an ORN. The 10-year disease-free, cancer-specific, and actuarial survival rates for the laparoscopic group were 94%, 97%, and 76% compared with 87%, 86%, and 58% in the open group, respectively. Hemal and colleagues [40] reported on their series of 132 patients having a laparoscopic nephrectomy for pT1 to pT2 RCC with a median follow-up of 56 months (range: 3–80 months). The survival analysis was grouped by T stage, with 5-year CSS rates and 5-year recurrence-free survival rates of 97.2% and 97.2%, 86.3% and 84.3%, and 82.2% and 82.2%, respectively, for pT1a, pT1b, and pT2 tumors. With a decade of follow-up in some series, LRN has now demonstrated oncologic equivalency to open surgery.

Technique

Approach

Transperitoneal, retroperitoneal, and hand-assisted approaches to LRN have all been reported. Similar to LPN, the choice often depends on surgeon experience and patient factors. One prospective study compared the three approaches and showed reduced operative time with the hand-assisted approach, whereas the incision size, hospital stay, and convalescence were less in the transperitoneal group [45]. A larger retrospective study confirmed these findings [46].

Morcellation

One of the benefits of laparoscopic surgery is the reduced invasiveness of the procedure and the improved cosmetic result. When a large incision is made for intact specimen removal, some of these benefits are lost. Specimen morcellation has been used to maintain these benefits. A nylon entrapment sack with a polyurethane inner coating is the only entrapment bag that has been routinely used for morcellation because it is the only entrapment device with the appropriate durability and proven impermeability available. Generally, morcellation is done with a ring forceps and suction; the authors routinely enlarge a 12-mm port site to 1 inch and use Sopher ring forceps because they are stronger with a broader ring than the traditional ring forceps in the general surgery tray. Before morcellation, the authors believe it is of paramount importance that the wound be meticulously triple draped (towel drape, plastic

Table 3
Summary of clinical series of laparoscopic radical nephrectomy

Authors	Institution	Type of surgery	Patients (N)	Tumor size (range)	Mean EBL (mL)	Length of follow-up [months] (range)	Complications	5-year survival			10-year survival		
								Recurrence-free (%)	Cancer-specific (%)	Overall (%)	Recurrence-free (%)	Cancer-specific (%)	Overall (%)
Colombo et al [39]	Cleveland Clinic	LRN	63	5.4	179	65 (19–92)	7%	91%	91%	78%	—	—	—
		ORN	53	6.4	501	76 (8–105)	—	93%	93%	84%	—	—	—
Hemal et al [40]	All India Institute	LRN	132	6.9 (3.6–14)	193	56 (3–80)	17%	87%	88%	86%	—	—	—
Kawauchi et al [41]	22 centers	HALRN	123	4.4	173	41	9%	92%	92%	—	—	—	—
		ORN	70	4.4	448	74	10%	91%	94%	—	—	—	—
Permpongkosol et al [42]	Johns Hopkins	LRN	67	T1–46 (69%) T2–21 (31%)	—	73 (12–164)	—	94%	97%	85%	94%	97%	76%
		ORN	54	T1–40 (74%) T2–14 (26%)	—	80 (8–157)	—	87%	89%	72%	87%	86%	58%
Saika et al [43]	Nagoya University	LRN	195	3.7	248	40 (2–121)	15%	91%	—	94%	—	—	—
		ORN	68	4.4	482	65 (11–126)	7%	87%	—	94%	—	—	—
Portis et al [44]	3 centers[a]	LRN	64	4.3 (2–10)	219	54 (0–94)	—	92%	98%	81%	—	—	—
		ORN	69	6.2 (2.5–15)	354	69 (8–114)	—	91%	92%	89%	—	—	—

[a] Washington University, University of Saskatchewan, Nagoya University.

adherent drape, and a nephrostomy drape), and once the removal of the specimen and entrapment sack is complete, all those in contact with the specimen regown and reglove. The wound from which the entrapment sack has been removed is then bathed in water or povidone iodine. This is to prevent seeding of the port site. Since the inception of laparoscopic nephrectomy by the authors more than 15 years ago using this approach, to the best of their knowledge, there has not been a single instance of wound seeding at Washington University or at the University of California–Irvine.

Cytoreductive laparoscopic nephrectomy

As the proficiency in performing LRN has improved, the indications for the laparoscopic management of renal tumors have expanded. Several groups have reported laparoscopic cytoreductive nephrectomy (LCN) before systemic therapy in patients who had stage IV RCC. Walther and colleagues [47] were the first to report a series of LCNs. The group of patients undergoing LCN whose tumor was morcellated had significantly reduced time to immunotherapy (interleukin [IL]-2 in this report) compared with patients undergoing open cytoreductive nephrectomy (OCN). With the introduction of the less toxic, oral, targeted therapies, patients undergoing laparoscopic cytoreductive surgery may benefit from improved recovery and even earlier initiation of therapy. Rabets and colleagues [48] confirmed the improved quality-of-life outcomes with LCN (n = 22) compared with OCN (n = 42) in the metastatic setting. The laparoscopic group had a shorter hospital stay (2.3 versus 6.1 days), decreased blood loss (288 versus 1228 mL), and a shorter time until receiving systemic therapy (36 versus 61 days). The 1-year survival rate was 61% in the laparoscopic group compared with 65% in the open group. Matin and colleagues [49] also reported the feasibility and safety of LCN in 38 patients. These reports support the role for a laparoscopic approach to nephrectomy in properly selected patients who have metastatic disease; however, no survival advantage from the earlier receipt of the planned immunotherapy has been demonstrated.

Regional lymphadenectomy

Historically, a lymph node dissection (LND) was included as part of a radical nephrectomy [50]. Whether this provides any benefit to the patient has been debated for many years, and no clear consensus has been reached. The only prospective randomized trial to assess the need for an LND detected unsuspected lymph node metastasis in 11 (3.3%) of 336 patients and did not find a difference in survival at 5-year follow-up [51]. Patients who had microscopic lymph node involvement with renal cancer are hypothetically most likely to benefit from an LND; however, given the low incidence of nodal involvement, demonstrating a survival advantage would require a large number of study patients. Improved staging is another argument for LND; however, without any effective adjuvant therapy to date, the need for this additional information is again questionable, plus there are data showing that the more distant nodes are merely reflective of the hilar node status [52]. In contrast, LND can be accomplished when one considers the chance of nodal involvement to be likely. To wit, Simmons and colleagues [53] reported successful LND in 14 patients. The LND added an average of approximately 30 minutes to the operative time. There was one complication in this group: postoperative ileus managed conservatively. These investigators emphasized the importance of patient selection, using the laparoscopic approach only if nodal masses were discrete and the tissue planes around the great vessels were preserved.

Conclusion

For most renal tumors, LRN, when compared with the open approach, produces superior morbidity outcomes while maintaining equivalent long-term oncologic results. When evaluating any of the options for treating small tumors with a nephron-sparing approach, it is important to remember that the outcomes should be measured against the current "gold standard" open approach. We are currently at a crossroad in the treatment of small renal tumors. Although many of the ablative therapies show tremendous promise, determining the most effective treatment that causes the least morbidity in potentially life-threatening tumors is in need of further clarification. To this end, well-done, meticulous, retrospective matched studies and prospective comparative studies are needed to determine which of the methods brings an efficacy level equivalent or possibly superior to open surgery while providing the most favorable morbidity and reasonable cost profile.

Transitional cell carcinoma

Upper tract TCC is an uncommon disease. Primary upper tract TCC represents approximately 5% of all urothelial carcinomas and 10% of all primary renal tumors. Like TCC of the bladder, upper tract urothelial carcinoma represents a field defect that can occur, recur, and progress in any location in the urinary tract. The most common location for ureteral TCC is the distal ureter (70%), followed by the middle ureter (25%) and proximal (5%) ureter [54]. Recurrence in the ipsilateral kidney is common and can be as high as 84%. Upper tract TCC is frequently multifocal (up to 44%). Recurrence rates in the contralateral ureter are less common. The incidence of contralateral synchronous and metachronous recurrence ranges from 1.8% to 5% [55,56]. The risk for contralateral recurrence persists even at 5 to 10 years. Surveillance for contralateral recurrence should continue for up to 10 years.

The diagnosis of upper tract TCC is most often made by contrast-enhanced imaging. Cytology is useful mostly in the setting of high-grade TCC or carcinoma in situ (CIS). Selective cytology for CIS of the upper tract has a reported accuracy rate as high as 80% [57]. Voided urine cytology for low-grade lesions (grade 1) can have a false-negative rate as high as 96%, however. The combination of a filling defect on CT scan, intravenous pyelogram, or retrograde urography with positive cytology often makes the diagnosis. The addition of ureteropyeloscopy and biopsy or ureteral brushings increases the diagnostic yield from 58% to 83% [58]. Prognosis is closely linked to location, stage, and grade. CT has often been inaccurate in determining the invasiveness of upper tract lesions. Therefore, ureteropyeloscopy is as essential to staging as it is to grading. Unlike bladder cancer, which typically has a thick muscle layer protecting against extravesicular extension, the smooth muscle covering the ureter and renal pelvis is much thinner. Tumors therefore have less time to remain organ confined, and there is less tissue to preserve a clear margin with extirpative procedures. Pathologic findings in large series of upper tract TCC revealed that upper tract tumors tend to present with a higher grade and stage than bladder cancer. Indeed, approximately 70% of upper tract TCCs were of moderate or high grade, and more than half had some degree of invasion [59].

Treatment options for upper tract TCC are numerous. Because of the high ipsilateral recurrence rate associated with upper tract TCC, nephroureterectomy with an open or laparoscopic technique remains the gold standard. In patients who cannot tolerate extirpative surgery because of serious comorbidities, however, or in patients who have renal insufficiency or solitary (or solitary functional) kidneys and may require dialysis after surgery, endoscopic management may be a reasonable alternative. As advances in endoscopy and ablative treatments have been made, the indications for endoscopic minimally invasive treatments have been increasing. The authors review all the minimally invasive treatment options for upper tract TCC.

Ureteroscopy

Along with solitary (or solitary functional) kidneys, contemporary indications for ureteroscopic treatment of upper tract TCC includes significant renal insufficiency, bilateral upper tract tumors, and patients who have comorbidities that preclude extirpative surgery. Experience, advances in technology, and our improved understanding of the biology of upper tract TCC have proved that a more conservative strategy can be successfully adopted in well-selected cases. The indications for ureteroscopy have expanded to include patients who have low-grade and low-stage tumors. In this patient population, meticulous and rigorous surveillance protocols must be maintained. Patients must be able and willing to follow up carefully with frequent urinary cytology and contrast-enhanced upper tract imaging to ensure prompt diagnosis and management of recurrence. Often, repeated and frequent endoscopic surveillance is appropriate in this population. Endoscopic therapy offers the advantages of minimally invasive surgery, and in highly selected patients, it may provide results equivalent to radical extirpative surgery [60,61].

In addition to patient characteristics, tumors amenable to ureteroscopic treatment are usually solitary, small (< 1.5 cm), low grade, and amenable to complete resection [62]. In contrast, higher grade tumors, larger size, and multifocality have been associated with tumor persistence and recurrence. Recently, Sowter and colleagues [63] found that the highest rate of patients needing nephroureterectomy after ureteroscopic resection was in patients who had grade III TCC. In their review, there was an overall survival rate of 80%, with a disease-specific survival rate of 100%.

Because it is less invasive and does not open any closed tissue planes, ureteroscopy is usually the preferred access technique for small upper tract TCC of the ureter, renal pelvis, and upper calices. Ureteroscopic treatment of focal low- and intermediate-grade superficial upper tract TCC is a safe alternative to nephroureterectomy in select patients when vigilant ureteroscopic follow-up is applied. Larger less accessible lesions that cannot be resected or fulgurated adequately can be treated percutaneously [64]. Primary tumors greater than 1 cm that are challenging to ablate or that result in bleeding or poor visibility can be treated in a staged manner with multiple ureteroscopic procedures.

Ureteroscopy can be performed in an ambulatory setting and requires minimal anesthesia and minimal postoperative analgesia. The disadvantages of ureteroscopic management are the challenges of long-term surveillance, patient anxiety, the potential for tumor seeding, and the requirement for multiple repeated procedures.

Technique

Midureteral or distal tumors can be accessed with a semirigid ureteral resectoscope, which offers excellent visualization and the ability to get deep resections, fulgurations, and negative margins. Tumor ablation is now an acceptable substitute for resection. Energy sources, such as the holmium:yttrium-aluminum-garnet (YAG) laser and neodymium:YAG laser delivered through small fibers (approximately 270 μ), can be used to ablate or coagulate tumors. Operative technique has been previously described by several researchers [64,65]. Although the initial experience with endourologic management of upper tract TCC made almost exclusive use of electrocautery and fulguration, more recent reports have emphasized the potential utility of lasers in this setting [66]. If an urothelial lesion is identified ureteroscopically, biopsy is usually the first management step. For papillary exophytic lesions, a small nitinol basket, a 2.4-French flat wire basket, or 3-French flexible cup biopsy forceps may be used to avulse a section of a tumor [64]. Other reported devices include the Segura helical, Bagley round-wire, Nitinol baskets, wire prong grasper, or 3-French Piranha biopsy forceps. More recently, the Bigopsy device has been introduced and may afford the surgeon the ability to obtain more robust endoscopic biopsies. After biopsy, the remaining tumor is ablated with laser or fulgurated with a 2-French electrode. In a comparative study evaluating local recurrences between tumors ablated with electrocautery and tumors treated with laser ablation, Krambeck

and colleagues [67] noted a recurrence rate of 38 (62.3%) in patients treated with cautery ablation compared with 14 (58.3%) in patients treated with laser ablation.

No standardized surveillance protocol for upper urinary tract TCC after endoscopic management has been established. In the authors' experience, however, surveillance includes urinary cytology and an endoscopic inspection of the bladder and upper urinary tract with urinary cytology on a 3- to 4-month schedule for the first 2 years. The upper urinary tract evaluation can be performed on an outpatient basis under sedation or regional or general anesthesia.

Ureteroscopic surveillance has been performed by urologists experienced with ureteroscopic technique in the office setting under topical lidocaine-based anesthetic in select patients with dilated systems [65]. More recently, Reisiger and colleagues [66] have reported on their long-term experience with the use of office-based ureteroscopy for upper tract TCC surveillance. In this series, these investigators performed ureteral unroofing after management of upper tract TCC that later facilitated the office surveillance. The most important aspect of office-based ureteroscopy is immediate termination of the procedure and rescheduling of the procedure in the operating room if any technical challenges are encountered. After the procedure, a quinolone antibiotic is given for 1 day. Patients can be followed up with a standard surveillance protocol, paralleling cystoscopic evaluation for bladder TCC (usually every 3 to 4 months for 2 years, every 6 months for 2 years, and annually thereafter), provided that no recurrence has developed [66].

Ultimately, treatment options and follow-up surveillance are based on tumor grade and stage. Unfortunately, with the limitations of upper tract ureteroscopic biopsy relating to depth of invasion, tumor staging information is limited. Therefore, clinical decision making is often determined by tumor grade alone. Low-grade (I) TCC is usually associated with a low stage, and superficial (Ta) TCC has a lower recurrence rate and does not frequently progress to muscle invasive or metastatic disease. As such, low-grade superficial TCC typically has an excellent outcome when treated endoscopically. Grade II TCC has more variable behavior and has a higher ipsilateral recurrence rate. Grade III tumors are often invasive, with significant metastatic potential, and have a poor prognosis regardless of the surgical approach.

Percutaneous

Percutaneous access allows larger tumors to be resected throughout the collecting system [68,69]. The percutaneous approach is best indicated for patients who have larger renal pelvic tumors, collecting system tumors (greater than 1.5 cm), or bulky proximal ureteral tumors. The percutaneous approach is advantageous because it permits a better working environment. The larger endoscopes provide better optics and irrigant flow for superior vision in addition to larger working instruments that facilitate the treatment of larger tumors. The percutaneous tract can be maintained for a "second look," and it provides an opportunity for the administration of adjuvant chemotherapy or immunotherapy through the matured tract.

The most important criterion for using the percutaneous approach is tumor grade. In a 13-year retrospective study, grade was the most important prognostic indicator in patients who had renal TCC regardless of the surgical approach. Grade III tumors were more aggressive, presenting in an advanced stage with invasion, and recurrences were usually associated with metastasis. Therefore, nephroureterectomy is most often indicated in this setting. The percutaneous option is best for grade I or II disease and may be extended beyond patients with solitary kidneys or chronic renal failure [70]. Percutaneous treatment can be offered to healthy individuals with normal contralateral kidneys who are willing to abide by a strict and lengthy follow-up [69].

The disadvantage to the percutaneous approach is the increased morbidity associated with percutaneous renal surgery compared with retrograde endoscopy. A second disadvantage is the unproved yet significant concern of a tumor-seeding tract through the access tract.

Technique

The percutaneous technique has been described previously [70–72]. The resection begins with obtaining proper access into the preferred calyx. The most direct accessible posterior calix should be punctured. Caliceal tumors are best approached as distal in the calyx as possible. Tumors in the pelvis are best approached through a midpole or upper pole calix [73]. It is useful to dilate up to a 30-French sheath to ensure minimal intrapelvic pressure. Endoscopy involves a resectoscope or flexible ureterorenoscopy under fluoroscopic guidance. To remove the bulk of the lesion, a cutting loop electrode using monopolar energy or biopsy forceps is commonly used. The neodymium:YAG and holmium:YAG lasers can ablate or resect the lesion as well. Typically, a second look procedure is performed within several days of the initial procedure, and any remaining tumor is treated. Intracavitary adjuvant therapy (bacille Calmette-Guérin [BCG] or mitomycin) can be administered 2 weeks after the resection, assuming that the access tract has matured and a nephrostogram is normal. Recently, the use of bipolar energy has been described for the resection of large renal pelvic tumors [74]. The advantage of bipolar energy is that normal saline can be used, limiting the incidence of dilutional hyponatremia secondary to water reabsorption.

The ipsilateral recurrence rate after percutaneous resection is 33%. Initially, 67% of the recurrences were grade 2 or 3 [71]. Only clinical stage and grade were prognostic factors for recurrence and survival. When carefully selected, the percutaneous approach can have comparably low recurrence rates to more aggressive therapies. Roupret and colleagues [75] performed a retrospective review of patients who underwent percutaneous surgery for upper tract TCC and reported 5-year disease-specific and tumor-free survival rates of 79.5% and 68%, respectively, for low-grade or superficial TCC localized in the kidney. Jabbour and colleagues [68] reported disease-free rates comparable to those of nephroureterectomy in patients who had grade II TCC treated percutaneously. After a mean follow-up of 51 months, these investigators described an overall tumor-specific survival rate of 84%; the rate was 100% for grade 1, 94% for grade 2, and 62% for grade 3 disease. Goel and colleagues [76] treated 20 patients who had TCC with percutaneous resection, with a mean of 64 months. All patients who had high-grade disease were treated with early nephroureterectomy. Six of the 15 patients who had low-grade noninvasive TCC went on to nephroureterectomy follow-up because of progression of disease, concomitant tumor, or as a result of complications. Sixty percent of the renal units with low-grade disease were preserved at a mean follow-up of 64 months. There was no evidence of any tumor seeding after a mean follow-up of 48 months. All excised tracks from patients undergoing nephroureterectomy were free of tumor. Tumor dissemination may be directly related to manipulation. As such, a single-stage percutaneous nephrostomy access tract dilation and maintaining a low renal pelvic pressure with a 30-French working sheath are advised. Still, there has been only one reported case of nephrostomy track seeding in the literature, which was of a high-grade lesion [77].

Laparoscopic nephroureterectomy

Since Clayman and colleagues [78] performed the first laparoscopic nephroureterectomy (LNU) in 1991, LNU with an excision of a bladder cuff has been rapidly replacing open nephroureterectomy (ONU) as the standard-of-care treatment of high-grade multifocal disease of the upper urinary tract for the extirpative management of upper tract TCC. When compared with its open counterpart, LNU offers patients the advantages of a laparoscopic access approach, minimizing the perioperative morbidity, decreasing the postoperative pain, and expediting convalescence, all while duplicating the oncologic outcome of open surgery. Table 4 compares the surgical outcomes for ONU and LNU. Shalhav and colleagues [79] reported that when compared with open surgery, patients who underwent LNU manifested half the estimated blood loss, required fourfold less morphine sulfate equivalents, resumed oral intake six times faster, were discharged three times earlier, and returned to normal activity two times more quickly. Despite these advantages, there are two limitations associated with LNU: longer operative time and the need for significant laparoscopic surgical experience. These disadvantages may be lessened by the use of the hand-assisted technique for nephroureterectomy. Indeed, hand-assisted nephroureterectomy (HALNU) is the most commonly reported technique for performing minimally invasive nephroureterectomy.

A series by Muntener and colleagues [85] reported that after LNU, tumor stage was the only factor significantly associated with death from the disease and that tumor location (ureter) was the only factor significantly associated with disease recurrence. Wolf and colleagues [86] published intermediate outcomes for HALNU. They demonstrated CSS rates of 94%, 86%, and 80% at 1, 2, and 3 years, respectively. When they stratified patients, patients who had stage 0 to I tumors had a 100% CSS at 26.5 months, whereas those who had stage II to IV tumors had rates of 53% and 36% at 2 and 3 years, respectively. Similarly, CSS in patients who had grade 1 to 2 tumors was 100% at 27 months of follow-up, whereas patients who had grade 3 tumors had CSS rates of 71% and 57% at 2 and 3 years, respectively.

Table 5 lists the most recent oncologic comparisons between ONU and LNU. Bariol and colleagues [87] found the 1- and 7-year metastasis-free survival rates were 80% and 72% for LNU compared with 87.2% and 82.1% for ONU ($P = .33$ and $P = .26$, respectively). Tumor grade and stage influenced the incidence of metastatic and contralateral disease but not the incidence of local or bladder recurrence.

Technique

Since the initial reports of LNU, there are several techniques that have been described for performance of the procedure. Regarding the nephrectomy component of the procedure, reports have described the application of a standard transperitoneal approach, a retroperitoneal approach, and a hand-assisted technique. All three are known to be safe and effective. Most of the controversy regarding LNU has been the optimal technique for management of the distal ureter and bladder cuff. Techniques for distal ureteral and bladder cuff management have included stapling and unroofing [89], a transvesical dissection [90], a pluck technique [91], and open distal ureteral management. Detailing the differences among these techniques is beyond the scope of this article. A complete extraction of the entire ureter with a bladder cuff is mandatory, however.

A second option, and the one that is most commonly used, is HALNU. The application of the hand-assisted device offers the urologic surgeon several advantages. First, by allowing one hand to remain in the realm of open surgery while the other hand and the surgeon's field of view are in a laparoscopic setting, the technique provides the newer laparoscopist a logical segue into minimally invasive surgery. The hand provides the surgeon with security, knowing that he or she can get out of trouble with his or her hand in the operative field. Thus, the hand-assisted technique decreases operative time and may allow less experienced laparoscopic surgeons to expand the scope of cases performed laparoscopically (ie, larger and more extensive tumors). Furthermore, removal of the kidney, ureter, and bladder cuff can easily be accomplished intact through a strategically placed hand-assisted device incision.

A disadvantage of LNU compared with ONU is exemplified by the two case reports on trocar site metastasis after LNU [92]. In a study of 97 patients, 54 had ONU, 27 had ureteroscopy, and 16 underwent percutaneous resection. The 5-year disease-specific survival rates after nephroureterectomy,

Table 4
Comparative nephroureterectomy trials (laparoscopic and hand-assisted laparoscopic versus open trials)

Series	Operative approach	N	OR time (hours)	EBL (mL)	Analgesic (mg MSO_4)	Hospital stay (days)	Complete convalescence (weeks)	Follow-up (years)	Major complications (%)
Shalhav et al [79]	LPN	25	7.7	199	37	3.6	2.8	2.0	8
	Open	17	3.9	441	144	9.6	10	3.6	29
Seifman et al [80]	HALN	16	5.3	557	48	3.9	2.5	1.5	19
	Open	11	3.3	345	81	5.2	7.5	1.2	27
Keeley and Tolley [81]	LNU	22	2.4	NA	NA	5.5	NA	NA	NA
	Open	26	2.3	NA	NA	10.8	NA	NA	NA
Hattori et al [82]	HALN	36	5.1	580	NA	NA	5	5	2
	LNU	53	4.3	354	NA	NA	4	5	1
	Open	60	5.4	665	NA	NA	8	5	3
Rassweiller et al [83]	LNU	23	3.3	450	18	10	NA	5	9
	Open	21	3.1	600	33	13	NA	5	10
Roupert et al [84]	LNU	20	2.7	274	NA	3.7	NA	5.75	15
	Open	26	2.6	338	NA	9.2	NA	6.5	15
Total	LNU	195	4.5	389	29.3	5.5	3.9	4.4	6.6
Total	Open	161	3.8	538	82	10.1	8.4	4.8	10.4

Table 5
Comparative of oncologic outcomes (laparoscopic and hand-assisted laparoscopic versus open trials)

Authors	Access	N	Tumor free	Port site metastasis	Short term disease-free survival	Intermediate disease-free survival
Bariol et al [87]	LNU	25	1 (4%)	0	80% at 1 year	72% at 7 years
	Open	40	6 (15%)	0	87.2% at 1 year	82% at 7 years
Hsueh et al [88]	HALN	66	23% at 2 years	NA	93.6% at 1 year	85% at 5 years
	Open	77	27% at 2 years	NA	82.9% at 1 year	77% at 5 years
Roupert et al [84]	LNU	20	71%	0	NA	90% at 5 years
	Open	26	51%	0	NA	61.5% at 5 years
Rassweiller et al [83]	LNU	23	65%	0	89% at 2 years	81% at 5 years
	Open	21	81%	0	83% at 2 years	63% at 5 years

ureteroscopy, and percutaneous resection were 84%, 80.7%, and 80%, respectively ($P = .89$); the corresponding 5-year tumor-free survival rates were 75.3%, 71.5%, and 72% ($P = .78$) [93].

Topical intracavitary therapy

Based on the well-characterized success of intravesical therapy in the treatment of bladder TCC and because of upper tract TCCs' similarly high rate of recurrence and progression, topical agents, such as thiotepa, mitomycin C, and BCG, have been used for the upper tract as well. First described by Herr [94] and Studer and colleagues [95] using BCG, topical therapy for upper tract TCC as an adjunct to ureteroscopic ablation has been used. Delivery of topical therapy accurately, reliably, and under low pressure to the upper tracts is much more complex than for bladder cancer, however. There are several techniques for instillation, which are briefly mentioned; however, no technique has emerged as a current standard. Agents can be instilled under gravity drainage by means of a preexisting or newly placed nephrostomy tube. A manometer is used to ensure that intrapelvic pressure remains less than 25 cm H_2O. In patients with double-J stents, which facilitate reflux, agents can be placed intravesically into the upper tract [96]. Finally, agents can be instilled in a retrograde fashion by means of an open-ended ureteral catheter.

Indications for the use of intracavitary chemotherapy or immunotherapy include bilateral disease, the presence of a solitary kidney (or solitary functional kidney), or significant renal insufficiency in which more aggressive surgical treatment risks placing the patient on permanent dialysis. A final indication is in patients at high operative risk, and alternative treatment forms are therefore necessary.

As in the bladder, the two most used agents are BCG and mitomycin. BCG is most commonly used for CIS, especially for higher risk patients who need close surveillance. Patel and Fuch [96] reported on 17 patients with a mean follow-up of 14.6 months. In 2 of 17 patients, multifocal tumors recurred within 12 months, which were ultimately treated with nephroureterectomy. The remaining 15 renal units have been preserved and remained tumor-free. In another series of 37 patients, the short-term efficacy of BCG perfusion therapy was reported to be 62.5% to 100%. Fourteen (38%) patients died of urothelial cancer, 11 died of other causes (29%), and 12 (33%) were still alive [97]. Katz and colleagues [98] studied 10 patients using a 6-week induction of BCG and interferon. With a median follow-up of 24 months, 8 patients (80%) demonstrated a complete response (CR) to therapy and 2 had a partial response (decrease in tumor size, number, or both). Six patients with a CR have continued on maintenance therapy. There were no side effects or complications with the instillation therapy. Among the disadvantages of BCG therapy is the fact that it is similar to the side affects of bladder instillation therapy. An additional disadvantage is the short dwell time, which is a result of our inability to keep it in sufficient contact with the urothelium to maximize its effect.

Mitomycin C has the same indications as BCG. These include multifocal disease, higher grade tumor, or rapid recurrence after previous treatment. Keeley and Bagley [99,100] reported their experience with mitomycin C in 19 patients during a 5-year period. They showed a 35% CR rate, a 27% partial response rate, and no response in 38%. With 30 months of follow-up, there was no progression, no dialysis, no systemic toxicity, and no deaths (Table 6). Despite the encouraging

Table 6
Results of intrapelvic therapy

Authors	No.patients	Agent	Access	Stage/grade	Recurrence (%)	Follow-up (months)
Sharpe et al	17	BCG	Retrograde	Ta,T1/CIS/G2–G4	28.5	11–64
Bellman	14	BCG	Percutaneous	n/a	12.5	n/a
Patel	13	BCG	Percutaneous	Ta low grade	13	6–36
Vasavada	8	BCG	Percutaneous	n/a	12.5	9–59
Nonomura	9	BCG	Retrograde	22	22	4–41
Eastham	7	Mitomycin C	Percutaneous	n/a	28.5	1–12
Keeley	20	Mitomycin C	Retrograde	G1–G3	54	30

Data from O'Donoghue JP, Crew, JP. Adjuvant topical treatment of upper urinary tract urothelial tumors, BJU Int 2004;94:483–5.

data, large prospective multicenter trials are needed to elucidate the role of intravesical therapy.

Summary

The number of available patients who meet the criteria for endoscopic treatment of upper tract TCC is small, and treatment algorithms are based more on experience than on large retrospective studies. Until such studies are available, experience reveals that minimally invasive options may be best suited for patients who have unifocal low-grade disease or for those patients who have bilateral disease, a solitary kidney, or comorbidities that contraindicate extirpative therapy. Upper tract TCC recurrences are to be expected after endoscopic resection, especially with high-grade and high-stage disease. Therefore, close endoscopic follow-up needs to part of the decision tree. Similar to TCC of the bladder, surveillance must be performed at regular intervals. The choice of endoscopic management must be offered on a case-by-case basis with the understanding that close surveillance is a requirement, and a key aspect of surveillance is the need for multiple and frequent procedures.

References

[1] Hollingsworth JM, Miller DC, Daignault S, et al. Rising incidence of small renal masses: a need to reassess treatment effect. J Natl Cancer Inst 2006; 98:1331–4.

[2] Clayman RV, Kavoussi LR, Soper NJ, et al. Laparoscopic nephrectomy: initial case report. J Urol 1991;146:278–82.

[3] Jeschke K, Peschel R, Wakonig J, et al. Laparoscopic nephron-sparing surgery for renal tumors. Urology 2001;58:688–92.

[4] Lane BR, Gill IS. 5-Year outcomes of laparoscopic partial nephrectomy. J Urol 2007;177:70–4.

[5] Permpongkosol S, Bagga HS, Romero FR, et al. Laparoscopic versus open partial nephrectomy for the treatment of pathological T1N0M0 renal cell carcinoma: a 5-year survival rate. J Urol 2006;176:1984–8.

[6] Marberger M, Schatzl G, Cranston D, et al. Extracorporeal ablation of renal tumours with high-intensity focused ultrasound. BJU Int 2005; 95(Suppl 2):52–5.

[7] Ponsky LE, Mahadevan A, Gill IS, et al. Renal radiosurgery: initial clinical experience with histological evaluation. Surg Innov 2007;14:265–9.

[8] Herr HW. Partial nephrectomy for unilateral renal carcinoma and a normal contralateral kidney: 10-year followup. J Urol 1999;161:33–5.

[9] Fergany AF, Hafez KS, Novick AC. Long-term results of nephron sparing surgery for localized renal cell carcinoma: 10-year followup. J Urol 2000;163: 442–5.

[10] Hafez KS, Fergany AF, Novick AC. Nephron sparing surgery for localized renal cell carcinoma: impact of tumor size on patient survival, tumor recurrence and TNM staging. J Urol 1999;162: 1930–3.

[11] Remzi M, Ozsoy M, Klingler HC, et al. Are small renal tumors harmless? Analysis of histopathological features according to tumors 4 cm or less in diameter. J Urol 2006;176:896–9.

[12] Frank I, Blute ML, Cheville JC, et al. Solid renal tumors: an analysis of pathological features related to tumor size. J Urol 2003;170:2217–20.

[13] Schachter LR, Cookson MS, Chang SS, et al. Second prize: frequency of benign renal cortical tumors and histologic subtypes based on size in a contemporary series: what to tell our patients. J Endourol 2007;21:819–23.

[14] Chawla SN, Crispen PL, Hanlon AL, et al. The natural history of observed enhancing renal masses: meta-analysis and review of the world literature. J Urol 2006;175:425–31.

[15] Kouba E, Smith A, McRackan D, et al. Watchful waiting for solid renal masses: insight into the natural history and results of delayed intervention. J Urol 2007;177:466–70.

[16] Winfield HN, Donovan JF, Godet AS, et al. Laparoscopic partial nephrectomy: initial case report for benign disease. J Endourol 1993;7:521–6.

[17] McDougall EM, Clayman RV, Anderson K. Laparoscopic wedge resection of a renal tumor: initial experience. J Laparoendosc Surg 1993;3:577–81.

[18] Moinzadeh A, Gill IS, Finelli A, et al. Laparoscopic partial nephrectomy: 3-year followup. J Urol 2006;175:459–62.

[19] Weld KJ, Venkatesh R, Huang J, et al. Evolution of surgical technique and patient outcomes for laparoscopic partial nephrectomy. Urology 2006;67: 502–6.

[20] Wille AH, Tullmann M, Roigas J, et al. Laparoscopic partial nephrectomy in renal cell cancer— results and reproducibility by different surgeons in a high volume laparoscopic center. Eur Urol 2006;49:337–42.

[21] Link RE, Bhayani SB, Allaf ME, et al. Exploring the learning curve, pathological outcomes and perioperative morbidity of laparoscopic partial nephrectomy performed for renal mass. J Urol 2005; 173:1690–4.

[22] Ramani AP, Desai MM, Steinberg AP, et al. Complications of laparoscopic partial nephrectomy in 200 cases. J Urol 2005;173:42–7.

[23] Abukora F, Nambirajan T, Albqami N, et al. Laparoscopic nephron sparing surgery: evolution in a decade. Eur Urol 2005;47:488–93.

[24] Allaf ME, Bhayani SB, Rogers C, et al. Laparoscopic partial nephrectomy: evaluation of long-term oncological outcome. J Urol 2004;172:871–3.

[25] Seifman BD, Hollenbeck BK, Wolf JS Jr. Laparoscopic nephron-sparing surgery for a renal mass: 1-year minimum follow-up. J Endourol 2004;18: 783–6.

[26] Gill IS, Kavoussi LR, Lane BR, et al. Comparison of 1,800 laparoscopic and open partial nephrectomies for single renal tumors. J Urol 2007;178:41–6.

[27] Gill IS, Matin SF, Desai MM, et al. Comparative analysis of laparoscopic versus open partial nephrectomy for renal tumors in 200 patients. J Urol 2003;170:64–8.

[28] Gill IS, Meraney AM, Schweizer DK, et al. Laparoscopic radical nephrectomy in 100 patients: a single center experience from the United States. Cancer 2001;92:1843–55.

[29] McDougall EM, Monk TG, Wolf JS Jr, et al. The effect of prolonged pneumoperitoneum on renal function in an animal model. J Am Coll Surg 1996;182:317–28.

[30] Lee HJ, Box GN, Deane LA, et al. Evaluation of laparoscopic vascular clamps using a load-cell device: are all clamps the same? J Endourol 2007; 21:A72.

[31] Finley DS, Lee DI, Eichel L, et al. Fibrin glue-oxidized cellulose sandwich for laparoscopic wedge resection of small renal lesions. J Urol 2005;173: 1477–81.

[32] Kane CJ, Mitchell JA, Meng MV, et al. Laparoscopic partial nephrectomy with temporary arterial occlusion: description of technique and renal functional outcomes. Urology 2004;63:241–6.

[33] Laven BA, Orvieto MA, Chuang MS, et al. Renal tolerance to prolonged warm ischemia time in a laparoscopic versus open surgery porcine model. J Urol 2004;172:2471–4.

[34] Nguyen MM, Gill IS. Halving ischemia time during laparoscopic partial nephrectomy. J Urol 2008;179: 627–32.

[35] Burak T, Rodrigo F, Kamoi D, et al. Risk factor analysis of complications in laparoscopic partial nephrectomy. J Endourol 2007;21:A278.

[36] Deane LA, Lee HJ, Box GN, et al. Laparoscopic partial nephrectomy: six degrees of hemostasis. J Endourol 2007;21:A275.

[37] Orvieto MA, Chien GW, Laven B, et al. Eliminating knot tying during warm ischemia time for laparoscopic partial nephrectomy. J Urol 2004;172: 2292–5.

[38] Phillips JM, Narula N, Deane LA, et al. Histologic evaluation of cold vs. hot cutting: clinical impact on margin status for laparoscopic partial nephrectomy. J Urol, submitted.

[39] Colombo JR Jr, Haber GP, Jelovsek JE, et al. Seven years after laparoscopic radical nephrectomy: oncologic and renal functional outcomes. Urology 2008;71(6):1149–54.

[40] Hemal AK, Kumar A, Gupta NP, et al. Oncologic outcome of 132 cases of laparoscopic radical nephrectomy with intact specimen removal for T1-2N0M0 renal cell carcinoma. World J Urol 2007; 25:619–26.

[41] Kawauchi A, Yoneda K, Fujito A, et al. Oncologic outcome of hand-assisted laparoscopic radical nephrectomy. Urology 2007;69:53–6.

[42] Permpongkosol S, Chan DY, Link RE, et al. Long-term survival analysis after laparoscopic radical nephrectomy. J Urol 2005;174:1222–5.

[43] Saika T, Ono Y, Hattori R, et al. Long-term outcome of laparoscopic radical nephrectomy for pathologic T1 renal cell carcinoma. Urology 2003; 62:1018–23.

[44] Portis AJ, Yan Y, Landman J, et al. Long-term followup after laparoscopic radical nephrectomy. J Urol 2002;167:1257–62.

[45] Nadler RB, Loeb S, Clemens JQ, et al. A prospective study of laparoscopic radical nephrectomy for T1 tumors—is transperitoneal, retroperitoneal or hand assisted the best approach? J Urol 2006;175: 1230–3.

[46] Matin SF, Dhanani N, Acosta M, et al. Conventional and hand-assisted laparoscopic radical nephrectomy: comparative analysis of 271 cases. J Endourol 2006;20:891–4.

[47] Walther MM, Lyne JC, Libutti SK, et al. Laparoscopic cytoreductive nephrectomy as preparation for administration of systemic interleukin-2 in the

treatment of metastatic renal cell carcinoma: a pilot study. Urology 1999;53:496–501.

[48] Rabets JC, Kaouk J, Fergany A, et al. Laparoscopic versus open cytoreductive nephrectomy for metastatic renal cell carcinoma. Urology 2004;64:930–4.

[49] Matin SF, Madsen LT, Wood CG. Laparoscopic cytoreductive nephrectomy: the M.D. Anderson Cancer Center experience. Urology 2006;68: 528–32.

[50] Robson CJ. Radical nephrectomy for renal cell carcinoma. J Urol 1963;89:37–42.

[51] Blom JH, van Poppel H, Marechal JM, et al. Radical nephrectomy with and without lymph node dissection: preliminary results of the EORTC randomized phase III protocol 30881. EORTC Genitourinary Group. Eur Urol 1999;36:570–5.

[52] Siminovitch JP, Montie JE, Straffon RA. Lymphadenectomy in renal adenocarcinoma. J Urol 1982; 127:1090–1.

[53] Simmons MN, Kaouk J, Gill IS, et al. Laparoscopic radical nephrectomy with hilar lymph node dissection in patients with advanced renal cell carcinoma. Urology 2007;70:43–6.

[54] Ho KL, Chow GK. Ureteroscopic resection of upper-tract transitional-cell carcinoma. J Endourol 2005;19(7):841–8.

[55] Murphy DM, Zincke H, Furlow WL. Management of high grade transitional cell cancer of the upper urinary tract. J Urol 1981;125:25–9.

[56] Babaian RJ, Johnson DE. Primary carcinoma of the ureter. J Urol 1980;123:357–9.

[57] Zincke H, Aquilo JJ, Farrow GM, et al. Significance of urine cytology in the early detection of transitional cell cancer of the upper urinary tract. J Urol 1976;116:781–3.

[58] Streem SB, Pontes J, Novick AC, et al. Ureteropyeloscopy in the evaluation of upper tract filling defects. J Urol 1986;136:383–5.

[59] Stewart GD, Bariol SV, Grigor KM, et al. A comparison of the pathology of transitional cell carcinoma of the bladder and upper urinary tract. BJU Int. 2005;95(6):791–3.

[60] Elliott DS, Segura JW, Lightner D, et al. Is nephroureterectomy necessary in all cases of upper tract transitional cell carcinoma? Long-term results of conservative endourologic management of upper tract transitional cell carcinoma in individuals with a normal contralateral kidney. Urology 2001;58:174–8.

[61] Liatsikos EN, Dinlenc CZ, Kapoor R, et al. Transitional-cell carcinoma of the renal pelvis: ureteroscopic and percutaneous approach. J Endourol 2001;15:377–83.

[62] Keeley FX Jr, Bibbo M, Bagley DH. Ureteroscopic treatment and surveillance of upper urinary tract transitional cell carcinoma. J Urol 1997;157(5): 1560–5.

[63] Sowter Steven J, Ilie Cristian P, Ioannis Efthimiou, et al. Endourologic management of patients with upper-tract transitional-cell carcinoma: long-term follow-up in a single center. J Endourol 2007; 21(9):1005–10.

[64] Chen GL, Bagley DH. Ureteroscopic management of upper tract transitional cell carcinoma in patients with normal contralateral kidneys. J Urol 2000;164:1173–6.

[65] Grasso M, Fraiman M, Levine M. Ureteropyeloscopic diagnosis and treatment of upper urinary tract urothelial malignancies. Urology 1999;54(2): 240–6.

[66] Reisiger K, Hruby G, Clayman RV, et al. Office-based surveillance ureteroscopy after endoscopic treatment of transitional cell carcinoma: technique and clinical outcome. Urology 2007;70(2):263–6.

[67] Krambeck AE, Thompson RH, Lohse CM, et al. Endoscopic management of upper tract urothelial carcinoma in patients with a history of bladder urothelial carcinoma. J Urol 2007;177(5):1721–6.

[68] Jabbour ME, Desgrandchamps F, Cazin S, et al. Percutaneous management of grade II upper urinary tract transitional cell carcinoma: the long-term outcome. J Urol 2000;163:1105–7.

[69] Lee BR, Jabbour ME, Marshall FF, et al. 13-Year survival comparison of percutaneous and open nephroureterectomy approaches for management of transitional cell carcinoma of renal collecting system: equivalent outcomes. J Endourol 1999;13: 289–94.

[70] Smith AD, Orihuela E, Crowley AR. Percutaneous management of renal pelvic tumors: a treatment option in selected cases. J Urol 1987;137:852–6.

[71] Clark PE, Streem SB, Geisinger MA. 13-Year experience with percutaneous management of upper tract transitional cell carcinoma. J Urol 1999;161: 772–5.

[72] Jarrett TW, Sweetser PM, Weiss GH, et al. Percutaneous management of transitional cell carcinoma of the renal collecting system 9-year experience. J Urol 1995;154:1629–35.

[73] Potter SR, Chow GK, Jarrett TW. Percutaneous endoscopic management of urothelial tumors of the renal pelvis. Urology 2001;58(3):457–9.

[74] Storm DW, Fulmer BR. Case report: percutaneous management of transitional-cell carcinoma of the upper urinary tract using the bipolar resectoscope. J Endourol 2007;21(9):1011–3.

[75] Roupret M, Traxer O, Tligui M, et al. Upper urinary tract transitional cell carcinoma: recurrence rate after percutaneous endoscopic resection. Eur Urol 2007;51(3):709–13.

[76] Goel MC, Mahendra V, Roberts JG. Percutaneous management of renal pelvic urothelial tumors: long-term followup. J Urol 2003;169:925–30.

[77] Huang A, Low RK, de VereWhite R. Nephrostomy tract tumor seeding following percutaneous

manipulation of a ureteral carcinoma. J Urol 1995; 153:1041–2.

[78] Clayman RV, Kavoussi LR, Firenshau RS, et al. Laparoscopic nephro-ureterectomy: initial case report. J Laparoendosc Surg 1991;1:343–9.

[79] Shalhav AL, Dunn MD, Portis AJ, et al. Laparoscopic nephroureterectomy for upper tract transitional cell cancer: the Washington University experience. J Urol 2000;163(4):1100–4.

[80] Seifman BD, Montie JE, Wolf JS. Prospective comparison between hand-assisted laparoscopic and open surgical nephroureterectomy for urothelial cell carcinoma. Urol 2001;57(1):133–7.

[81] Keeley FX, Tolley DA. Laparoscopic nephroureterectomy: making management of upper-tract transitional cell carcinoma entirely minimally invasive. J Endourol 1998;12:139–41.

[82] Hattori R, Yoshino Y, Gotoh M, et al. Laparoscopic nephroureterectomy for transitional cell carcinoma of renal pelvis and ureter: Nagoya experience. Urology 2006;67(4):701–5.

[83] Rassweiler JJ, Schulze M, Marrero R, et al. Laparoscopic nephroureterectomy for upper urinary tract transitional cell carcinoma: is it better than open surgery? Eur Urol 2004;46(6):690–7.

[84] Roupret M, Hupertan V, Sanderson KM, et al. Oncologic control after open or laparoscopic nephroureterectomy for upper urinary tract transitional cell carcinoma: a single center experience. Urology 2007;69(4):656–61.

[85] Muntener M, Nielsen ME, Romero FR, et al. Long-term oncologic outcome after laparoscopic radical nephroureterectomy for upper tract transitional cell carcinoma. Eur Urol. 2007;51(6): 1639–44.

[86] Wolf JS Jr, Dash A, Hollenbeck BK, et al. Intermediate followup of hand assisted laparoscopic nephroureterectomy for urothelial carcinoma: factors associated with outcomes. J Urol 2005;173: 1102–7.

[87] Bariol SV, Stewart GD, McNeill SA, et al. Oncological control following laparoscopic nephroureterectomy: 7-year outcome. J Urol. 2004;172(5 Pt 1):1805–8.

[88] Hsueh TY, Huang YH, Chiu AW, et al. Survival analysis in patients with upper urinary tract transitional cell carcinoma: a comparison between open and hand-assisted laparoscopic nephroureterectomy. BJU Int 2007;99(3):632–6.

[89] Baughman SM, Sexton W, Bishoff JT. Multiple intravesical linear staples identified during surveillance cystoscopy after laparoscopic nephroureterectomy. Urology 2003;62:351.

[90] Gill IS, Soble JJ, Miller SD, et al. A novel technique for management of the en bloc bladder cuff and distal ureter during laparoscopic nephroureterectomy. J Urol 1999;161:430–4.

[91] Jones DR, Moisey CU. A cautionary tale of the modified "pluck" nephroureterectomy. Br J Urol 1993;71:486–7.

[92] Tsivian A, Sidi AA. Port site metastases in urological laparoscopic surgery. J Urol 2003;169:1213–8.

[93] Roupret M, Hupertan V, Traxer O, et al. Comparison of open nephroureterectomy and ureteroscopic and percutaneous management of upper urinary tract transitional cell carcinoma. Urology 2006;67(6):1181–7.

[94] Herr HW. Durable response of a carcinoma in situ of the renal pelvis to topical bacillus Calmette Guerin. J Urol 1985;134:531–2.

[95] Studer UE, Casanova G, Kraft R, et al. Percutaneous bacillus Calmette-Guerin perfusion of the upper urinary tract for carcinoma in situ. J Urol 1989;142:975–7.

[96] Patel A, Fuch GJ. New techniques for the administration of topical adjuvant therapy after endoscopic ablation of upper urinary tract transitional cell carcinoma. J Urol 1998;159(1):71–5.

[97] Thalmann GN, Markwalder R, Walter B, et al. Long-term experience with bacillus Calmette-Guérin therapy of upper urinary tract transitional cell carcinoma in patients not eligible for surgery. J Urol 2002;168:1381–5.

[98] Katz MH, Lee MW, Gupta M. Setting a new standard for topical therapy of upper-tract transitional-cell carcinoma: BCG and interferon-alpha2B. J Endourol 2007;21(4):374–7.

[99] Keeley FX Jr, Bagley DH. Adjuvant mitomycin C following endoscopic treatment of upper tract transitional cell carcinoma. J Urol 1997;158(6): 2074–7.

[100] O'Donoghue JP, Crew JP. Adjuvant topical treatment of upper urinary tract urothelial tumors. BJU Int 2004;94(4):483–5.

ELSEVIER
SAUNDERS

Urol Clin N Am 35 (2008) 385–396

UROLOGIC
CLINICS
of North America

Laparoscopic Partial Nephrectomy: an Update on Contemporary Issues

Sero Andonian, MD[a], Günter Janetschek, MD[b],
Benjamin R. Lee, MD[a],*

[a]Smith Institute for Urology, North Shore–Long Island Jewish Health System, 450 Lakeville Road, Suite M-41,
New Hyde Park, New York, NY 11040, USA
[b]Department of Urology, Elisabethinen Hospital, Fadingerstrasse 1, 4010 Linz, Austria

Renal cell carcinoma (RCC) is the most common malignancy of the kidney and accounts for approximately 3% of adult cancers [1]. It comprises 85% of newly diagnosed malignancies of the kidney, with an age-adjusted incidence of 12.8 cases per 100,000 population and age-adjusted mortality rate of 4.2 deaths per 100,000 population [2]. Incidence rates have been increasing over the last 30 years in the United States, particularly among African Americans [3]. During 2007, it was estimated that approximately 51,190 new cases of kidney cancer would be diagnosed, and 12,890 people would die of the disease in the United States [4]. Factors such as increased resolution and application of imaging modalities have led to an increase in the incidental detection of renal masses. Classically, radical nephrectomy has been described as the standard surgical therapy for renal masses. Several studies, however, have indicated that partial nephrectomy provides cancer control similar to radical nephrectomy [5]. Furthermore, partial nephrectomy has been shown to decrease risk of end-stage renal failure requiring renal replacement therapy when compared with radical nephrectomy [6–8]. Laparoscopic partial nephrectomy (LPN), introduced in 1993, has become an acceptable alternative to open partial nephrectomy for expert laparoscopic

urologists [9–11]. Initially, LPN was used for benign disease such as lower-pole calyceal diverticulum containing a calculus, or atrophic hydronephrotic moiety [9,10]. Laparoscopic hemi-nephrectomy also has been successful for nonfunctioning renal moieties in the pediatric population [12,13]. This article presents some of the earliest series and the latest largest series (Table 1).

Indications and contraindications

Initially, absolute indications for partial nephrectomy included localized enhancing renal masses in solitary kidneys, bilateral synchronous renal masses, or chronic renal insufficiency [5,21–23]. Relative indications for partial nephrectomy are hereditary forms of renal cell carcinoma such as von Hippel-Lindau disease (VHL), hereditary papillary renal cell carcinoma, Birt-Hogg-Dubé syndrome, or tuberous sclerosis, where there is increased risk of metachronous renal malignancies. These tumors often present at a younger age and are more likely to be multifocal and bilateral [21]. Relative indications for partial nephrectomy also exist when the contralateral kidney is at increased risk of failure because of hypertension, diabetes mellitus, nephrolithiasis, or chronic pyelonephritis [24]. Finally, elective indications include localized incidental renal-enhancing masses with a normal contralateral kidney. These indications originally were described for open partial nephrectomy, but they are also applicable to LPN. Contraindications to partial nephrectomy include renal vein or inferior vena

This work was supported in part by grants from the Quebec Urological Association Foundation and Frank McGill Travel Fellowship to Sero Andonian.

* Corresponding author.
E-mail address: blee@lij.edu (B.R. Lee).

Table 1
Comparison of operating room time, ischemia time, pathology, and follow-up data

Senior author	Years	#	Age	Size (cm)	Trans/ retro	Operating room (minutes)	Ischemia (minutes)	EBL (mL)	Histology	Stage	LOS (days)	Follow-up (months)	Local Rec	Mets
Clayman [9]a	93–98	3	68	1.2 (1–1.5)	1 Trans; 2 retro	210 (120–324)	0	92 (75–100)	2 (66%) Benign; 1 (33%) RCC	N/A	2.7	46	0	0
Abbou [14]	95–98	13	42.9	3.2 (2–6)	Retro	113 (60–200)	7.4 (2–10)	72 (0–400)	8 (61%) Benign; 5 (39%) RCC	3 pT1a	6.1	22	0	0
Janetschek [15]	94–99	25	62.9	1.9 (1–5)	15 Trans; 10 retro	163.5 (90–300)	N/A	287 (20–800)	6 (24%) Benign; 19 (76%)RCC	18pT1 1pT3a	N/A	22.2 (1–65)	0	0
Janetschek [16]	04–05	25	60.4 (40–74)	2.6 (1.1–3.9)	Trans	211.7 (155–260)	28.9 (19–40)	177.4 (50–1500)	6 (24%) Benign; 19 (76%) RCC; 0% +M	24pT1a 1pT1b	8.3 (5–13)	6.2 (1–15)	N/A	N/A
Gill [11,17]	99–01	58	64 (30–85)	2.9 (1.3–7)	Trans and retro	180 (45–348)	23 (9.8–40)	270.4 (40–1500)	37 (66%) RCC	32pT1 2pT2	2.2 (1–9)	68.4 (60–82.8)	1/37 (2.7%)	0
Gill [18]	01–04	100	64	3.2 ± 1.5	Trans	208 ± 52	31.1 ± 9.2	221 ± 226	75%RCC; 2% +M	N/A	2.9 ± 1.7	N/A	N/A	N/A
Gill [18]	01–04	63	60	2.5 ± 0.9	Retro	173 ± 54	28.0 ± 9.0	217 ± 285	67% RCC	N/A	2.2 ± 1.6	N/A	N/A	N/A
Kavoussi [19]	99–04	217	56.6	2.6 (1–10)	199 Trans; 18 retro	186 (75–400)	27.6 (5–60)	385 ± 377	66% RCC; 3.5% +M	N/A	3.1 ± 1.6	24 ± 12	2 (1.4%)	0
Ramon [20] (2nd group)	02–06	110	62	3.9 (1.4–6.2)	Trans	100 (75–140)	30 (18–49)	510 (20–1200)	15 (14%) Benign; 95 (86%) RCC; 3.6% +M	N/A	N/A	16 (4–42)	0	0
Average (range)	93–06	614	60 (30–85)	3.1 (1–10)	449 Trans; 91 retro	171 (45–400)	27.8 (2–60)	332 (0–1500)	178 (29%) Benign; 436 (71%) RCC; 3.2% +M	77pT1 2pT2 1pT3a	3.2 (1–13)	26.8 (1–83)	1.7% (1.4–2.7)	0

Abbreviations: EBL, estimated blood loss; LOS, length of stay; Mets, metastasis; +M, positive surgical margin rate; RCC, renal cell carcinoma; Rec, recurrence; Retro, retroperitoneal; Trans, transperitoneal.

a Patients with exophytic renal masses who underwent wedge resection were included in the table.

cava tumor thrombus, massive tumor size, and local invasion. Relative contraindications include lymphadenopathy and bleeding diathesis [21]. Although initially partial nephrectomy was limited to 4 cm masses because of lower risk of local recurrence and multifocality, recently size criterion has been abolished as long as the tumor can be resected effectively with a negative margin [25,26]. This has been shown for open partial nephrectomy (OPN) versus radical nephrectomy, and it also may be applicable for LPN versus laparoscopic radical nephrectomy. This remains a controversial issue.

When there is a normal contralateral kidney, increased risks of peri-operative complications of partial nephrectomy, local recurrence, and tumor multifocality have to be balanced with decreased risk of developing chronic renal insufficiency [6–8,27]. In a review of 878 patients who had OPN, the rate of operative mortality was 1%, urine leak 7%, abscess 1%, bleeding 2%, and reoperation 2% [24]. In addition, the overall risk of local recurrence in partial nephrectomy series has been found to be 0% to 10% depending on tumor size, histology, and stage. For tumors 4 cm or less, the local recurrence risk is even lower, at 0% to 3% [5]. Furthermore, histologic pattern, such as papillary, rather than tumor size, has proven to be the most reliable predictor of multicentricity [28,29].

As with any new laparoscopic procedure, patient selection is crucial for success. Initially, LPN focused on those patients who had unifocal, small, polar, exophytic lesions, with a limited depth of penetration of less than 1 cm through the renal cortex. With evolution of the technique and improved methods of hemostasis, hilar and endophytic lesions, and masses abutting the collecting system can be resected [30].

Comparison with open partial nephrectomy

There are several retrospective series demonstrating advantages of LPN over the traditional OPN. These include lower narcotic requirements, improved cosmesis, earlier resumption of diet, shorter hospitalization, and lower expense [31,32]. Furthermore, in a larger series from the Cleveland Clinic, LPN, as compared with OPN, was associated with a shorter surgical time, lower blood loss, longer warm ischemia (27.8 minutes versus 17.5 minutes), and higher rate of intra-operative complications (5% versus 0%) [33].

In a multicenter comparison of 771 LPNs versus 1028 OPNs, LPN was associated with longer ischemia time and more postoperative complications (especially urological), in addition to its benefits of shorter operative time, decreased blood loss, and shorter hospital stay [34]. Selection bias of more complicated patients for OPN is evident from these retrospective studies. The advantages of lower blood loss, shorter hospitalization, and convalescence, however, are evident. To provide level 1 evidence, randomized trials comparing the two procedures are needed.

Technique

The technique of LPN, both transperitoneal and retroperitoneal, has been detailed in schematic form in a recently published atlas [21,22]. The authors would like to emphasize certain points. Knowledge of the tumor in relationship to the collecting system, renal hilum, as well as proximity to the vascular structures, will help guide dissection, isolation, and resection of the mass. Three-dimensional reconstruction following helical CT scan or magnetic resonance angiography allow high-quality images of the renal artery and vein and provide multiple views of the intrarenal anatomy [35]. Preoperative knowledge of the number and location of renal arteries and veins improves intraoperative planning and surgical dissection.

No hilar clamping

The earliest LPN series was performed on small (less than 2 cm) exophytic lesions without hilar dissection or clamping. Janetschek and colleagues [15] reported on 25 patients who underwent wedge resection of small (less than 2 cm) exophytic lesions with an average blood loss of 287 mL (range of 20 to 800 mL). In this technique, bipolar coagulation forceps were used for simultaneous dissection and hemostasis. In this series, there was 8% rate of urinary fistula postoperatively. This technique of resection without hilar clamping may be applicable for small exophytic lesions with depth of invasion less than 1 cm from the surface [36]. For larger and central lesions, however, hilar control is essential. A novel technique of clamping the renal parenchyma with a Satinsky clamp (Aesculap Inc., Center Valley, Pennsylvania) inserted through a separate 1 cm stab incision has been described [37]. Preliminary results in five patients with polar lesions averaging 3 cm showed the mean blood loss was 250 mL, and none required transfusions. This technique, however, is not applicable to renal masses involving the hilum or deeper invasion into the collecting system.

Habib radiofrequency technique

Another way of minimizing warm ischemia time without clamping the renal hilum is the use of a laparoscopic Habib probe (AngioDynamics, Queensbury, New York). It is a four-pronged bipolar radiofrequency device that ablates tissue between the probes in a bipolar fashion. Using the Habib probe, an avascular plane is created 10 mm away from the renal lesion. Its use has been shown to reduce transfusions in liver resections [38]. The Habib probe was evaluated in a pilot study of three patients undergoing LPN without hilar clamping. The mean estimated blood loss was 100 mL, and none of the patients required transfusions [39]. Cautery artifact, however, can cause difficulty in interpreting the frozen section margin. Randomized studies are needed to further evaluate its impact on blood loss, frozen section analysis, and long-term renal function.

Methods of hilar clamping and warm ischemia

To replicate OPN and perform LPN on larger (greater than 2 cm), endophytic, central, or hilar lesions, it is essential to control the renal hilum (either the renal artery alone or together with the renal vein). The advantage of hilar control is the ability to tackle lesions that once were thought to

be only amenable to OPN. This has two primary functions: decreasing intraoperative hemorrhage and improving access to the renal collecting system for repair [40]. There are three techniques of hilar control.

Gill was the first to demonstrate that LPN can duplicate open surgical principles [11]. Laparoscopic bulldog clamps are the most widely used instruments to clamp the renal artery alone, or together with the renal vein (Aesculap Incorporated, Center Valley, Pennsylvania) (Fig. 1 A, B). The advantages include ability to individually clamp the artery, and the ease of applying and removing. It also frees up a port for the most crucial part of the surgery: reconstruction of the nephrotomy defect. It is the personal preference of the authors to use the same instrument to place and remove the bulldog clamp. Disadvantages include difficulty in removing the clamp if not aligned well with the applicator.

Another option of clamping the renal vessels laparoscopically is the use of laparoscopic Satinsky clamps, which allow en bloc clamping of the entire renal hilum (Fig. 2). The advantage is that the renal artery and vein can be taken en bloc and do not have to be dissected individually. The disadvantage is that an additional port must be employed to place the instrument. In addition, the assistant must take care not to exert excessive traction or pressure on the clamp inadvertently to avoid stretch or intimal injury to the vessel.

Finally, a Rumel tourniquet can be used to efficiently achieve vessel control and occlusion.

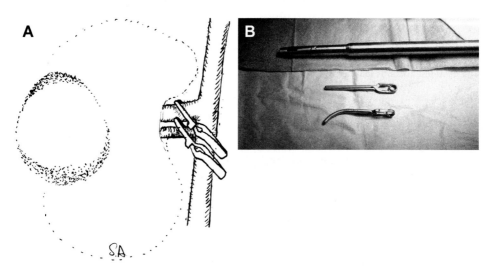

Fig. 1. *A*: A schematic diagram of laparoscopic bulldog clamps on the right renal artery and vein. The right kidney has an exophytic mass. *B*: A photograph of laparoscopic straight and curved bulldog clamps and the applicator.

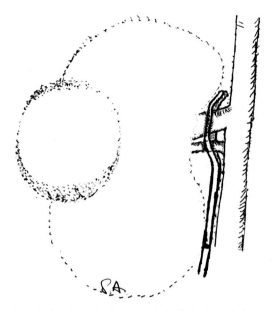

Fig. 2. A schematic diagram of the Satinsky technique of hilar clamping on the right kidney with an exophytic mass.

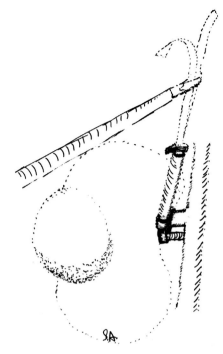

Fig. 3. A schematic diagram of the Rumel technique of hilar clamping on the right kidney with an exophytic mass.

The renal vein and artery are secured en bloc by an umbilical tape (Bard PTFE, Braided tape, 4 mm × 61 cm) (Bard Inc., Murray Hill, New Jersey), inserted through a 10 mm trocar. The tape is left in place until the end of the procedure and can achieve rapid reocclusion of the vessels if needed. To free the trocar from the umbilical tape, the trocar is removed and repositioned with the tape on the outside of the trocar. The Rumel tourniquet consists of a 5 cm piece of silicone drainage tube (10F) and a 20 cm vascular loop folded over once to form a U loop (Fig. 3).

Besides being able to perform LPN on more complex renal lesions, the advantages of hilar control also include lower rates of urinary fistula (1.4% to 4%) (Table 2). The most significant disadvantage of hilar control, however, is ischemia. Prolonged periods of ischemia result in acute tubular necrosis and renal failure. Intravenous mannitol 12.5 g is often administered before clamping. This has several protective mechanisms, such as: free radical scavenger, decreased intracellular edema, decreased intrarenal vascular resistance, increased blood flow and glomerular filtration rate of superficial nephrons, and osmotic diuresis [43,44]. Furthermore, furosemide is administered to promote diuresis after unclamping of the renal vessels.

One way of decreasing ischemic injury is early unclamping after a running suture on the tumor bed [45]. The vascularized renal parenchyma then is closed over a surgical bolster. With this technique, the warm ischemia time was reduced from 27.2 minutes to 13.7 minutes, without increasing intraoperative bleeding or postoperative complications. The decreased ischemia time also may be attributed to increased expertise, as the early unclamping group was performed later on. Another method of reducing ischemia time is on-demand clamping of the hilum [46]. In this technique, the hilum is dissected early but clamped only in the case of excessive bleeding. Out of 39 patients, 31 required on-demand clamping, with a mean ischemia time of 9 minutes. There was a high rate of blood transfusions (8 of 39 patients, or 21%), however, and two patients required open conversion because of excessive bleeding.

Animal studies have shown that clamping of the renal artery alone during open surgery better protects the kidney from warm ischemia compared with renal artery and vein clamping. This benefit, however, was not observed in laparoscopic surgery [47]. The authors speculated that this could be because of partial occlusion of the

Table 2
Complications rate

Senior author	Years	#	Trans/retro	Overall complications	Open conversion	Bowel injury	Urinary fistula (%)	Hemorrhage (%)	Number reoperation (%)	ARF
Clayman [9]	93–98	3	1 Trans; 2 retro	0	0	0	0	0	0	0
Abbou [14]	95–98	13	Retro	N/A	0	0	2 (15%)	0	1 (8%) Completion nephrectomy	0
Gill [41]	99–01	200	Trans and retro	66 (33%)	2 (1%)	1 (0.5%)	9 (4.5%)	19 (9.5%)	4 (2%)	4 (2%)
Gill [18]	01–04	100	Trans	18 (18%)	1 (1%)	1 (1%)	4 (4%)	2 (2%)	N/A	3 (3%)
Gill [18]	01–04	63	Retro	6 (10%)	0	0	2 (3%)	2 (3%)	N/A	0
Gill [30]	03–05	200	146 Trans; 54 retro	38 (19%)	3 (1.5%)	0	4 (2%)	9 (4.5%)	3 (1.5%)	1 (0.5%)
Kavoussi [19,42]	99–04	217	199 Trans; 18 retro	23 (10.6%)	4 (1.6%)	0	3 (1.4%)	4 (1.9%)	N/A	2 (0.9%)
Average	93–05	796	Laparoscopic	151 (19%)	10 (1.3%)	2 (0.3%)	24 (3%)	36 (4.5%)	8 (1.9%)	10 (1.3%)

Abbreviations: ARF, acute renal failure; Retro, retroperitoneal; Trans, transperitoneal.

renal vein secondary to pneumoperitoneum, thus negating any benefit of clamping only the renal artery. In a similar study in a porcine model, warm ischemia of up to 90 minutes resulted in an initial renal dysfunction. However, this was not statistically different by 2 weeks postoperatively [48]. Therefore, at least in the porcine model, clamping of the renal artery alone or artery and vein together has similar effects in laparoscopic approach. Similarly, warm ischemia of up to 90 minutes is tolerated well.

Thirty minutes of warm ischemia arbitrarily have been designed as the safe warm ischemia time in LPN. Even though there is no absolute cut-off for warm ischemia time, the longer it is, the worse the renal dysfunction. This cut off has been examined in terms of long-term renal injury. For example, Bhayani and colleagues [49] compared patients who had no hilar clamping versus two groups of patients who had hilar clamping of less than and more than 30 minutes. The median creatinine did not change significantly postoperatively, and none of the 118 patients required dialysis. Porpiglia and colleagues [50] confirmed these results. The glomerular filtration rate (GFR) was not significantly different 3 months after LPN with warm ischemia of more than 30 minutes in 18 patients. On renal scintigraphy, however, the contribution of the affected kidney decreased from 48% to 36% on postoperative day 5, then increased to 40% at 3 months and 43% at 1 year postoperatively. Therefore, in these limited retrospective studies, despite decreasing contribution of the affected renal moiety, the overall GFR was maintained, and no patients required dialysis in the presence of a normal contralateral kidney. Furthermore, patients who have renal dysfunction (creatinine greater than 2 mg/dL), hypertension, or diabetes mellitus do not tolerate warm ischemia well and may be more susceptible to ischemic injury when this exceeds 30 minutes. The authors agree with Bhayani and colleagues [49], in that efforts to minimize warm ischemia are important but should not jeopardize cancer control, hemostasis, or collecting system closure. In particular, when more complex renal lesions are tackled and the surgeon feels that the ischemia time to resect and reconstruct the kidney would be longer than 30 minutes, then the following techniques of cold ischemia should be contemplated.

Cold ischemia

There have been three methods of inducing cold ischemia in an effort to minimize the ischemic injury to the kidney. Gill and colleagues [51] described the ice slush technique that replicates OPN. A laparoscopic Endocatch II (US Surgical, Norwalk, Connecticut) was placed through a 12 mm port site around the mobilized kidney. A Satinsky clamp was used to en bloc clamp the renal artery and vein. After placement of 600 mL of ice slush around the kidney, LPN was performed in 12 patients, with an average ischemia time of 43.5 minutes (range 25 to 55 minutes). Renal parenchymal temperature was kept between 5°C to 19°C. Postoperative renal scans confirmed functional renal moieties. There were two intra-operative complications, however, partial bag slippage in one and Satinsky clamp malfunction in another patient [51].

A second technique of cold ischemia during LPN uses a 7F ureteral catheter and cold (4°C) saline irrigation [52]. This technique also identified the open collecting system secondary to saline outflow. Although the postoperative creatinine was higher in the group with cold ischemia as compared with no ischemia (1.45 mg/dL versus 1.26 mg/dL), this was not statistically significant.

Janetschek and colleagues [53] described another technique of cold ischemia using an angiocatheter inserted through a percutaneous femoral puncture and advanced under fluoroscopic guidance to the renal artery. Two hundred milliliters of 20% mannitol are administered 15 minutes before the renal artery occlusion. The renal artery is occluded using the Rumel tourniquet technique. At this point, 1 L of Ringer's lactate with 100 mL of 20% mannitol at a temperature of 4°C is infused at a rate of 50 mL/min. Parenchymal temperature is monitored and kept at 25°C. This technique has been used in 28 patients with mean ischemia time of 40.8 minutes (25 to 101). Parenchymal transit time on Technetium-99m mercaptoacetyltriglycine (MAG-3) renal scan has been shown to be a good indicator of ischemic damage to the kidney [54]. MAG-3 clearance decreased on the operated side, but the peak concentration times were not different pre- and postoperatively, indicating no postoperative dysfunction of the remnant moiety [55]. In a retrospective comparison of 12 patients who had warm ischemia with 14 patients who had cold ischemia, there was one loss of function in the group with cold ischemia. Therefore, LPN even with short periods of cold ischemia can lead to loss of function in that moiety [54].

Renal function

In a large comparative study, the renal functional outcomes at 3 months postoperatively were similar in LPN and OPN, with 97.9% and 99.6% of renal units retaining function [34]. In another study, despite a lower mean calculated postoperative split, MAG-3 clearance on the operated side (74.0 mL/min versus 110.7 mL/min), there was no difference in the mean postoperative concentration time between the two sides, indicating absence of renal dysfunction on the operated side [56,57].

Hemostasis of the nephrotomy defect

There are three ways of achieving hemostasis of the nephrotomy defect. The first is by using the bipolar coagulation forceps [15]. Its advantages include simultaneous dissection and hemostasis. The second is the argon beam coagulator. In addition to the cost and nonavailability in some centers, one disadvantage is the sudden rise of peritoneal pressure, which can lead to pneumothorax. Therefore, it is important to vent the trocar while activating the argon beam, and to closely monitor the intra-abdominal pressure [15]. It is also important to note that it can only handle superficial (interlobular) vessels and is unlikely to handle interlobar or segmental branches very effectively.

Hemostatic agents such as fibrin gel (Tisseel) (Baxter, Deerfield, Illinois), gelatin matrix thrombin (FloSeal) (Baxter, Deerfield, Illinois), bovine serum albumin (BioGlue) (CryoLife Inc., Kennesaw, Georgia), cyanoacrylate glue (Glubran) (GEM, Viareggio, Italy), and oxidized regenerated cellulose (Surgicel) (Ethicon Inc., Somerville, New Jersey) have all been used to cover the nephrotomy defect and to reconstruct the kidney after resection. Their use varies by surgeon preference. One study comparing Fibrin glue with sutured bolster repair of the collecting system found that there was 41% postoperative hemorrhage or urinary leakage after Fibrin glue, compared with 11% when sutured bolsters were used [36]. A retrospective survey of 18 centers with 1347 cases of LPN found that 16 centers used haemostatic agents in addition to performing concomitant suturing of the nephrotomy bed. The overall postoperative hemorrhage requiring transfusion was 2.7%, and the rate of urinary leakage was 1.9% [58].

Histologic results/positive margins

Table 1 lists the percentage of benign and malignant tumors in the earliest and the most recent largest series. In the early series, most (61% to 66%) lesions resected were benign [9,14]. In more recent series, most (66% to 86%) lesions resected have proven to be malignant, reflecting the etiology of renal masses determined from open partial and radical nephrectomy series [17,20].

The positive margin rate in the final pathology has ranged from 2% to 3.6% (see Table 1). During OPN, when a positive margin is found on frozen sectioning, a deeper resection margin is obtained before reconstructing the nephrotomy and unclamping the vessels. In LPN, however, by the time the results of a frozen section are obtained, the nephrotomy defect already is closed, and the hilum is unclamped to minimize warm ischemia. Taking down the nephrotomy repair is difficult and may warrant conversion to open surgery to safely complete the partial nephrectomy to negative margins. The classical teaching after a positive margin with a partial nephrectomy is to consider proceeding with completion radical nephrectomy as a measure of cancer control. In retrospective multi-institutional survey of 17 centers performing laparoscopic partial nephrectomy, the rate of positive margins on frozen sections was 2.4%. Out of 21 cases that had positive margins, 14 underwent immediate radical nephrectomy based on positive frozen sectioning, and the rest were followed. Data regarding recurrence, however, were not obtained [59]. A positive margin may not indicate residual disease. In a multicenter study of 511 LPNs, there were nine patients (1.8%) who had positive margins. Two underwent completion radical nephrectomies revealing no residual tumor. One patient who had VHL died of metastatic RCC 10 months postoperatively. The rest of the six patients were disease-free at a median follow-up of 32 months [60]. The authors recommend vigilant monitoring with CT every 6 to 12 months. Recently, data from OPN with 10-year follow-up has shown that positive surgical margins were not associated with an increased risk of local recurrence or metastatic disease [61]. Therefore, patients should be given the option of completion radical nephrectomy versus close monitoring until long-term rate of recurrence post LPN is determined.

Risk of tumor spillage/port site metastasis

Laparoscopic port site metastasis is defined as early recurrent malignant lesions developing locally in the abdominal wall within the scar tissue of one or more trocar sites, without evidence of peritoneal carcinomatosis [62]. In a retrospective review of over 1000 laparoscopic cases, there were only two cases (0.18%) of port site metastases [63]. There have been five reported cases of port site metastasis after LRN [62]. Recently, the first case of port site metastasis after a LPN was reported [64]. Several correctable factors have been identified from animal models. The following precautions have resulted in decreased recurrence from 63.8% to 13.8% [65]. These are:

Smallest skin incisions as possible
Trocar fixation to prevent trocar dislodgement and gas leak
Disinfection of instruments with povidone–iodine
Meticulous surgical technique
Use of entrapment sacks to remove specimens
Addition of heparin to irrigation solution or alternatively irrigation of the surgical field with sterile water to lyse floating tumor cells
Exsufflation of pneumoperitoneum through the trocar valve rather than through the skin incisions
Peritoneal closure as a protective barrier
Rinsing of trocar sites with povidone–iodine [62,65]

The most important factors remain avoiding direct contact of instruments and trocars with tumor cells and removal of tumors within an entrapment bag [15].

Survival outcomes

Cancer-specific survival rates in patients without metastases were 91% at 5 years and 80% at 10 and 20 years. In an aggregate review of 1800 patients, after a mean follow-up of 2 to 6 years, the cancer-specific survival rate exceeded 90% [5]. Negative predictors of survival include: high tumor grade, high tumor stage, bilateral disease, and tumors greater than 4 cm [66]. Location of the tumor (central versus peripheral, endophytic versus exophytic) is a significant technical consideration for nephron-sparing surgery; it has a less important biological role for determining cancer-specific outcomes [67].

Multifocality risk increases with larger tumors (greater than 4 cm) and stage pT3 disease. In a review of 1800 cases, the incidence of multifocal tumors with primary renal masses 4 cm or less was found to be 4.9% [5]. Furthermore, the risk of local recurrence was found to be 0% to 10%, and lowest for patients who underwent nephron-sparing surgery for lesions less than or equal to 4 cm [5].

In one retrospective series, the 3-year cancer-specific survival for cT1N0M0 tumors was 99.3% for LPN and 99.2% for OPN [34]. Another study found the 3-year cancer- specific survival to be 100% and overall survival to be 96.2% [65]. Similarly, there was no difference in 5-year cancer-specific survival (91.4% versus 97.4%) and actuarial survival (93.8% versus 95.8%) between LPN and OPN, respectively [68].

Complications

Table 2 lists the complications reported in LPN series. In a review of 878 patients, the rate of operative mortality was 1%, urine leak 7% (1.4% to 17.4%), abscess 1%, bleeding 2%, and reoperation 2% [24]. In LPN, the rate of urinary leak varies from 0% to 15%. Urinary fistula usually is managed conservatively with insertion of ureteral stent and Foley catheter. Alternatively, percutaneous nephrostomy may be placed. The diagnosis is made with biochemical evaluation of the drainage fluid, which demonstrates elevated creatinine (drainage fluid to serum ratio greater than 2).

With OPN, the need for temporary or permanent dialysis occurs in 4.9% of patients, postoperative hemorrhage in 2.8% of cases, injury to adjacent organs such as spleen in 0.6%, and the overall reoperative rate after nephron-sparing surgery is 1.9%. Bleeding after partial nephrectomy may be acute or delayed and presents typically with hypotension, distended abdomen, and decreased hematocrit. In a retrospective series examining predictors of hemorrhage following LPN, Ost and colleagues [69] found that older patients (age greater than 64 years) who have renal insufficiency are at increased risk of transfusion. Interestingly, increased tumor size, obesity, hypertension, diabetes, and smoking do not predispose patients who have LPN to increased risk of bleeding. Furthermore, certain tumor characteristics strongly correlate with risk of technical complications in other series. For example, patients at highest risk include those who have functionally solitary kidney, bilateral lesions, and large or centrally located tumors [70]. There recently has been a shift in management of postoperative bleeding, with a greater role of percutaneous embolization of pseudoaneurysms that develop.

Cost of laparoscopic partial nephrectomy

Recently, two groups have studied the comparative costs of nephron-sparing surgeries. OPN was found to be more expensive than LPN (1.2 times more expensive) [19]. OPN could achieve cost equivalence to LPN, when the operative time of the OPN is less than 2.8 hours, or when the length of hospitalization of OPN patients was less than 3 days [19]. Similarly, LPN was found to cost less than OPN in another study ($7013 versus $7767). There was no statistical significance, however [71]. Whereas surgical supply costs were significantly higher for LPN than OPN, LPN had less than a third of the room and board costs of OPN. Therefore, LPN is cost-equivalent to OPN, as the shorter stay compensates for significantly higher surgical supply costs [71].

Robotic-assisted laparoscopic partial nephrectomy

There are two small series on robotic-assisted LPN [72,73]. So far, there is limited experience with this mode of laparoscopic partial nephrectomy. The advantages of three-dimensional vision, 540° movement, motion scaling, and tremor elimination have not translated into lower rates of complications or shorter ischemia [72,74]. The disadvantages include the extra cost of the disposables, use of the robot surgical platform, and the requirement of two laparoscopic surgeons, who are expert in robotic techniques [74]. Randomized trials are needed to better evaluate this technology in terms of its added costs compared with decreased ischemia time.

Summary

LPN is a technically challenging procedure, successfully performed by expert urologic laparoscopists in centers of excellence. The advantages of lower cost, decreased postoperative pain and early recovery have to be balanced with prolonged warm ischemia, which may not result in long-term morbidity of increased renal insufficiency or hemodialysis requirements. Randomized clinical trials comparing OPN versus LPN are needed.

References

[1] Linehan WM, Zbar B, Bates SE, et al. Cancer of the kidney and ureter. In: DeVita VT Jr, Hellman S, Rosenberg SA, editors. Cancer: principles and

practice of oncology. 6th edition. Philadelphia: Lippincott Williams & Wilkins; 2001. p. 1362–96.

[2] Surveillance, Epidemiology, and End Results (SEER) program SEER*stat database: incidence — SEER 9 regs limited-use, Nov 2006 Sub (1973–2004), National Cancer Institute, DCCPS, Surveillance Research Program, Cancer Statistics Branch, released April 2007, based on the November 2006 submission. Available at: www.seer.cancer.gov. Accessed November 1, 2007.

[3] Chow WH, Devesa SS, Warren JL, et al. Rising incidence of renal cell cancer in the United States. JAMA 1999;281(17):1628–31.

[4] Jemal A, Siegel R, Ward E, et al. Cancer statistics, 2007. CA Cancer J Clin 2007;57:43–66.

[5] Uzzo R, Novick A. Nephron-sparing surgery for renal tumors: indications, techniques, and outcomes. J Urol 2001;166(1):6–18.

[6] Lau WK, Blute ML, Weaver AL, et al. Matched comparison of radical nephrectomy vs nephron-sparing surgery in patients with unilateral renal cell carcinoma and a normal contralateral kidney. Mayo Clin Proc 2000;75(12):1236–42.

[7] McKiernan J, Simmons R, Katz J, et al. Natural history of chronic renal insufficiency after partial and radical nephrectomy. Urology 2002;59(6):816–20.

[8] Sorbellini M, Kattan MW, Snyder ME, et al. Prognostic nomogram for renal insufficiency after radical or partial nephrectomy. J Urol 2006;176(2):472–6.

[9] McDougall EM, Clayman RV, Anderson K. Laparoscopic wedge resection of a renal tumor: initial experience. J Laparoendosc Surg 1993;3(6): 577–81.

[10] Winfield HN, Donovan JF, Godet AS, et al. Laparoscopic partial nephrectomy: initial case report for benign disease. J Endourol 1993;7(6):521–6.

[11] Gill IS, Desai MM, Kaouk JH, et al. Laparoscopic partial nephrectomy for renal tumor: duplicating open surgical techniques. J Urol 2002;167(2 Pt 1) 469–76.

[12] Janetschek G, Seibold J, Radmayr C, et al. Laparoscopic heminephroureterectomy in pediatric patients. J Urol 1997;158(5):1928–30.

[13] Wang DS, Bird VG, Cooper CS, et al. Laparoscopic upper-pole heminephrectomy for ectopic ureter: surgical technique. J Endourol 2003;17(7):469–73.

[14] Hoznek A, Salomon L, Antiphon P, et al. Partial nephrectomy with retroperitoneal laparoscopy. J Urol 1999;162(6):1922–6.

[15] Janetschek G, Jeschke K, Peschel R, et al. Laparoscopic surgery for stage T1 renal cell carcinoma: radical nephrectomy and wedge resection. Eur Urol 2000;38:131–8.

[16] Hacker A, Albadour A, Jauker W, et al. Nephron-sparing surgery for renal tumours: acceleration and facilitation of the laparoscopic technique. Eur Urol 2007;51(2):358–65.

[17] Lane BR, Gill IS. 5-year outcomes of laparoscopic partial nephrectomy. J Urol 2007;177(1):70–4.

[18] Ng CS, Gill IS, Ramani AP, et al. Transperitoneal versus retroperitoneal laparoscopic partial nephrectomy: patient selection and perioperative outcomes. J Urol 2005;174(3):846–9.

[19] Link RE, Bhayani SB, Allaf ME, et al. Exploring the learning curve, pathological outcomes, and perioperative morbidity of laparoscopic partial nephrectomy performed for renal mass. J Urol 2005;173(5):1690–4.

[20] Nadu A, Mor Y, Laufer M, et al. Laparoscopic partial nephrectomy: single-center experience with 140 patients—evolution of the surgical technique and its impact on patient outcomes. J Urol 2007;178(2): 435–9.

[21] Williams CS, Pinto PA. Laparoscopic partial nephrectomy. In: Bishoff JA, Kavoussi LR, editors. Atlas of laparoscopic urologic surgery. Philadelphia: WB Saunders; 2007. p. 110–20.

[22] Janetschek G. Laparoscopic partial nephrectomy: how far have we gone? Curr Opin Urol 2007;17(5): 316–21.

[23] Novick AC. Renal-sparing surgery for renal cell carcinoma. Urol Clin North Am 1993;20(2):277–82.

[24] Oakley NE, Hegarty NJ, McNeill A, et al. Minimally invasive nephron-sparing surgery for renal cell cancer. BJU Int 2006;98(2):278–84.

[25] Hafez KS, Fergany AF, Novick AC. Nephron-sparing surgery for localized renal cell carcinoma: impact of tumor size on patient survival, tumor recurrence, and TNM staging. J Urol 1999;162(6): 1930–3.

[26] Mitchell RE, Gilbert SM, Murphy AM, et al. Partial nephrectomy and radical nephrectomy offer similar cancer outcomes in renal cortical tumors 4 cm or larger. Urology 2006;67(2):260–4.

[27] Fergany AF, Saad IR, Woo L, et al. Open partial nephrectomy for tumor in a solitary kidney: experience with 400 cases. J Urol 2006;175(5):1630–3.

[28] Kletscher BA, Qian J, Bostwick DG, et al. Prospective analysis of multifocality in renal cell carcinoma: influence of histological patterns, grade, number, size, volume, and deoxyribonucleic acid ploidy. J Urol 1995;153(3 Pt 2):904–6.

[29] Ornstein DK, Lubensky IA, Venzon K, et al. Prevalence of microscopic tumor in normal - appearing renal parenchyma of patients with hereditary papillary renal cancer. J Urol 2000;163(2):431–3.

[30] Simmons MN, Gill IS. Decreased complications of contemporary laparoscopic partial nephrectomy: use of a standardized reporting system. J Urol 2007;177(6):2067–73.

[31] Beasley KA, Al Omar M, Shaikh A, et al. Laparoscopic versus open partial nephrectomy. Urology 2004;64(3):458–61.

[32] Schiff JD, Palese M, Vaughan ED Jr, et al. Laparoscopic vs open partial nephrectomy in consecutive patients: the Cornell experience. BJU Int 2005; 96(6):811–4.

[33] Gill IS, Matin SF, Desai MM, et al. Comparative analysis of laparoscopic versus open partial

nephrectomy for renal tumors in 200 patients. J Urol 2003;170(1):64–8.

[34] Gill IS, Kavoussi LR, Lane BR, et al. Comparison of 1800 laparoscopic and open partial ephrectomies for single renal tumors. J Urol 2007;178(1):41–6.

[35] Coll DM, Uzzo RG, Herts BR, et al. 3-dimensional volume-rendered computerized tomography for pre-operative evaluation and intraoperative treatment of patients undergoing nephron sparing surgery. J Urol 1999;161(4):1097–102.

[36] Johnston WK III, Montgomery JS, Seifman BD, et al. Fibrin glue v sutured bolster: lessons learned during 100 laparoscopic partial nephrectomies. J Urol 2005;174(1):47–52.

[37] Verhoest G, Manunta A, Bensalah K, et al. Laparoscopic partial nephrectomy with clamping of the renal parenchyma: initial experience. Eur Urol 2007;52(5):1340–6.

[38] Ayay A, Jiao LR, Habib NA. Bloodless liver resection using radiofrequency energy. Dig Surg 2007; 24(4):314–7.

[39] Andonian S, Adebayo A, Okeke Z, et al. Habib laparoscopic bipolar radiofrequency device: A novel way of creating an avascular resection margin in laparoscopic partial nephrectomy. J Laparoendosc Adv Surg Tech A, in press.

[40] Novick AC. Renal hypothermia: in vivo and ex vivo. Urol Clin North Am 1983;10(4):637–44.

[41] Ramani AP, Desai MM, Steinberg AP, et al. Complications of laparoscopic partial nephrectomy in 200 cases. J Urol 2005;173(1):42–7.

[42] Rais-Bahrami S, Lima GC, Varkarakis IM, et al. Intraoperative conversion of laparoscopic partial nephrectomy. J Endourol 2006;20(3):205–8.

[43] Lang F. Osmotic diuresis. Ren Physiol 1987;10(3–4):160–73.

[44] Nosowsky EE, Kaufman JJ. The protective action of mannitol in renal artery occlusion. J Urol 1963;89:295–9.

[45] Baumert H, Ballaro A, Shah N, et al. Reducing warm ischaemia time during laparoscopic partial nephrectomy: a prospective comparison of two renal closure techniques. Eur Urol 2007;52(4):1164–9.

[46] Bollens R, Rosenblatt A, Espinoza BP, et al. Laparoscopic partial nephrectomy with on-demand clamping reduces warm ischemia time. Eur Urol 2007;52(3):804–9.

[47] Orvieto MA, Zorn KC, Mendiola F, et al. Recovery of renal function after complete renal hilar versus artery alone clamping during open and laparoscopic surgery. J Urol 2007;177(6):2371–4.

[48] Laven BA, Orvieto MA, Chuang MS, et al. Renal tolerance to prolonged warm ischemia time in a laparoscopic versus open surgery porcine model. J Urol 2004;172(6 Pt 1):2471–4.

[49] Bhayani SB, Rha KH, Pinto PA, et al. Laparoscopic partial nephrectomy: effect of warm ischemia on serum creatinine. J Urol 2004;172(4 Pt 1):1264–6.

[50] Porpiglia F, Renard J, Billia M, et al. Is renal warm ischemia over 30 minutes during laparoscopic partial nephrectomy possible? One-year results of a prospective study. Eur Urol 2007;52(4):1170–8.

[51] Gill IS, Abreu SC, Desai MM, et al. Laparoscopic ice slush renal hypothermia for partial nephrectomy: the initial experience. J Urol 2003;170(1):52–6.

[52] Guillonneau B, Bermudez H, Gholami S, et al. Laparoscopic partial nephrectomy for renal tumor: single-center experience comparing clamping and no clamping techniques of the renal vasculature. J Urol 2003;169(2):483–6.

[53] Janetschek G, Abdelmaksoud A, Bagheri F, et al. Laparoscopic partial nephrectomy in cold ischemia: renal artery perfusion. J Urol 2004;171(1):68–71.

[54] Abukora F, Albqami N, Nambirajan T, et al. Long-term functional outcome of renal units after laparoscopic nephron-sparing surgery under cold ischemia. J Endourol 2006;20(10):790–3.

[55] Beri A, Lattouf J-B, D'Ambros OFJ, et al. Partial nephrectomy using renal artery perfusion for cold ischemia: functional and oncologic outcomes. J Endourol 2008;22(6):1285–90.

[56] Lattouf J-B, Beri A, D'Ambros OFJ, et al. Laparoscopic partial nephrectomy: functional and oncologic outcomes with up to 6 years follow-up. Manuscript in preparation.

[57] Lattouf J-B, Beri A, D'Ambros OFJ, et al. Laparoscopic partial nephrectomy for hilar tumors: technique and results. Eur Urol, in press.

[58] Breda A, Stepanian SV, Lam JS, et al. Use of haemostatic agents and glues during laparoscopic partial nephrectomy: a multi-institutional survey from the United States and Europe of 1347 cases. Eur Urol 2007;52(3):798–803.

[59] Breda A, Stepanian SV, Liao J, et al. Positive margins in laparoscopic partial nephrectomy in 855 cases: a multi-institutional survey from the United States and Europe. J Urol 2007;178(1):47–50.

[60] Permpongkosol S, Colombo JR Jr, Gill IS, et al. Positive surgical parenchymal margin after laparoscopic partial nephrectomy for renal cell carcinoma: oncological outcomes. J Urol 2006;176(6 Pt 1):2401–4.

[61] Yossepowitch O, Thompson RH, Leibovich BC, et al. Positive surgical margins at partial nephrectomy: predicors and oncological outcomes. J Urol 2008;179(6):2158–63.

[62] Lee BR, Tan BJ, Smith AD. Laparoscopic port site metastases: incidence, risk factors, and potential preventive measures. Urology 2005;65(4):639–44.

[63] Rassweiler J, Tsivian A, Kumar AV, et al. Oncological safety of laparoscopic surgery for urological malignancy: experience with more than 1000 operations. J Urol 2003;169(6):2072–5.

[64] Castillo OA, Vitagliano G, Diaz M, et al. Port-site metastasis after laparoscopic partial nephrectomy: case report and literature review. J Endourol 2007; 21(4):404–7.

[65] Schneider C, Jung A, Reymond MA, et al. Efficacy of surgical measures in preventing port-site recurrences in a porcine model. Surg Endosc 2001;15(2):121–5.

[66] Bostwick DG, Murphy GP. Diagnosis and prognosis of renal cell carcinoma: highlights from an international consensus workshop. Semin Urol Oncol 1998;16(1):46–52.

[67] Black P, Filipas D, Fichtner J, et al. Nephron-sparing surgery for central renal tumors: experience with 33 cases. J Urol 2000;163(3):737–43.

[68] Permpongkosol S, Bagga HS, Romero FR, et al. Laparoscopic versus open partial nephrectomy for the treatment of pathological T1N0M0 renal cell carcinoma: a 5-year survival rate. J Urol 2006;176(5):1984–8.

[69] Ost MC, Montag S, Permpongkosol S, et al. Predictors of hemorrhage following laparoscopic partial nephrectomy [abstract VP2-21]. J Endourol 2006;20(Suppl 1):A12.

[70] Campbell SC, Novick AC, Streem SB, et al. Complications of nephron-sparing surgery for renal tumors. J Urol 1994;151(5):1177–80.

[71] Lotan Y, Cadeddu JA. A cost comparison of nephron-sparing surgical techniques for renal tumour. BJU Int 2005;95(7):1039–42.

[72] Caruso RP, Phillips CK, Kau E, et al. Robot-assisted laparoscopic partial nephrectomy: initial experience. J Urol 2006;176(1):36–9.

[73] Kaul S, Laungani R, Sarle R, et al. da Vinci-assisted robotic partial nephrectomy: technique and results at a mean of 15 months of follow-up. Eur Urol 2007;51(1):186–91.

[74] Phillips CK, Taneja SS, Stifelman MD. Robot-assisted laparoscopic partial nephrectomy: the NYU technique. J Endourol 2005;19(4):441–5.

ELSEVIER
SAUNDERS

Urol Clin N Am 35 (2008) 397–414

UROLOGIC
CLINICS
of North America

Renal Thermal Ablative Therapy

Samuel P. Sterrett, DO[a], Stephen Y. Nakada, MD[a],*,
Marshall S. Wingo, MD[b], Steve K. Williams, MD[b],
Raymond J. Leveillee, MD, FRCS-G[b]

[a]Department of Urology, G5/339 Clinical Science Center, University of Wisconsin, 600 Highland Drive,
Madison, WI 53792-7375, USA
[b]Radiology and Biomedical Engineering, Department of Urology, University of Miami Miller School of Medicine,
Dominion Tower, 5th Floor, 1400 NW 10th Avenue, Miami, FL 33136, USA

Widespread use of abdominal imaging has increased the number of incidental tumors found in greater than 38,000 renal masses diagnosed in the United States in 2006 [1]. It is estimated that as many as 51,190 cases of renal cancer were diagnosed in 2007 and that the disease would cause 12,890 deaths [2]. By the mid-1990s, incidental lesions accounted for 60% of all renal masses [3]. These incidental lesions present at a lower stage, grade, and likelihood of metastasis and have improved survival outcomes compared with tumors detected in symptomatic patients [3–5]. The frequency of detection of small, asymptomatic, solid renal masses with low biologic activity continues to increase [6]. The management of these tumors over the past decade has shifted from radical nephrectomy to NSS. The potential "overtreatment" of incidental small renal lesions with radical nephrectomy, along with a desire to reduce patient morbidity and preserve renal function, led to the development of nephron-sparing techniques and minimally invasive methods to manage renal tumors. Nephron-sparing surgery (NSS) was initially indicated for patients who have localized renal cell carcinoma (RCC) combined with a compromised contralateral kidney and a need to preserve overall renal function but now has become applicable in patients who have single, unilateral, localized RCC with a normal contralateral renal unit [7].

Partial nephrectomy has proved to be effective for patients who have small single renal tumors that do not involve the collecting system. It is also associated with significant morbidity, however, including longer operative time, increased blood loss, and prolonged hospital stay compared with radical nephrectomy [8–10]. Minimally invasive approaches, such a laparoscopic partial nephrectomy, are rapidly gaining acceptance for treatment of small localized renal tumors; however, laparoscopic partial nephrectomy is associated with increased complications compared with open partial nephrectomy [11]. Renal ablative techniques were developed to offer widespread application, improved patient procedural morbidity, and reduced potential for complications. A large variety of generators, ablation probes, and energy delivery systems are now commercially available. In addition to their efficacy and safety, oncologic outcomes have been excellent to date, which supports the rationale of in situ tumor destruction to reduce morbidity and invasiveness further [12,13]. In situ thermal destruction of RCC uses techniques that destroy tumor tissue through freezing (cryotherapy) or heating (radiofrequency ablation [RFA], microwave ablation, laser interstitial therapy, high-intensity focused ultrasound [HiFU]), and radiosurgery). Each of these techniques relies on controlled energy delivery in an attempt to minimize collateral damage to normal renal parenchyma and other surrounding structures.

* Corresponding author.
  E-mail address: nakada@surgery.wisc.edu
(S.Y. Nakada).

Cryotherapy

The term *cryotherapy* refers to the therapeutic use of cold. Cryosurgery is the use of cold as a means of tissue destruction. The Egyptians began using cold to treat injuries and inflammation around 2500 BC [14]. The first application of cryotherapy to treat malignancy was described in the mid-nineteenth century by Arnott [15], who used a salt solution containing crushed ice at −18°C to −24°C to shrink breast, cervical, and skin cancers. Technologic advances leading to the invention of an automated cryosurgical apparatus in the early 1960s and vacuum-insulated liquid nitrogen or argon-cooled probes led to a renewed interest in cryosurgery and its possible application in renal cancer [14,16].

Animal models of renal cryoablation were first published in 1974 [17]. Human literature was not reported until more than 2 decades later when Uchida and colleagues [18] first published their reports of percutaneous cryoablation of renal lesions. Soon after, reports on open and laparoscopic approaches appeared in 1996 [19] and 1998 [20], respectively. Many of these early studies demonstrated that renal cryoablation was technically feasible, safe, and initially efficacious. As new 5-year postoperative data emerge, cryoablation is finally gaining acceptance as a standard option for the treatment of patients who have localized renal masses less than 4 cm.

Principles of cryotherapy (freezing)

The key factors involved in freezing injury include direct mechanical shock, osmotic shock, and cellular hypoxia. Cryotherapy-induced necrosis is essentially a three-step process. Initially, extracellular ice formation increases the osmolarity in the extracellular space, leading to a shift of fluid from the intracellular to extracellular space. As a result, changes in pH lead to protein denaturation and accumulation of toxins within the cell. Next, intracellular ice forms with lower temperatures, and disruption of cellular membranes occurs. Finally, delayed microcirculatory failure occurs with the thaw phase of the freeze-thaw cycle, resulting in further cell disruption, endothelial damage, microvascular thrombosis, and eventual tissue ischemia. This last process may take days to weeks and is ultimately responsible for the coagulative necrosis, fibrosis, and collagen deposition seen by 1 month [21].

The lethal temperature for achieving reliable deaths of normal and cancerous renal cells is near −20°C. Investigators have shown that exposure of renal cancer cell lines to −10°C for 60 minutes resulted in cell death in only 5% of cells. Exposure to −20°C, however, resulted in 85% cell death [22]. Despite the low temperatures created near the tip of the cryoprobe, or center of the ice ball, there is rapid warming of the tissue toward the periphery of the ice ball (Fig. 1). Campbell and colleagues [23] showed in a canine model that the edge of the ice ball had to extend at least 3.1 mm beyond the edge of the target lesion for adequate cell death to occur. We routinely extend the ice ball at least 10 mm beyond the edge of the tumor to ensure an adequate margin of tissue death. In addition to the temperature that should be achieved, the duration of freezing has been demonstrated to be an important factor leading to tissue destruction. Once the tissue temperature reaches a certain level, more cellular destruction can be achieved by prolonged freezing at this temperature [24]. Not all structures are equally cryosensitive. The renal collecting system has been shown to remain intact after ice ball involvement if the tissue has not been lacerated mechanically [25].

As outlined, thawing of the cryoablated tissue is as instrumental as the freezing process to ensure

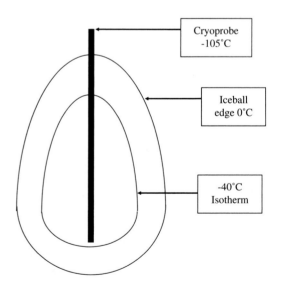

Fig. 1. Cryoprobe isotherm. The temperature within the cryolesion is not uniform. From cryoprobe to ice ball edge, the temperature continues to increase in a predictable pattern. The −40°C isotherm should completely cover the tumor to ensure complete ablation.

tumor destruction. It has been reported that repeating the freeze-thaw cycle exacerbates tissue damage and increases liquefaction necrosis [26]. The authors currently use two freeze-thaw cycles. Optimal freeze times have also been studied in swine. Five-minute freeze times were shown to be inadequate to cause tissue necrosis and were associated with excessive bleeding, whereas 15-minute freeze times produced consistent necrosis but were associated with renal fracture. It was concluded that the 10-minute freeze time seems to be optimal to produce necrosis without complications [27]. Still debated, however, is whether a slow passive thaw is more effective than a rapid active thaw. Finally, clamping the renal artery before cryotherapy to avoid the heat sink effect of renal blood flow has been shown to increase the size of the cryolesion only marginally [28].

Cryoprobes and cryogens

The goal of cryotherapy is to freeze a specified volume of tissue resulting in necrosis without significant damage to the surrounding healthy tissue. With this in mind, cryoprobes have been developed with characteristics, such as variable diameter and length of the freeze zone, to produce a specific size of cryolesion. In addition, the velocity of the temperature change and the nadir probe temperature affect the dimensions and temperature gradient of the ice ball. Finally, thermal conductivity of the target tissue affects the volume of tissue that is ablated. For example, a 3.4-mm probe cooling at the rate of 50°C per minute to a nadir probe tip temperature of −175°C creates a cryolesion 4 cm in diameter in 20 minutes. In comparison, an 8-mm probe cooling at the rate of 100°C per minute to a nadir tip temperature of −190°C results in a cryolesion 7 cm in diameter in 20 minutes [29]. Knowing this, a cryoprobe may be chosen on the basis of the size of the lesion to be ablated. Alternatively, a single probe may be placed repeatedly to achieve a larger cryolesion in large or irregular tumors.

Various clinically relevant cryogens are available, with the boiling point of each determining the nadir temperature that the specific cryoprobe can produce. Liquid argon and liquid nitrogen, the two most commonly used cryogens, have boiling points of −186°C and −196°C, respectively. Liquid nitrogen–based systems circulate the compressed nitrogen within the cryoprobe, allowing it to boil at the tip, thereby extracting the latent heat of boiling from its surrounding environment. Liquid argon–based systems rely on the Joule-Thompson effect, in which compressed gas or liquid under high pressure is allowed to expand rapidly through a narrow orifice in the tip cavity of the cryoprobe. The rapid cooling that results creates an ice ball [30].

Surgical technique

Cryotherapy can be delivered by means of an open, laparoscopic, or percutaneous surgical approach. Open cryotherapy requires an incision large enough for kidney mobilization and tumor exposure. This approach is typically entertained when a concomitant open abdominal procedure is being performed. Although invasive, the open approach allows for excellent sonographic monitoring with ultrasound.

Laparoscopy has been the preferred method for renal cryoablation, especially for anterior and anteromedial tumors. The transperitoneal approach offers the advantages of familiarity to most urologic surgeons and a distensible cavity to provide a large working space. Retroperitoneoscopy offers the advantages of working away from other organs and limitation of hematoma spread with the protection of the perirenal fat and Gerota's fascia. Advantages of laparoscopy include careful visual monitoring of probe placement and ice ball progression in relation to the mass under laparoscopic ultrasound guidance; mobilization of vital structures away from the treatment area, including bowel, liver, and spleen; and easy establishment of hemostasis.

The percutaneous approach can also be used successfully under cross-sectional imaging or ultrasound guidance. The advantages of a percutaneous approach over the laparoscopic approach include less invasiveness, shorter hospitalization, excellent ice ball monitoring with cross-sectional imaging, less pain medication requirement, decreased operating time, and cost-effectiveness. Disadvantages include the lack of visual cues for probe placement, inability to separate vital structures from the treatment area, and radiation exposure during CT treatment.

Regardless of the approach used, the fundamentals are the same. The procedure involves real-time imaging of the tumor, needle biopsy of the tumor, insertion of the cryoprobe perpendicular to the tumor, placement of the distal tip of the probe at the deep margin of the tumor, ensuring that the probe is not in contact with surrounding viscera, creation of an ice ball extending approximately 10 mm beyond the tumor, and achievement of adequate hemostasis after removal of the cryoprobe.

In most series, the investigators follow the ablated lesion using contrast-enhanced CT or MRI every 3 to 6 months initially. Lack of enhancement on CT or MRI, with stable or decreased tumor size, can be considered a sign of successful cryoablation (Fig. 2). Signs of recurrent cancer include increased tumor size, lack of tumor shrinkage, and nodular or lesion enhancement greater than 10 Hounsfield units (HU).

At the University of Wisconsin, select patients are offered cryoablation or laparoscopic partial nephrectomy for most localized renal tumors 4 cm or less in size. Laparoscopy is the preferred technique for anterior and lateral tumors, and percutaneous cryoablation is preferred for posterior tumors with a clear window for probe placement. Cryotherapy is administered under general anesthesia, although some centers use local sedation, and is performed using an argon gas–based system that operates on the Joule-Thompson principle. Cryoprobes are available in diameters of 1.4 mm, 2.4 mm, 3.4 mm, and 3.8 mm. The number and size of cryoprobes used in individual cases vary because of differences in tumor size and location. Most probes can typically be passed percutaneously or laparoscopically, because variable lengths are offered with each probe size. For

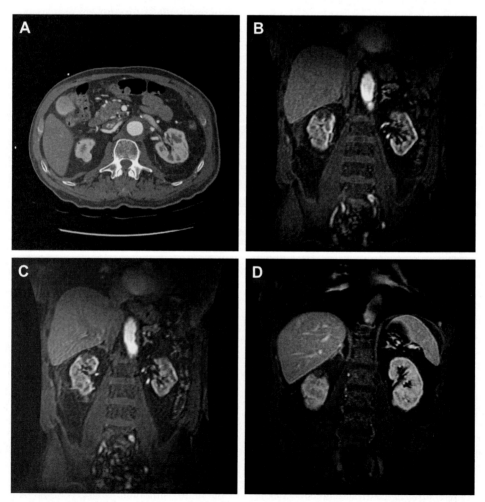

Fig. 2. (A) CT and (B) MRI scans of a 2-cm right upper pole renal mass before treatment. MRIs demonstrate lack of enhancement over a previous tumor site 3 months (C) and 7 months (D) after cryoablation.

the laparoscopic approach, we now leave Gerota's fascia intact to tamponade the bleeding from the cryoablated site and minimize tumor spillage. Laparoscopic ultrasound is used to confirm tumor and proper probe placement, and cryotherapy is initiated using two 10-minute freeze cycles (Fig. 3). The freeze cycles are monitored so that the ice ball extends 1 cm beyond the tumor margin. The cryolesion is monitored with real-time sonography performed by a radiologist experienced in laparoscopic ultrasound, which we believe better confirms adequate treatment of the margin. A passive thaw is allowed between the freezing cycles, and an active thaw is allowed after the second freeze. The authors allow the probe to loosen spontaneously before removing it during the active thaw. Hemostatic matrix is then injected into the cryoprobe defect (Fig. 4) and covered with absorbable hemostat. Direct pressure is applied for 10 minutes. With the insufflation pressure decreased, the cryolesion is observed for 15 minutes to confirm hemostasis. For the percutaneous approach, the cryoprobes are placed under ultrasound or CT guidance with the patient in the prone position. After the cryoprobe is removed, images are routinely obtained to rule out postoperative hemorrhage.

All patients are admitted overnight after surgery for observation. Serum creatinine and hematocrit are measured on the day after surgery, and patients are discharged home once they tolerate diet with their pain controlled on oral analgesics. The ablated lesions are followed using contrast-enhanced CT or MRI every 3 months during the first year, every six months during the second year, and then yearly. If a lesion does not shrink appropriately, more diligent follow-up is required.

Outcomes

Three clinical series have recently matured to provide us with 5-year follow up data for renal cryoablation. Hegarty and colleagues [31] reported on 194 patients undergoing laparoscopic renal cryoablation since 1997, with 66 patients having more than 5 years of follow up with MRI surveillance. Of the 66 patients with long-term follow-up, the indication for treatment was a solitary sporadic renal lesion in 48 (73%). Mean patient age was 66 years. Mean tumor size was 2.3 cm (range 1–4.5 cm). Three patients (6%) developed tumor recurrence requiring nephrectomy. One patient was diagnosed with metastatic RCC shortly after treatment and died 19 months later. The authors report an overall 5-year survival of 81% and a 5-year cancer-specific survival of 98% [31].

The second series with a 5-year follow-up included 48 patients, all with more than a 3-year follow-up (median of 64 months). Twenty-four patients were treated with the open technique, whereas the other 24 were treated with the laparoscopic technique. The median lesion size was 2.6 cm (range: 1.1–4.6 cm). The overall survival rate was 89.5%. Five patients (12.5%) were diagnosed with persistent disease and treated with repeat renal cryoablation (n = 1), laparoscopic nephrectomy (n = 2), laparoscopic partial nephrectomy (n = 1), and observation (n = 1). The cancer-specific survival rate was 100%, and

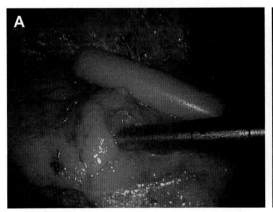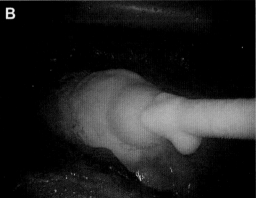

Fig. 3. (*A*) Cryoprobe is inserted into the renal mass under laparoscopic ultrasound guidance. (*B*) After confirming proper probe placement at the deep margin of the tumor, cryotherapy is initiated.

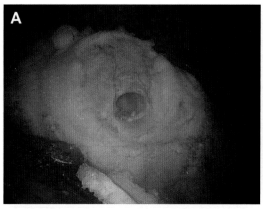 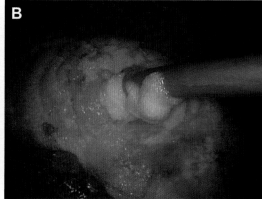

Fig. 4. (*A*) The cryoprobe loosens spontaneously during the active freeze of the second freeze thaw cycle and is removed. (*B*) Hemostatic matrix is placed into the cryoprobe defect with the aid of a laparoscopic applicator.

the cancer-free survival rate after a single cryoablation procedure was 87.5%. This improved to 97.5% after repeat treatment. No complications were observed [32].

Bandi and colleagues [33] recently reported the first series with 5-year data using percutaneous cryoablation. A total of 78 patients had 88 small renal masses treated by laparoscopic cryoablation (n = 58) and percutaneous cryoablation (n = 20). Mean tumor size was 2.6 cm. Mean follow-up was 19 months. The overall, cancer-specific, and recurrence-free survival rates were 88.5%, 100%, and 98.7%, respectively. Four patients required a repeat treatment because of persistent disease, and 1 had progression to locally advanced disease. Five patients had complications during cryoablation, and 7 had complications afterward [33].

Table 1 summarizes the largest cryotherapy trials (>20 patients) to date. These studies suggest that cryotherapy is a safe minimally invasive treatment option for patients who have small renal masses at the intermediate follow-up.

Complications

The complications of renal cryotherapy are rare and have rates similar to those of other laparoscopic and percutaneous procedures. Complications stem from the technical approach and from the ablation. Pain or paresthesia at the probe site seems to be the most common complication, occurring in approximately 5% of all patients [41]. Because the entire probe is cooled in cryotherapy, care must be taken to avoid injury to the sensory nerves at the body surface. Other complications include hemorrhage, urinary infection, pneumonia,

renal insufficiency, wound infection, ileus, adjacent organ injury, and respiratory difficulty. The complications of the larger cryotherapy series are listed in Table 2.

In a multi-institutional study evaluating complications after 139 cryoablation procedures, with 2 major and 18 minor complications, was reported. Overall, 4 complications were reported in the laparoscopic group and 16 were reported in the percutaneous group. Of these 20 complications, only 2 were reported as major complications and no deaths were reported. The investigators also reported that all major complications occurred early in the series, suggesting that experience with laparoscopy and percutaneous procedures is important for preventing and managing these complications [41].

Radiofrequency ablation

Indications for radiofrequency ablation treatment

RFA is a heat-based method of tissue destruction originally developed for the treatment of aberrant cardiac pathways. The first oncologic application involved the treatment of primary and metastatic liver tumors [42,43]. Current applications include the treatment of breast malignancy, aberrant cardiac pathways, gynecologic tumors, prostate disease, bone lesions, pancreatic cancer, renal tumors [44], and metastatic lesions.

With reports of RFA success in renal tumors ranging from small incidental lesions to metastatic deposits, how do we determine who is appropriate for renal RFA treatment? Prospective randomized clinical series to identify patients appropriate for

Table 1
Largest cryotherapy studies (>20 patients) to date with associated outcomes

Study (year)	Approach	Patients	Tumor size (cm)	Follow-up (months)	OR time (minutes)	EBL (mL)	Complications	Hospital stay (days)	Recurrence
Shingleton and Sewell (2001) [34]	Perc	20	3.2	9.1	97	NA	1	1	0
Cestari et al (2004) [35]	Lap	37	2.6	20.5	194	165	7	3.8	1
Gill et al (2005) [36]	Lap	56	2.3	NA (all >3 years)	180	87	4	NA	2
Hegarty et al (2006) [31]	Lap	66	2.3	NA	NA	NA	NA	NA	3
Schwartz (2006) [37]	Open/Lap	85	2.6	10	NA	58	3	3	2
Davol et al (2006) [32]	Open/Lap	48	2.6	64	NA	NA	7	3	5
Polascik et al (2007) [38]	Lap	26	2.5	7	NA	NA	2	2	0
Tillet et al (2006) [39]	Lap	41	3.1	12.5	NA	NA	3	NA	3
Beemster and De la Rosette (2006) [40]	Lap	31	2.4	NA	204	NA	3	5.1	1
Bandi et al (2007) [33]	Lap/Perc	78	2.6	19	220	NA	11	2.1	4

Abbreviations: Lap, laparotomy; NA, not available; Perc, percutaneous.

RFA therapy have not been performed to date. Phase II trials have included patients receiving RFA simultaneously with open or laparoscopic nephrectomy before nephrectomy, in patients deemed inappropriate for extirpative surgery because of comorbidities, and in patients who had hereditary RCC. Most clinicians agree that patients with a solitary kidney, multiple synchronous RCC, von Hippel-Lindau disease, familial RCC, or limited renal function are appropriate candidates for RFA treatment, but controversy exists in younger patients without significant comorbid conditions, normal contralateral renal function, and minimal future risk for renal function loss. As experience with RFA accumulates and intermediate and long-term oncologic results become available, favorable outcomes may justify the treatment of smaller and potentially less aggressive tumors in younger and healthier patients with RFA.

Principles of radiofrequency ablation (heat)

RFA techniques convert radiant energy into thermal energy in the tissues, ultimately leading to coagulative necrosis. The results are less dramatic than with cryoablation, but there is no evidence that RFA is less effective. Damage is believed to manifest through protein denaturation, DNA/RNA chain disruption, and vascular congestion. Effective ablation and cell damage are time- and temperature-dependent processes. (Fig. 5) Various ranges of temperature (heat) damage tissue and result in cell death equivalently, but more time is required at lower temperatures. High temperatures ($>100°C$) result in immediately identifiable cellular changes, including obvious structural damage, desiccation, vaporization, and carbonization. Lower temperatures ($45°C–55°C$) are associated with less grossly apparent changes, including denatured cellular enzymes; damaged membrane channels; and cellular edema, organelle swelling, and blebbing after several hours. Elevated temperatures cause the intracellular buffering capacity and transport mechanisms to fail, resulting in an overload of intracellular calcium and cell death. Disruption of the delicate intracellular balance causes localized inflammatory changes to appear, followed by an ischemic response, leading to acidosis and eventual coagulative necrosis.

Table 2
Major and minor complications reported in large cryotherapy trials

Study (year)	Major complications	Minor complications
Shingleton and Sewell (2001)	None	Wound infection
Cestari et al (2004)	UPJO	Fever (3) Hematoma (2) Hematuria
Schwartz (2006)	Renal fracture CVA	Hydronephrosis (resolved)
Gill et al (2005)	Splenic hematoma CHF	Pleural effusion Herpetic esophagitis
Davol et al (2006)	None	Capsular fracture (4) Transfusion (2) Ileus
Polascik et al (2007)	None	Transfusion Ileus
Tillet et al (2006)	None	Transfusion (2) Urinary fistula (resolved)
Beemster and De la Rosette (2006)	None	Pneumonia Skin paresthesia Urinary tract infection
Bandi et al (2007)	Bowel injury Atrial fibrillation Respiratory failure	Hematoma (4) Neuropathic pain (2) Urine leak Narcotic overdose

Abbreviations: CVA, cerebrovascular accident; CHF, congestive heart failure; UPJO, ureteropelvic junction obstruction.

After thermal injury, the basic structure of the cell is preserved. Three to 7 days after RFA treatment, the damaged tissue begins to show signs of coagulative necrosis with interspersed

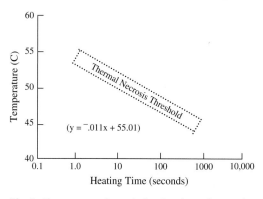

Fig. 5. Temperature-time relation for thermal necrosis.

inflammatory cells. The necrotic debris is then removed by fragmentation or phagocytosis. Concomitant apoptosis can increase the total area of cell kill through the promotion of nuclear pyknosis in cells adjacent to directly injured cells [45]. All evidence of organized renal cellular architecture disappears by 30 days. The necrotic tissue absorbed with fragmentation and phagocytosis transforms into avascular scar tissue that may become smaller in size and does not enhance on contrasted imaging [46,47].

"Heat-sink" considerations

Tissue vascularity within and surrounding the renal tumor may affect the volume of the ablated area. Adjacent blood flow may dissipate the generated heat, resulting in a "heat-sink" phenomenon, making it more challenging to treat highly vascular lesions and lesions adjacent to larger blood vessels, such as the renal hilum. Attempts have been made by researchers to reduce this effect by clamping the renal hilum during treatment. Corwin and colleagues [48] used clamping of the renal hilum in a swine model and demonstrated that the ablated lesion size was larger in the ischemic kidneys than in the normally perfused cohort. When researchers examined the kidneys 1 month after treatment, however, no difference in lesion size was detectable. Although clamping of the renal hilum is not possible in percutaneous procedures, research examining selective arterial constriction and embolization of renal tumor vasculature before RFA is ongoing.

Radiofrequency ablation technology background

Radiofrequency energy is composed of an alternating electrical current (alternating current [AC]) with a wavelength between 10 kHz and 900 MHz. Commercially available radiofrequency generators typically produce current at frequencies from 400 to 500 kHz [45]. Energy is typically delivered through a monopolar circuit. Current emanates from the radiofrequency generator through the electrode, passes through the patient's tissues, and returns to the generator through a grounding pad on the skin. Bipolar systems for which no grounding pad is required exist but are not commonly used. Impedance (Ω) or resistance to flow of current exists within the circuit and varies depending on the tissue density and composition. Alternatively, radiofrequency energy delivered through a bipolar circuit begins at the electrode and returns through an additional electrode in close proximity to the point of origin. This circuit type minimizes the amount of tissue traversed by the electrical current and offers advantages and disadvantages but is not discussed here.

Plain or "dry" electrodes

Plain electrode RFA involves the delivery of current through a single, expandable, or bipolar electrode. Conventional plain radiofrequency electrodes are limited in tissue ablation efficiency by high-current densities at the metal electrode–tissue interface. High-current densities result in high temperatures ($>100°C$) followed by tissue desiccation and charring close to the electrode surface (<1 mm) as described previously [49]. In attempts to improve the propagation of radiofrequency energy and reduce high electrode tissue density, investigators have tried to manipulate several variables in the radiofrequency circuit. Engineers have developed a negative feedback circuit limiting the applied power when the impedance increases and have installed a thermal sensor at the electrode tip to maintain the temperature at less than $100°C$ by reducing the power applied to the circuit. These maneuvers have resulted in mixed success. Attempts to reduce the electrode temperature and tissue impedance through reduction of the power applied to the circuit limit the amount, rate, and total volume of tissue treated.

Strategies to manipulate the tissue-electrode interface resulted in the development of alternative radiofrequency probe configurations. Single-shaft radiofrequency electrodes include plain, cooled, expandable, bipolar, and wet configurations. Multiple electrode systems are also available and classified according to probe number, electric mode, activation mode, and electrode type (ie, plain, wet, cooled, expandable). Detailed descriptions of these numerous systems are beyond the scope of this article [50].

Predicting the size of the "zone of kill"

The goal of therapy should be the creation of a zone of heat that includes the entire volume of the mass and extends beyond the tumor edge to achieve an acceptable treatment margin. Adequacy of partial nephrectomy is considered if the entire tumor is removed (ie, as long as the margin

is negative). At the University of Miami, the authors perform ablations with the goal of achieving at least a 5-mm zone of "adequate" thermal intensity and duration (ie, $60°C$ for 1 second).

Electrode systems

Mulier and colleagues [50] proposed a standardized nomenclature for radiofrequency electrode systems. Single-shaft radiofrequency electrodes are described as plain, cooled, expandable, bipolar, or wet. Cooled electrodes are further classified as single or clustered. Expandable electrodes include the subcategories multitined and coiled. Some of these features can occur simultaneously along a single-shaft electrode and are referred to as double-and triple-combination designs. Multiple electrode systems are classified by the number of probes, circuit type (monopolar or bipolar), activation mode (consecutive, simultaneous, or switching), site of insertion, and electrode system (wet, cooled, or expandable) [50]. A standardized nomenclature system allows more accurate comparison of technologies and a better understanding of published radiofrequency techniques. Almost all the published literature regarding renal RFA has primarily involved centers using two systems. Further detailed discussion of the other types of electrode systems is beyond the scope of this article.

Radiofrequency ablation surgical technique

Laparoscopic-assisted technique

Much like cryoablation, radiofrequency treatment may be performed through a percutaneous or laparoscopic approach. Anteriorly or laterally oriented renal tumors are best approached by laparoscopic mobilization of the bowel, exposure of the tumor surface, and direct visualized insertion of the ablation probe into the tumor parenchyma for efficacy and safety (Fig. 6). Laparoscopic exposure reduces the risk for thermal injury to adjacent organs, such as the liver, spleen, and bowel, in addition to other vital structures, including the ureter and renal pelvis from the ablation zone. Posterior tumors can also be accessed through retroperitoneal laparoscopic approaches. Laparoscopy requires small port incisions, and abdominal insufflation. Multiple percutaneous core biopsies are done with a spring-loaded (16- or 18-gauge) needle before ablation. This is guided

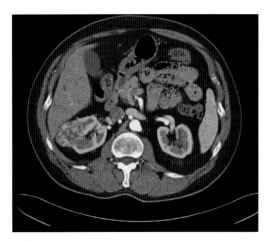

Fig. 6. Laterally oriented renal tumor for laparoscopic-assisted RFA.

visually and confirmed with laparoscopic ultrasonography. Because heat is not detectable with ultrasound, the authors use temperature monitoring at the tumor margin. If peripheral temperature monitoring is performed, they then place three and four fiberoptic temperature sensors at the peripheral (superior, inferior, lateral, and medial) and deep margins of the tumor, 5 mm from the tumor-parenchymal interface (Fig. 7A).

The RFA probe(s) is then positioned under direct visualization and ultrasound guidance toward the center of the tumor. The ablation is complete after a specified time interval; the temperature or impedance goal is reached; or in the case of peripheral temperature monitoring, when all temperature monitors reach the target temperature (see Fig. 7B, C). Manipulation and alternate targeting of the radiofrequency probe and repeat application of radiofrequency energy may be necessary to achieve complete thermal coverage of the lesion. After the completion of the ablation procedure, all the probes are removed. Because the heat acts to coagulate blood vessels, unlike cryoablation, we have not found it necessary to add any topical hemostatic agents.

CT-guided radiofrequency ablation treatment

CT-guided RFA can be performed under general anesthesia, under intravenous sedation, or after infiltration of a local anesthetic. At the University of Miami, general anesthesia is preferred for all treatments because of the precision with which all probes must be positioned to ensure effective tumor ablation and to minimize

collateral damage. In the authors' unit, the ablation "team" consists of the urologic surgeon, interventional radiologist, anesthesiologist, surgical nurse, and CT technician. Purely percutaneous radiofrequency treatment with the assistance of radiologic imaging may be performed in posteriorly oriented tumors (Fig. 8). Several methods of bowel manipulation have been described. Saline solution or CO_2 injection has been used with RFA to increase the separation between vital structures and the renal lesion. The patient is placed in a prone or full-flank position to provide percutaneous access to the retroperitoneum. After preoperative imaging is reviewed by the team, probe type, location, and circuit type are determined based on tumor characteristics, size, and anatomic relation to other structures.

If peripheral temperature monitoring is performed (as is the case for all the authors' treatments), a minimum of three fiberoptic temperature sensors are placed under CT guidance at the peripheral (superior, inferior, lateral, and medial) and deep margins of the tumor, 5 mm from the tumor-parenchymal interface (Fig. 9). The probes are inserted through nonconducting 18-gauge sheaths. These are placed before biopsy to avoid the possibility of bleeding, obscuring the radiographic planes. Contrast is not routinely used if the preoperative imaging done with contrast demonstrates a well-defined border. The radiofrequency probe(s) is positioned under CT guidance percutaneously and directed toward the center of the tumor and advanced until the deep margin is reached with the probe tip. Conversely, for those who use expandable ablation needles, the needles are deployed according to the manufacturer's algorithm. After the ablation needle is properly positioned the radiofrequency cycle is initiated. The ablation is complete after a specified time interval, when a target temperature or impedance is reached at the probe tip or, in the case of peripheral temperature monitoring, when all the target temperatures have been achieved at the tumor margins (>5 mm, 60°C). Manipulation and alternate targeting of the radiofrequency probe and repeat application of radiofrequency energy may be necessary to achieve a compete ablation. Based on the authors' experience, we recommend that all tumors positioned within 1 cm of the bowel should be considered for a laparoscopic approach to provide definitive separation between the tumor and all vital structures. After the CT-guided RFA, patients are discharged home the same day and resume normal activities within 1 week.

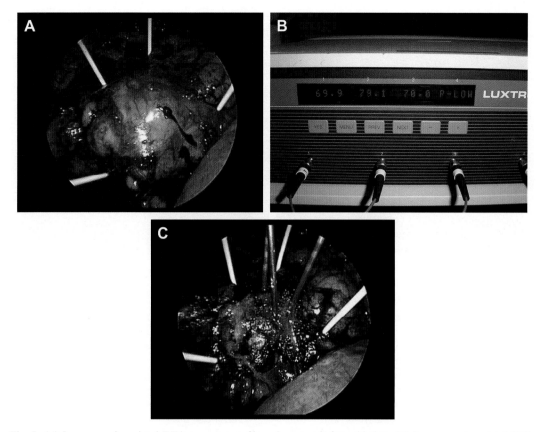

Fig. 7. (*A*) Laparoscopic-assisted RFA temperature fiber placement before ablation. (*B*) Laparoscopic-assisted RFA temperature fiber placement: three fibers exceed the 60°C targeted area adequately treated requirement, and the procedure can be terminated. (*C*) Laparoscopic-assisted RFA ablation tumor surface immediately after ablation.

MRI-guided technique

Lewin and colleagues [51] described the application of RFA using MRI guidance. Radiofrequency energy is delivered through custom-fabricated MRI-compatible "cooled-tip" radiofrequency electrodes using a temperature-controlled system. Treatments are administered for 12 to 15 minutes at 90°C with real-time temperature monitoring of the radiofrequency lesion identified by changes in the MRI enhancement patterns. If intraoperative imaging suggests incomplete treatment, the electrode is repositioned and additional radiofrequency cycles are performed. Follow-up is obtained through serial MRI scans to confirm the absence of persistent enhancement or radiographic recurrence.

Monitoring treatment area and ablated lesion size

You cannot see heat. Determining the size of the radiofrequency lesion in real-time is difficult,

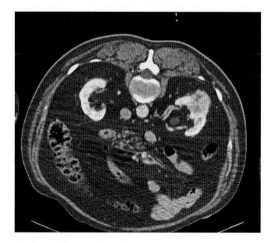

Fig. 8. Posteriorly oriented renal tumor for CT-guided RFA (prone position).

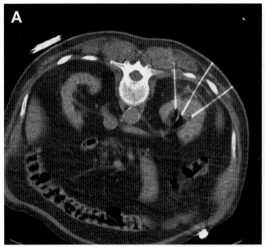
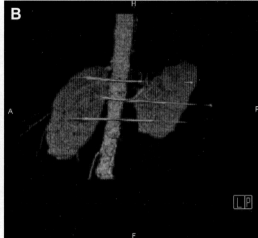

Fig. 9. (*A, B*) CT-guided placement of peripheral temperature-sensing probes.

because most tissue changes are not immediately visible. Ultrasound, CT, and MRI have been investigated in RFA therapy.

Peripheral fiberoptic temperature monitoring has been developed as a means to perform real-time monitoring during the RFA treatment as described previously [52]. Continuous temperature measurements are returned from each probe during the ablation. RFA continues until all peripheral temperatures exceed the predetermined level and duration. RFA probes can be repositioned and a treatment cycle repeated if a region of the tumor periphery does not reach the desired temperature. Carey and Leveillee [52], have demonstrated that large tumors, up to 3 to 5 cm in diameter, can be treated successfully with infrequent need for retreatment.

Postablation imaging and follow-up

Success is defined in many series by radiographic follow-up imaging. After RFA treatment, tumors are monitored by contrasted MRI with "no lesion enhancement" or CT (preferable and quantifiable) lack of enhancement by an increase in HU less than 20 HU and no evidence of growth indicative of a treatment success (Fig. 10). Long-term experience with following ablated tumors radiographically is lacking and optimal surveillance intervals are yet to be determined. Unlike cryoablated lesions, RFA lesions tend not to shrink in size. Matsumoto and colleagues [53] described the typical characteristics of the RFA

mass. These characteristics include a nonenhancing wedge-shaped lesion, frequently with a thin rim of fat between the lesion and the normal parenchyma. Exophytic tumors tend to retain their preablation shape and size. Imaging characteristics can change at any time and a regimented follow-up protocol is encouraged in all patients. Recurrences have been documented as late as 31 months. Table 3 summarizes single treatment success with renal RFA in larger series. Mixed success in these studies emphasizes the need to perform RFA in a meticulous manner with excellent targeting and lesion monitoring. Full ablation

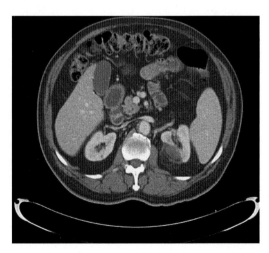

Fig. 10. Postoperative CT scan 1 month after posterior RFA.

Table 3
Single treatment success with renal radiofrequency ablation series with 10 or more patients

Authors	Tumor no.	Tumor size (cm)	Approach	Single treatment success
Pavlovich et al [55]	24	2.4	Perc (US and CT)	19/24 (79%)
Roy-Choudhury et al [56]	11	3.0	Perc (US and CT)	9/11 (82%)
Gervais et al [57]	42	3.2	Perc (US and CT)	36/42 (86%)
Su et al [58]	35	2.2	Perc (CT)	33/35 (94%)
Mayo-Smith et al [59]	36	2.6	Perc (US and CT)	26/32 (81%)
Farrell et al [60]	35	1.7	Perc (US and CT)	35/35 (100%)
Hwang et al [61]	24	2.2	Perc (CT) and lap	23/24 (96%)
Matsumoto et al [62]	64	N/A	Perc (CT), lap, and open	62/64 (97%)
Zagoria [63]	24	3.5	Perc (CT)	20/24 (83%)
Lewin et al [51]	10	2.3	Perc (MR)	10/10 (100%)
Varkarakis et al [64]	56	N/A	Perc (CT)	47/56 (84%)
McGovern et al [65]	62	1–5.5	Perc (CT)	55/62 (89%)
Ogan and Cadeddu [66]	13	2.4	Perc (CT)	12/13 (92%)
Jacomides et al [67]	17	1.96	Lap (US)	17/17 (100%)
Park et al [68]	109	N/A	Perc (CT) and lap	106/109 (97%)
Carey and Leveillee [52]	134	2.6 (1–5.3)	Perc (CT) and lap (US)	128/134 (96%)

Abbreviations: Lap, laparotomy; Perc, percutaneous; US, ultrasound.

should always be performed, and multiple probes should be used when necessary to ablate completely beyond the interface between tumor and normal parenchyma in larger tumors. The authors advocate the use of peripheral temperature monitoring to ensure that lethal temperatures reach beyond the tumor margin.

Complications

Although patients and clinicians expect minimal morbidity, complications are still possible. Uzzo and Novick [54] reviewed the literature from 1980 to 2000 and found a complication rate for nephron-sparing procedures (most were partial nephrectomies) ranging from 4% to 30%, with an average of 13.7%. To become an accepted form of nephron-sparing therapy, RFA must demonstrate equivalent oncologic efficacy with lower complication rates.

Most complications reported in the literature are minor and include subcapsular or perinephric hematomas that do not require treatment. Ureteropelvic junction (UPJ) obstructions have been described requiring pyeloplasty in one and nephrectomy secondary to pain and loss of renal function in another [69,70].

A multi-institutional review of complications of cryoablation and RFA was performed. [41] Eleven complications were seen in 133 cases (8.3%) of RFA. Eight complications were listed as minor, requiring no intervention, and 3 were considered major. Minor complications were

described as pain and paresthesias at the probe puncture site in addition to transiently increased serum creatinine. Major complications included an ileus, a UPJ obstruction that ultimately led to renal loss and nephrectomy, and a urinary leak.

The 8.3% complication rate is certainly comparable to the 13.7% overall experience with partial nephrectomy and is more impressive considering that many patients who underwent RFA were deemed inappropriate for more invasive surgical therapies.

Other energy ablative technologies

High-intensity focused ultrasound

HiFU focuses ultrasonic waves that pass through human tissues onto a target lesion within the body. The aim of HIFU technology is the "noncontact" destruction of tissues by extracorporeally applied ultrasound energy by means of an acoustic window. HiFU applies the same principles as diagnostic ultrasound (frequencies in the range of 1–20 MHz), which can propagate harmlessly through living tissue. Unlike diagnostic ultrasound, HiFU uses frequencies several orders of magnitude greater with focal zones that are cigar shaped, measuring a height of 12 to 32 mm and a width of 3 to 4 mm [71,72] with depths limited to 10 to 16 cm [73].

HiFU causes tissue insult by two mechanisms: a thermal effect and a mechanical effect [74]. As the power intensity increases, heat is generated as a result of absorption of the acoustic energy.

This causes an increase in the tissue temperature, leading to protein denaturation and cell death. This is the primary mechanism for tumor cell destruction in HiFU therapy.

Focusing also results in high intensities at a specific location and over a small volume (eg, 1-mm diameter and 9-mm length). With high-intensity energy over shorter periods, mechanical effects are achieved by bubble implosion, leading to mechanical disruption. Mechanical effects include cavitation, microstreaming, and radiation forces [75,76]. This occurs because of alternating compression and expansion of tissue as an ultrasound field passes through it. If the tissue disruption is of sufficient magnitude, gas may be extracted from the tissue, resulting in the formation of bubbles. These bubbles may remain relatively stable and simply oscillate, or they may collapse spontaneously, causing mechanical stresses and generating temperatures of 2000 to 5000 K in the microenvironment [77]. Microstreaming may produce high shear forces close to the bubble, leading to the disruption of cell membranes [78].

Conclusion

HiFU represents an attractive modality for the noninvasive treatment of tumors. The main advantage of HiFU is its ability to deposit large amounts of energy to targeted tissue, with millimeter accuracy and little or no damage to intervening tissue. Insufficient long-term data exist, although emerging data suggest that extracorporeal HiFU ablation is possibly facing severe technical challenges with recent evolution toward laparoscopic HiFU applications.

Clinical studies have all been preliminary, and further investigation is necessary before the widespread use of HiFU can be recommended.

Radiosurgery

The CyberKnife is a frameless image-guided radiosurgery device that uses a linear accelerator mounted on a robotic arm and divides the high-dose radiation into up to 1200 beams. Thus, the individual dose of each beam is relatively benign to adjacent tissue, although at the focal point of these beams, the dose is additive and the desired ablative dose is attained. Radiotherapy exerts its effect at the cellular level by induction of single- and double-stranded DNA breaks, which induce apoptosis and prevent successful cell division. Programmed cell death is not the only method

of tissue destruction possible by radiotherapy, however [79]. High enough doses of radiotherapy, when applied to a tumor or any tissue, can completely ablate the tumor or tissue. The use of external beam radiotherapy allows the delivery of high-energy radiation to tumor tissue and kills cancer cells. Such an approach subjects the surrounding tissue to the deleterious effects of radiation as well, however, and the treatment margins are indistinct.

Conclusion

Initial preclinical and clinical series of the Cyberknife for extracorporeal renal tissue ablation seem to be promising and demonstrate its ability to ablate a targeted area with relative sparing of the surrounding tissue precisely and completely, because no acute toxicities have been reported. It is still, however, not "noninvasive," because there is a need for biopsy and placement of fiducial markers. Further research is necessary before the role of radiosurgery in the management of renal tumors can be established.

Microwave thermotherapy: insufficient human data

For solid renal masses there are few data currently available pertaining to microwave thermotherapy. Energy is delivered by means of an antenna placed directly into the target lesion. The antenna generates an electromagnetic filed, causing rapid ion oscillation resulting in frictional heat. In principle, it is similar to RFA but has the advantage of delivering heat 100 times faster. Preclinical data exist and have been summarized by Wen and Nakada [80].

Clark and colleagues [81] recently published their work in humans. A phase I study was performed in humans evaluating ablation zones before surgery just before radical or partial nephrectomy. Ten tumors were ablated with no "skip" areas (visual, histologic, and NADH staining used) seen within the ablated zones. Further studies allowing for "ablate and leave" rather than resect are warranted.

Laser interstitial thermal therapy: inadequate human data, paucity of preclinical data

The first clinical series of laser thermal ablation was reported by Dick and colleagues [82] in 2002. Using MRI guidance, they performed real-time thermal mapping in nine patients who had renal masses and were not surgical candidates. They used a neodymium-yttrium-argon laser delivered with a 600-μm fiber for 10 to 30 minutes (one or two sessions). Mean tumor size was 3.7 cm, and mean follow-up was 16.9 months. Metrics were a percentage of enhancement change (73.7% before ablation to 29.5% after ablation). A second subset of patients was reported by Williams and Swishchuck [83] in abstract form. Data on 10 patients demonstrated in an "ablate and resect" study that coagulative necrosis could be achieved at 85°C. No pathologic findings were reported. There are no other instances of laser interstitial renal ablation that the authors are aware of.

Pulsed cavitational ultrasound: no human data

Pulsed cavitational ultrasound, also known as "histotripsy," is the transcutaneous noninvasive delivery of ultrasound energy that uses cavitational effects to damage target tissue by varying acoustic parameters. The nonthermal mechanical effects attributable to ultrasound are thought to have advantage over temperature-based ablation systems, whereby lesion precision is limited because of local factors. There is no thermal collateral damage to the surrounding tissue and skin or to the collecting system. A potential theoretic complication is the dissemination of malignant cells from the shear forces generated by the procedure, although this has not been seen experimentally. Two studies are available in rabbit and porcine kidneys. [84,85] There are no human data to date; thus, this form of ablation is still considered experimental.

Summary

Renal cryoablation is an excellent minimally invasive treatment option for small renal masses in appropriately selected patients. The ability to monitor the ice ball is a distinct advantage. Radiofrequency, likewise, has distinct procedural advantages and favorable outcomes. Five-year outcomes are now available confirming it as efficacious and with low morbidity.

Energy targeting is greatly enhanced through imaging modalities, which greatly assist needle placement or energy delivery to the optimal location for maximal effectiveness. When vital structures obscure access to the renal lesion, laparoscopic mobilization of these structures with direct visualization of the tumor can increase the likelihood of ablation success and minimize complication risk. Monitoring the size and

geometry of the ablation lesion ensures that the outermost reaches of the renal tumor have been completely treated. For most of the newer technologies (HiFU, radiosurgery, interstitial laser, microwave, and pulsed cavitational ultrasound), there is insufficient evidence to make them the forerunners currently. Independent of the ablation type or control method, when sustained lethal temperatures are verified at the tumor margins, the clinician can be confident that the treatment is complete. Ablative therapies are attractive because of their minimal impact on patient quality of life in addition to their morbidity and cost. Although they show promise of efficacy, they must be evaluated with long-term follow-up before they are considered the standard of oncologic care. Safety profiles thus far are excellent, and as technology and techniques advance, ablative therapies should gain more widespread use and acceptance. Renal masses can be treated with a laparoscopic or percutaneous approach depending on tumor location, size, and the available technology and experience of the center.

References

[1] Jemal A, Siegel R, Ward E, et al. Cancer statistics, 2006. CA Cancer J Clin 2006;56:106.
[2] Jemal A, Siegel R, Ward E, et al. Cancer statistics, 2007. CA Cancer J Clin 2007;57:43.
[3] Luciani LG, Cestari R, Tallarigo C. Incidental renal cell carcinoma—age and stage characterization and clinical implications: study of 1092 patients (1982–1997). Urology 2000;56:58.
[4] Hafez KS, Fergany AF, Novick AC. Nephron sparing surgery for localized renal cell carcinoma: impact of tumor size on patient survival, tumor recurrence and TNM staging. J Urol 1999;162:1930.
[5] Pantuck AJ, Zisman A, Rauch MK, et al. Incidental renal tumors. Urology 2000;56:190.
[6] Marshall FF, Stewart AK, Menck HR. The National Cancer Data Base: report on kidney cancers. The American College of Surgeons Commission on Cancer and the American Cancer Society. Cancer 1997;80:2167.
[7] Novick AC. Laparoscopic and partial nephrectomy. Clin Cancer Res 2004;10:6322S.
[8] Herr HW. Partial nephrectomy for unilateral renal carcinoma and a normal contralateral kidney: 10-year follow up. J Urol 1999;161:33.
[9] Parekh DJ, Chiang LW, Herrell SD. In vivo assessment of radio frequency induced thermal damage of kidney using optical spectroscopy. J Urol 2006; 176:1626.
[10] Yip SK, Cheng WS, Tan BS, et al. Partial nephrectomy for renal tumours: the Singapore General

Hospital experience. J R Coll Surg Edinb 1999;44: 156.

[11] Ramani AP, Desai MM, Steinberg AP, et al. Complications of laparoscopic partial nephrectomy in 200 cases. J Urol 2005;173:42.

[12] Gill IS, Kavoussi LR, Lane BR, et al. Comparison of 1,800 laparoscopic and open partial nephrectomies for single renal tumors. J Urol 2007;178:41.

[13] Novick AC, Derweesh I. Open partial nephrectomy for renal tumours: current status. BJU Int 2005; 95(Suppl 2):35.

[14] Gage AA. History of cryosurgery. Semin Surg Oncol 1998;14:99.

[15] Arnott J. Practical illustrations of the remedial efficacy of a very low or anaesthetic temperature I. Lancet 1850;2:257.

[16] Cooper Is LA. Cryostatic congelation: a system for producing a limited controlled region of cooling or freezing of biologic tissues. J Nerv Ment Dis 1961; 133:259.

[17] Breining H, Helpap B, Minderjahn A, et al. The parenchymal reaction of the kidney after local freezing. Urol Res 1974;2:29.

[18] Uchida M, Imaide Y, Sugimoto K, et al. Percutaneous cryosurgery for renal tumours. Br J Urol 1995; 75:132.

[19] Delworth MG, Pisters LL, Fornage BD, et al. Cryotherapy for renal cell carcinoma and angiomyolipoma. J Urol 1996;155:252.

[20] Gill IS, Novick AC, Soble JJ, et al. Laparoscopic renal cryoablation: initial clinical series. Urology 1998;52:543.

[21] Chosy SG, Nakada SY, Lee FT Jr, et al. Monitoring renal cryosurgery: predictors of tissue necrosis in swine. J Urol 1998;159:1370.

[22] Stephenson RA, King DK, Rohr LR. Renal cryoablation in a canine model. Urology 1996; 47:772.

[23] Campbell SC, Krishnamurthi V, Chow G, et al. Renal cryosurgery: experimental evaluation of treatment parameters. Urology 1998;52:29.

[24] Hoffmann NE, Bischof JC. The cryobiology of cryosurgical injury. Urology 2002;60:40.

[25] Sung GT, Gill IS, Hsu TH, et al. Effect of intentional cryo-injury to the renal collecting system. J Urol 2003;170:619.

[26] Auge BK, Santa-Cruz RW, Polascik TJ. Effect of freeze time during renal cryoablation: a swine model. J Endourol 2006;20:1101.

[27] Collyer W, Venkatesh R, Vanlangendonck R, et al. Enhanced renal cryoablation with hilar clamping and intrarenal cooling in a porcine model. Urology 2004;63:1209.

[28] Orihuela E, vanSonnenberg E, Motamedi M, et al. Thermodynamics of RCC during cryotherapy: effect of warm renal arterial blood flow [abstract]. J Urol 1999;161:144.

[29] Gage AA, Baust J. Mechanisms of tissue injury in cryosurgery. Cryobiology 1998;37:171.

[30] Carvalhal EF, Novick AC, Gill IS. Renal cryoablation application in nephron sparing treatment. Brazilian Journal of Urology 2000;26:558–70.

[31] Hegarty NJ, Kaouk JH, Remer EM, et al. Laparoscopic renal cryoablation: oncological outcomes at 5 years [abstract]. J Endourol 2006;20:A12.

[32] Davol PE, Fulmer BR, Rukstalis DB. Long-term results of cryoablation for renal cancer and complex renal masses. Urology 2006;68:2.

[33] Bandi G, Wen CC, Hedican SP, et al. Cryoablation of small renal masses: assessment of the outcome at one institution. BJU Int 2007;100:798.

[34] Shingleton WB, Sewell PE Jr. Percutaneous renal tumor cryoablation with magnetic resonance imaging guidance. J Urol 2001;165:773.

[35] Cestari A, Guazzoni G, dell'Acqua V, et al. Laparoscopic cryoablation of solid renal masses: intermediate term follow up. J Urol 2004;172:1267.

[36] Gill IS, Remer EM, Hasan WA, et al. Renal cryoablation: outcome at 3 years. J Urol 2005;173:1903.

[37] Schwartz BF, Rewcastle JC, Powell T, et al. Cryoablation of small peripheral rean masses: a retrospective analysis. Urology 2006;68(Suppl 1):14–8.

[38] Polascik TJ, Nosnik I, Mayes JM, et al. Short term clinical outcome after laparoscopic cryoablation of the renal tumor ≤3.5 cm. Technol Cancer Res Treat 2007;6:621.

[39] Tillet J, Ogan K, Nieh P, et al. Laparoscopic assisted cryoablation of renal tumors: temperature based model [abstract]. J Endourol 2006;20(Suppl 1):A174.

[40] Beemster PW, Lagerveld BW, de la Rosette JJ, et al. Laparoscopic cryosurgery of small renal tumours: clinical results and complications in The Netherlands [abstract]. J Endourol 2006;20(Suppl 1):A176.

[41] Johnson DB, Solomon SB, Su LM, et al. Defining the complications of cryoablation and radio frequency ablation of small renal tumors: a multi-institutional review. J Urol 2004;172:874.

[42] Lau WY, Leung TW, Yu SC, et al. Percutaneous local ablative therapy for hepatocellular carcinoma: a review and look into the future. Ann Surg 2003; 237:171.

[43] Lencioni R, Crocetti L, Cioni D, et al. Percutaneous radiofrequency ablation of hepatic colorectal metastases: technique, indications, results, and new promises. Invest Radiol 2004;39:689.

[44] Mirza A, Fornage B. Radiofrequency ablation of solid tumors. Cancer J 2001;7.

[45] Leveillee RJ, Hoey MF. Radiofrequency interstitial tissue ablation: wet electrode. J Endourol 2003;17: 563.

[46] Hsu TH, Fidler ME, Gill IS. Radiofrequency ablation of the kidney: acute and chronic histology in porcine model. Urology 2000;56:872.

[47] Crowley JD, Shelton J, Iverson AJ, et al. Laparoscopic and computed tomography-guided percutaneous radiofrequency ablation of renal tissue: acute and chronic effects in an animal model. Urology 2001;57:976.

[48] Corwin TS, Lindberg G, Traxer O, et al. Laparo-scopic radiofrequency thermal ablation of renal tissue with and without hilar occlusion. J Urol 2001;166:281.

[49] Organ LW. Electrophysiologic principles of radio-frequency lesion making. Appl Neurophysiol 1976; 39:69.

[50] Mulier S, Miao Y, Mulier P, et al. Electrodes and multiple electrode systems for radiofrequency abla-tion: a proposal for updated terminology. Eur Radiol 2005;15:798.

[51] Lewin JS, Nour SG, Connell CF, et al. Phase II clin-ical trial of interactive MR imaging-guided intersti-tial radiofrequency thermal ablation of primary kidney tumors: initial experience. Radiology 2004; 232:835.

[52] Carey RI, Leveillee RJ. First prize: direct real-time temperature monitoring for laparoscopic and CT-guided radiofrequency ablation of renal tumors between 3 and 5 cm. J Endourol 2007; 21:807.

[53] Matsumoto ED, Watumull L, Johnson DB, et al. The radiographic evolution of radio frequency ablated renal tumors. J Urol 2004;172:45.

[54] Uzzo RG, Novick AC. Nephron sparing surgery for renal tumors: indications, techniques and outcomes. J Urol 2001;166:6.

[55] Pavlovich CP, Walther MM, Choyke PL, et al. Per-cutaneous radio frequency ablation of small renal tumors: initial results. J Urol 2002;167:10.

[56] Roy-Choudhury SH, Cast JE, Cooksey G, et al. Early experience with percutaneous radiofrequency ablation of small solid renal masses. AJR Am J Roentgenol 2003;180:1055.

[57] Gervais DA, McGovern FJ, Arellano RS, et al. Re-nal cell carcinoma: clinical experience and technical success with radio-frequency ablation of 42 tumors. Radiology 2003;226:417.

[58] Su LM, Jarrett TW, Chan DY, et al. Percutaneous computed tomography-guided radiofrequency abla-tion of renal masses in high surgical risk patients: preliminary results. Urology 2003;61:26.

[59] Mayo-Smith WW, Dupuy DE, Parikh PM, et al. Im-aging-guided percutaneous radiofrequency ablation of solid renal masses: techniques and outcomes of 38 treatment sessions in 32 consecutive patients. AJR Am J Roentgenol 2003;180:1503.

[60] Farrell MA, Charboneau WJ, DiMarco DS, et al. Imaging-guided radiofrequency ablation of solid re-nal tumors. AJR Am J Roentgenol 2003;180:1509.

[61] Hwang JJ, Walther MM, Pautler SE, et al. Radio frequency ablation of small renal tumors: intermedi-ate results. J Urol 2004;171:1814.

[62] Matsumoto ED, Johnson DB, Ogan K, et al. Short-term efficacy of temperature-based radiofrequency ablation of small renal tumors. Urology 2005;65:877.

[63] Zagoria RJ. Imaging-guided radiofrequency ablation of renal masses. Radiographics 2004; 24(Suppl 1):S59.

[64] Varkarakis IM, Allaf ME, Inagaki T, et al. Percuta-neous radio frequency ablation of renal masses: re-sults at a 2-year mean followup. J Urol 2005;174: 456.

[65] McGovern FJ, Wood BJ, Goldberg SN, et al. Radio frequency ablation of renal cell carcinoma via image guided needle electrodes. J Urol 1999;161:599.

[66] Ogan K, Cadeddu JA. Re: percutaneous radio fre-quency ablation of small renal tumors: initial results. J Urol 2002;168:660, author reply 660.

[67] Jacomides L, Ogan K, Watumull L, et al. Laparo-scopic application of radio frequency energy enables in situ renal tumor ablation and partial nephrec-tomy. J Urol 2003;169:49.

[68] Park S, Anderson JK, Matsumoto ED, et al. Radio-frequency ablation of renal tumors: intermediate-term results. J Endourol 2006;20:569.

[69] Michaels MJ, Rhee HK, Mourtzinos AP, et al. In-complete renal tumor destruction using radio fre-quency interstitial ablation. J Urol 2002;168:2406.

[70] Johnson DB, Saboorian MH, Duchene DA, et al. Nephrectomy after radiofrequency ablation-induced ureteropelvic junction obstruction: poten-tial complication and long-term assessment of ablation adequacy. Urology 2003;62:351.

[71] Kohrmann KU, Michel MS, Steidler A, et al. Tech-nical characterization of an ultrasound source for noninvasive thermoablation by high-intensity focused ultrasound. BJU Int 2002;90:248.

[72] Marberger M, Schatzl G, Cranston D, et al. Extra-corporeal ablation of renal tumours with high-intensity focused ultrasound. BJU Int 2005; 95(Suppl 2):52.

[73] Weld KJ, Landman J. Comparison of cryoablation, radiofrequency ablation and high-intensity focused ultrasound for treating small renal tumours. BJU Int 2005;96:1224.

[74] Dubinsky TJ, Cuevas C, Dighe MK, et al. High-intensity focused ultrasound: current potential and oncologic applications. AJR Am J Roentgenol 2008;190:191.

[75] Yang R, Reilly CR, Rescorla FJ, et al. High-intensity focused ultrasound in the treatment of experimental liver cancer. Arch Surg 1991;126: 1002.

[76] Chen W, Wang Z, Wu F, et al. [High intensity focused ultrasound alone for malignant solid tumors]. Zhonghua Zhong Liu Za Zhi 2002;24: 278.

[77] Clement GT. Perspectives in clinical uses of high-intensity focused ultrasound. Ultrasonics 2004;42: 1087.

[78] Holland CK, Apfel RE. Thresholds for transient cavitation produced by pulsed ultrasound in a controlled nuclei environment. J Acoust Soc Am 1990;88:2059.

[79] Chang SD, Adler JR. Robotics and radiosurgery—the Cyberknife. Stereotact Funct Neurosurg 2001; 76:204.

[80] Wen CC, Nakada SY. Energy ablative techniques for treatment of small renal tumors. Curr Opin Urol 2006;16:321.

[81] Clark PE, Woodruff RD, Zagoria RJ, et al. Microwave ablation of renal parenchymal tumors before nephrectomy: phase I study. AJR Am J Roentgenol 2007;188:1212.

[82] Dick EA, Joarder R, De Jode MG, et al. Magnetic resonance imaging-guided laser thermal ablation of renal tumours. BJU Int 2002;90:814.

[83] Williams Jc MP, Swishchuck PN, et al. Laser induced thermotherapy of renal cell carcinoma in mandosimetry, ultrasound and histopathologic correlation [abstract]. J Urol 2000;163: 2000.

[84] Roberts WW, Hall TL, Ives K, et al. Pulsed cavitational ultrasound: a noninvasive technology for controlled tissue ablation (histotripsy) in the rabbit kidney. J Urol 2006;175:734.

[85] Kieran K, Hall TL, Parsons JE, et al. Refining histotripsy: defining the parameter space for the creation of nonthermal lesions with high intensity, pulsed focused ultrasound of the in vitro kidney. J Urol 2007;178:672.

ELSEVIER
SAUNDERS

Urol Clin N Am 35 (2008) 415–424

UROLOGIC
CLINICS
of North America

Laparoscopic Donor Nephrectomy

David A. Duchene, MD[a],*, Howard N. Winfield, MD[b]

[a]Department of Urology, University of Kansas Medical Center,
MS 3016, 3901 Rainbow Boulevard, Kansas City, KS 66160, USA
[b]Department of Urology, University of Iowa Hospitals & Clinics,
RCP 3235, 200 Hawkins Drive, Iowa City, IA 52242, USA

Renal transplantation is the definitive therapy for patients who have end-stage renal disease. The number of patients awaiting renal transplantation, however, far exceeds the number of cadaveric organs available. Approximately 74,000 patients are on the renal transplant waiting list in the United States (based on the United Network of Organ Sharing Web site, which provides frequently updated data: http://www.unos.org). In 2006, 13,615 renal transplants were performed, of which nearly half (6434) were from living donors (http://www.unos.org). In fact, since 2001, the number of living persons donating kidneys in the United States exceeded that of cadaveric donors, but a higher number of cadaveric kidneys still exist. Living donor kidneys have excellent graft survival rates at 1, 3, and 5 years of 95%, 88%, and 80% respectively [1]. This is compared with cadaveric donors graft survival rates of 87%, 77%, and 65% [1]. The differences in graft survival are caused by decreased ischemia time between procurement and transplantation into a recipient and ability to optimize the recipient's and donor's medical status before transplantation.

Ratner and associates [2] first performed laparoscopic donor nephrectomy (LDN) in 1995. This first case was attempted 5 years following the first laparoscopic nephrectomy [3] and after the feasibility of donor nephrectomy was demonstrated in a porcine model [4]. Early in the experience, concerns were raised concerning early graft dysfunction, ureteral complications, and loss of

right-sided donor kidneys [5,6]. Experience with the LDN technique, however, has demonstrated equivalent outcomes for the grafts [7]. LDN now is considered the standard of care in most transplant centers in the United States.

This article reviews the current indications, selection criteria, surgical approaches, outcomes, and complications of LDN.

Indications and selection criteria

Prospective kidney donors represent unique surgical candidates. The donor patient is an otherwise healthy individual with a solely altruistic motive to undergo a potentially harmful operation. Therefore, extreme care must be taken by all providers to minimize the risk to the donor. Likewise, the donor organ is essential to benefit the quality of life of another individual, so everything must be done to preserve the best function of the kidney. Preoperative evaluation is the first essential step in selecting kidney donors.

It is recommended that each transplant center organizes a transplant committee to discuss all cases of live organ donation. Potential donors must go through extensive medical and psychological evaluation in accordance with guidelines published by the American Society of Transplant Physicians [8]. Patients undergo a comprehensive history and physical, complete blood count, metabolic panel, chest radiograph, electrocardiogram, and screening for potentially transmissible diseases. In addition to the medical examination, all patients are required to have a preoperative psychological examination. To emphasize the importance of the psychological aspect, the Live

* Corresponding author.

E-mail address: dduchene@kumc.edu
(D.A. Duchene).

Organ Donor Consensus Group published recommendations for organ donation [9]. The statement emphasizes the need for full informed consent of the procedure the patient will undergo to include all the immediate possible peri-operative complications and potential unforeseeable or long-term complications. Ample time should be provided between the initial discussion and the actual surgery, so donors have time to consider their decision. Psychological stressors surrounding donation and the patient's motivation for donation need to be defined. Family and interpersonal relationships may have long-term consequences on both the donor and recipient, and any hint of coercion renders a donor ineligible [9].

Preoperative imaging

LDN requires accurate preoperative radiographic imaging to identify any vascular or anatomic variations that may influence operative technique and/or exclude a potential donor. MR imaging angiogram and CT angiogram have replaced standard renal arteriography in defining the vascular anatomy [10,11]. Both modalities also allow evaluation of the kidneys for any stones, lesions, malformations, and approximate estimates of differential renal function [10,11]. Bhatti and colleagues [12] prospectively compared CT and MR imaging angiography for evaluating the renal vascular anatomy in potential living donors and found that both had good sensitivity for detecting major arteries and veins (100% for CT, 97% for MR imaging). CT angiography, however, did much better at detecting small accessory renal arteries and accessory renal veins. Bhatti and colleagues felt a multidetector CT angiography should be the study of choice [12]. Either modality, however, requires three-dimensional reconstruction of the images, which can be labor-intensive for radiology technicians/radiologists. Schlunt and colleagues [10] found that the sensitivity of CT angiogram also was improved when the films were reviewed by the radiologist and operative surgeon together. Therefore, the decision on preoperative imaging choice often depends on the resources available at the institution and the radiologist's and urologist's preference to obtain the most accurate imaging.

Kidney selection (left versus right)

The selection of which kidneys are acceptable for transplantation and the donor side varies widely among transplant centers. The left donor kidney generally is preferred because of the longer renal vein length in both open and laparoscopic donor nephrectomy. This facilitates implanting the kidney into the recipient. The favored use of left kidneys was especially true during the early LDN experience because of a high rate of vascular complications, such as renal vein thrombosis and graft loss in the initial attempts at right-sided LDN [13]. Many centers in the early experience (and some currently) offered left-sided laparoscopic procedures, but obtained right kidneys in an open fashion [14].

At the same time that right-sided LDN was being approached cautiously, several studies demonstrated arterial and venous anomalies were not a contraindication to left-sided LDN. Lin and colleagues [15] demonstrated that circumaortic or retro-aortic renal veins in left-sided LDN had similar surgical variables such as operative time, warm ischemia time, blood loss, and length of vessels. Likewise, Troppman and colleagues [14] showed that multiple renal arteries in left-sided kidneys undergoing laparoscopic donation were not associated with significant changes in ischemia time or recipient function, although operative time was longer in those patients. Many laparoscopic surgeons felt that multiple left renal arteries were less problematic than obtaining a right donor kidney [16].

Subsequently, experience with right-sided LDN has made it an option for laparoscopic donation [17,18]. Buell and colleagues [17] reported on a multicenter review of 97 attempted right-sided LDNs. Ninety-four were completed laparoscopically with 98% graft success rate and no major complications after overcoming the initial learning curve. The authors found the same patient benefits and no increased risk of complications when compared with left-sided laparoscopic donors. Therefore, when evaluating patients for LDN, the goal to leave the best kidney with the donor patient should be applied. Typical indications to require a right-sided nephrectomy include: smaller right kidney, right renal cysts, multiple left renal arteries, left renal vein anomaly, right nephrolithiasis, and right renal artery stenosis [17–19] (Movie 1: Laparoscopic Right Donor Nephrectomy*) (Courtesy of Iowa Hospitals & Clinics, Iowa City, IA; with permission.).

---

* Videos for this article can be accessed by visiting www.urologic.theclinics.com. In the online table of contents for this issue, click on "add-ons."

Surgical approaches

The term laparoscopic donor nephrectomy actually encompasses a large variety of surgical approaches. LDN can be performed either transperitoneally or retroperitoneally, and by a pure-laparoscopic, hand-assisted, robotic, or a combination of these techniques.

Initial dissection (transperitoneal versus retroperitoneal)

Most institutions use a transperitoneal technique, because it provides a large working space that is familiar to the laparoscopist. The patient is placed in the modified flank position, with the planned extraction site facing upwards at approximately 70°. This allows access to both the flank and the abdomen for specimen retrieval. The patient must be supported with the assistance of an axillary roll and beanbag device cushioned with a Gelpad (Keomed Inc., Minnetonka, Minnesota). The patient is secured to the table with wide-cloth tape. All pressure points are padded. A pneumoperitoneum is achieved with Veress (Covidien, Norwalk, Connecticut) needle access for a pure-laparoscopic approach, or a hand-assistant port is placed.

A pneumoperitoneum of 12 to 15 mm Hg pressure is created. It is important to attempt to keep the pneumoperitoneum at the minimal possible working pressure, because elevated intra-abdominal pressure has been shown in animal models to decrease the renal blood flow and theoretically could decrease renal function and lead to delayed graft function [20]. An argument against LDN is the potential for delayed graft function from the intraperitoneal pressures during the laparoscopic case. Although more recent animal studies have demonstrated no delirious effect of pneumoperitoneum on kidney function, most surgeons still attempt to keep low intraperitoneal pressure [21]. To counteract the pneumoperitoneum, patients generally are given a large amount of intravenous crystalloids (up to 2 L/h) to maintain adequate kidney perfusion. Donors also may benefit and have less vascular compromise to the kidney if given an overnight intravenous infusion of fluids and a fluid bolus before the creation of pneumoperitoneum [22]. Bergman and colleagues [23], however, recently challenged the fluid dogma and found no difference in short- or long-term graft function between aggressive (greater than 10 mL/kg/h) or conservative (less than 10 mL/kg/h)

intraoperative fluid management, but this needs confirmation with a prospective study.

Ports are placed in standard laparoscopic fashion. This includes either:

A periumbilical hand port versus 10 mm camera port
A 5 (or 10) mm port in the midclavicular line two finger breaths below the costal margin
A 12 mm port in the lower quadrant in the midclavicular line
An optional 5 mm port in the anterior axillary line just above the umbilical line for assistant retraction
A 5 mm trocar in the midaxillary line at the umbilical level for liver retraction (right side only)

The colon is reflected medially by incising along the white line of Toldt. Wide mobilization of the colon is necessary to provide maximal exposure of the kidney and renal vessels. Proponents of a retroperitoneal approach believe that mobilization of the colon during transperitoneal surgery may risk injury to the intestine and lead to prolonged postoperative ileus [24]. A retroperitoneal technique may lead to less ileus and shorter operative times due to not requiring colon mobilization. Ruszat and colleagues [25] compared the retroperitoneal approach with hand-assisted, pure laparoscopy, and open techniques. The authors confirmed a lower incidence of ileus and shorter operative time for retroperitoneal approach versus the other laparoscopic techniques. Overall complications, however, were similar among the different modalities [25]. Experience with retroperitoneal laparoscopic donor nephrectomy varies greatly between institutions and remains less used than a transperitoneal approach. Surgeons should perform the technique most likely in their hands to provide good results without complications.

Once the colon has been reflected to enter the retroperitoneal space, the gonadal vein generally is identified and followed up to the left renal vein or inferior vena cava (IVC). The renal vein should be identified and cleared of all surrounding adventitial tissue. All lumbar and other accessory veins also are identified at this time. To gain maximal length of the renal vein, the gonadal vein, lumber veins, and adrenal vein (on left) are isolated, clipped, and divided. This is especially important on right-sided donor nephrectomy to obtain maximal vein length. The artery then is identified and cleared of surrounding tissue to the junction of the aorta (on the left), or the level the artery goes posterior to the IVC (on the right).

Ureteral dissection

The ureter and its associated attachments are dissected away from the psoas muscle. Care must be taken not to compromise the vascular supply of the ureter. Careful retraction should be used, and the ureter should be grasped (only if necessary) gently with laparoscopic bowel graspers. The gonadal vein also can be mobilized without detaching it from the ureter to minimize risk of vascular compromise [26]. The ureter is dissected down to the level of the iliac vessels.

The kidney then is mobilized completely by incising through Gerota's fascia and dissecting it free from the surrounding perirenal fat. The kidney then is rotated anteriorly, and the posterior attachments of the renal vein and artery are completely freed to ensure maximal vessel length.

Once the dissection is completed, the ureter is clipped distally and divided to observe for adequate urine output. Most surgeons administer 12.5 g of mannitol and 20 mg of furosemide in addition to the crystalloid fluids to ensure a brisk diuresis.

Transecting the vessels

Proper handling of the vessels is a key step in LDN. Multiple variations of vessel division have been reported. The essential aspects include properly securing the vessel stump remaining with the donor, preservation of maximal arterial and venous length of the donor organ, and avoidance of vessel damage [24]. As in a radical nephrectomy, the renal artery should be divided first. Although renal artery length is not generally the limiting factor in transplanting the organ into the recipient, care should be taken to preserve maximal length, especially on the left side. Early experience with nonlocking 10 mm titanium clips resulted in nonsufficient vessel occlusion [27]. Animal studies confirmed that three clips needed to be placed 2.5 mm apart to secure the vessel [28]. Obviously, this limited artery length.

Therefore, many surgeons routinely and successfully have used 10 mm Hem-o-Lok clips (Weck Closure Systems, Research Triangle Park, North Carolina) for the artery, leaving the graft end unclipped [29]. The authors have placed two clips on the arterial stump approximately 2 mm apart, although some authors only use one clip for the arterial stump [30]. Unfortunately, in April 2006, Teleflex Medical (the manufacturer of Hem-o-lok clips) issued a product safety warning stating that the clips were contraindicated for ligating the renal artery during LDN because of nine reported cases of severe hemorrhage from the renal hilum. The US Food and Drug Administration, however, did not issue a statement on the issue. Good data do not exist on the technique used to apply the clip or numbers of clips in these cases. The decision to continue to use this device for LDN is difficult, however, and must be discussed openly by each individual surgeon's hospital and applied against the standard of care in the surrounding community [31]. Most surgeons have switched to alternative forms of vascular division.

The renal vein is generally too large to undergo division with titanium clips or Hem-o-lok clips, so vascular staplers are used. The vascular staplers now also usually are employed for arterial ligation. The choice of staplers can be an Endo-TA or an Endo-GIA vascular stapler (Autosuture, Covidien, Norwalk, Connecticut). The Endo-GIA stapler can lead to a loss of 1 cm of vessel length and requires a row of staples to be removed before perfusion of the donor kidney. It is not recommended to remove the lateral rows of the Endo-GIA clips before stapling because of increased likelihood of stapler misfire [24]. The Endo-TA stapler does not articulate and sometimes is difficult to get flush with the aorta and/or IVC. It will get additional length, however, because it does not leave a lateral row of staples. This is very important to get extra length on the right renal vein during a right LDN. The Endo-TA also has been used in conjunction with Hem-o-loc clips to get maximal occlusion of the renal artery [32].

Alternatively, for right-sided donors, an endoscopic Satinsky atraumatic vascular clamp (Aesculap Inc, Center Valley, PA) can be placed on the side of the caval vein, so the renal vein can be excised in full length [33]. It is important to pay meticulous attention to any method used to transect the vessels to prevent significant intraoperative and postoperative hemorrhage. Linear stapling devices can lead to multiple complications. Primary stapler malfunction is rare (0.3% in review of donor nephrectomy stapler complications), but interposition of titanium clips or improper usage leads to most failures [34]. Friedman and colleagues [35] reported on hemorrhagic complications of LDN and found that the use of nonlocking clips on the renal artery was associated with the most frequent and severe hemorrhages, but that locking clips and staplers also caused occasional significant hemorrhage in the postoperative period. The important point all these findings show is that the vessels should be skeletonized completely and the tips of the stapling or clipping device must be visualized clearly before engaging the instrument. Proper use will limit complications, and the surgeon should confirm correct placement of the device before activation. Although the extra confirmation time may increase warm ischemia time slightly, it may save a major hemorrhagic complication.

Kidney extraction site (hand-assisted versus pure-laparoscopic)

The site of organ extraction largely depends on the approach used for the LDN. During a retroperitoneal approach, it generally is removed through a lower quadrant incision just off the anterior superior iliac spine [36].

For hand-assisted laparoscopy, the kidney is removed through the hand port. Wolf and colleagues [37] first described hand-assisted LDN in 1998. Proponents of the hand-assisted technique argue that using the already-placed hand port will decrease warm ischemia time, and the extraction incision is used better during the procedure [38]. The hand assistance also gives the surgeon better tactile sensation for dissection, retraction, and controlling the vascular structures. Comparative studies have shown an overall decrease in operative time with the hand-assisted technique, but the operative times achieved in the comparative studies varied widely and more likely reflected the surgeons' experience with their chosen technique [24].

Extraction site, however, may be a disadvantage for the hand-assisted technique and favors the pure-laparoscopic approach. In a pure-laparoscopic approach, the kidney may be extracted through an upper flank, subumbilical midline, or Pfannenstiel incision per the patient's preference. A low transverse Pfannestiel incision is too low to perform a hand-assisted LDN through, and the hand port usually is placed in the para-umbilical region. An increased number of hernias and postoperative ileus has also been found with the hand-assisted technique, felt to be caused by more stretching of the incision during hand assistance and manipulation of the intestines with the use of the hand [38,39].

Experience with robotic-assisted LDN remains limited. One of the major concerns is anticipated increased warm ischemia time and difficulty removing the specimen with the robotic platform docked. The kidney usually is removed through a low midline incision with the robotic technique. One of the largest published series on robotic LDN reports using a hand-assist port from the beginning of the case in the low midline, which allows for specimen extraction at the conclusion of the case [40].

Regardless of the approach, all attempts should be made to limit warm ischemia time. Prolonged warm ischemia has been criticized as a risk factor during LDN. Early experience with the pure laparoscopic technique involved placing the specimen in an extraction bag and then removing the specimen. The kidney therefore was detached from its blood supply, placed in a bag, and then removed. Several reports of bag breakage and difficult entrapment led to occasional prolonged warm ischemia times [41]. Therefore, many authors use a technique described by Shalhav and colleagues [42] during pure LDN. The technique also addresses important points that can be used with retroperitoneal, robotic, or hand-assisted extraction. The technique involves placing an assistant's hand through a small Pfannenstiel incision (to maintain pneumoperitoneum) before dividing the vessels. The kidney is secured by the assistant's hand, and the ureter is retracted away from the vessels. Once the hilum is confirmed to be free of surrounding tissue and ready to divide, the artery and vein are divided, hemostasis confirmed, and the kidney is removed quickly by the assistant and passed off the back table. With this technique, Shalhav demonstrated a significant decrease in warm ischemia time (101 seconds versus 173 seconds; $P < .001$). The key features are the ability to perform a desirable low Pfannenstiel incision and complete control of the donor kidney during the crucial steps of vessel division and retrieval.

Outcomes

Ratner and colleagues [2] were attempting to decrease kidney donor morbidity and increase live kidney donation when they applied concepts of laparoscopy to donor nephrectomy in 1995. The goal was to provide a donor nephrectomy technique to cause less pain, shorter hospital stay, reduced time away from work, and a better cosmetic result. The technique, however, also had to demonstrate equal outcomes from a donor, graft, and recipient standpoint. Numerous studies have been published demonstrating the advantages of laparoscopic over open donor nephrectomy. Several of these studies have had high levels of evidence-based results, either randomized, controlled trials or prospective, nonrandomized trials [43–49]. The studies find that compared with open donor nephrectomy, LDN provides equal graft function, rejection rate, urological complications, and patient and graft survival. LDN has the advantage of decreased pain, decreased analgesic requirement, shorter hospital stay, and earlier time to return to work. These studies, however, suggest slightly increased operative time, marginally increased warm ischemia time, and increased major complications requiring reoperation (especially in the early learning phase) in the laparoscopic cases compared with the open approach [43–49].

Current anticipated outcomes for LDN at an experienced, high-volume center can be highlighted in a large series from the University of Maryland, in which 738 consecutive patients undergoing LDN were reviewed [50]. The study found that 57% of donors were female. Nephrectomy was left-sided in 96% of patients; operative time was 202 minutes, and mean warm ischemia time was 169 seconds, Additionally, extraction site length was 6.6 cm; estimated blood loss was 128 cc, and mean number of arteries was 1.3 [50]. Average hospital stay was 64.4 hours, with clear liquid diet beginning at 26.5 hours, regular diet at 46.8 hours, bowel sounds recorded at 32.1 hours, flatus recorded at 48.1 hours, and bowel movements recorded at 63.5 hours after surgery [50]. Postoperative donor serum creatinine level was 1.5 times the preoperative level [50]. A summary of outcomes from current series of LDN is shown in Table 1.

In attempts to further decrease pain and length of stay after donor nephrectomy, Breda and colleagues [51] recommended a strict implementation of preoperative bowel rest combined with ketorolac for pain control. All patients underwent a bowel preparation regimen to include clear liquid diet beginning 2 days before surgery, two bottles of magnesium citrate orally the day before surgery, and a self-administered Fleets enema the evening before surgery. Postoperatively, the patients received ketorolac 30 mg intravenously every 6 hours for a maximum of 48 hours. The mean donor stay was only 1.1 days, with no readmissions for ileus. Many surgeons are reluctant to administer ketorolac in the postoperative setting to a patient who has a solitary kidney, but the authors found no instances of long-term kidney

dysfunction caused by the short-term administration [51].

Lind and colleagues [52] explored the effect LDN had in time to return to work. They found laparoscopic donors returned to work at some capacity at 6 weeks after surgery (5 weeks earlier than open or hand-assisted donors) and had complete return to work 9 weeks earlier than the open or hand-assisted groups [52]. Much of the difference, however, was accounted for by expectations given to the patients by the physician. It emphasizes the need to discuss realistic expectations about activity restrictions with potential donors before surgery and the power of positive suggestion in the recovery process.

Complications

Complications occur with all laparoscopic procedures, but the consequences of subjecting an otherwise healthy individual to a potential long-term problem causes extra scrutiny of a technique. The learning curve definitely attributed to some early complications, with reports from 20% major complications occurring in the first 50 cases decreasing to 6% in cases 200 to 250, to 30% complications in the first 30 cases with no complications during the next 50 [41,53]. Others reported series without significant effect of the learning curve as long as experienced laparoscopists with a dedicated team performed the procedure [54].

Two large series from the United States examined major and minor complications and found rates of 2.8% to 6.8% of major intraoperative complications and 10.3% to 17.1% postoperative complications [50,55]. The rate of open conversion was 1% to 2%. One series found that obesity increased operative time, but neither series showed increased complication rate because of obesity [50,55]. The rate of delayed graft function was 2.6% to 4.4% [50,55].

A critical analysis of delayed graft function after LDN found that female donor kidneys into male recipients and highly HLA- mismatched donors were significant factors in delayed graft function, but that no variable related to the laparoscopic procedure itself (prolonged carbon dioxide pneumoperitoneum, warm ischemia time, renal artery length, use of right kidney) affected the functional outcome of the allografts [56].

An interesting topic that rarely is reported because of lack of extended follow-up is the effect of kidney donation on long-term donor kidney

Table 1
Laparoscopic donor nephrectomy experience: recent results

Author/ institution	Pts (n)	Left/right	WIT (min)	OR time (min)	EBL (mL)	Conversion (n) (%)	LOS (days)	Complications (major/minor)	DGF (n) (%)	Recipient Cr (mg/dL)	Graft survival
Breda et al [61]/ University of California Los Angeles 2007	300	297/3	4 ± 2	180 ± 55	80 ± 50	3 (1%)	1.1 (1–3)	5 (1.6%)/ 7 (2.3%)	—	—	—
Sundaram et al [55]/ Indiana University 2007	253	237/16	2.2 ± 1.05	199 ± 50	115 ± 285	3 (1.2%)	2.8 ± 0.9	10 (3.9%)/ 16 (6.3%)	11 (4.4%)	1.90 ± 1.87 (7 days) 1.39 ± 0.53 (1 year)	—
Simforoosh et al [46]/ Tehran, Iran 2005	100	100/0	8.7 (4–17)	270.8 ± 58.5	—	1 (1%)	2.26 (2–5)	4 (4%)/ 19 (19%)	11 (11%)	2.01 (0.7–12.5) (3 days) 1.32 (0.8–2.8) (1 year)	93.8% (1 year)
Jacobs et al [50]/ University of Maryland 2004	738	709/29	2.28 ± 1.5	202.1 ± 52.4	128 ± 179	12 (1.6%)	2.68 ± 1.6	5 (2.0%)/ 50 (6.8%)	19 (2.6%)	2.0 ± 1.5 (7 days) 1.6 ± 1.4 (1 year)	—
Su et al [62]/ Johns Hopkins 2004	381	362/19	4.9 ± 3.4	253 ± 55.7	334 ± 690	8 (2.1%)	3.3 ± 4.5	29 (7.6%)/ 34 (8.9%)	17 (4.5%)	2.6 ± 2.3 (4 days)	65.5 ± 25.8 (5 years)
Rawlins et al [54]/ Virginia Mason 2002	100	100/0	2.3	231	102	1 (1%)	3.3	0 (0%)/6 (6%)	—	1.47 (5 days) 1.64 (6 months)	97% (6 months)

Abbreviations: Cr, creatinine; DGF, delayed graft function; EBL, estimated blood loss; LOS, length of stay; OR, operating room; Pts, patients; WIT, warm ischemia time.

function. A retrospective study of 736 patients with mean time since donation of 3 years showed that serum creatinine, systolic and diastolic blood pressure, and urinary protein excretion all increased significantly from preoperative values. Twenty-four percent developed proteinuria, and 10% developed hypertension. Obese donors had a higher rate of hypertension and new-onset diabetes [57]. Another smaller study of 162 living donors with a mean of 8-year follow-up, however, found normal residual kidney function and the same incidence of diabetes and hypertension in donors as in the normal population [58].

The true complication rates are difficult to completely ascertain because of a lack of a centralized donor registry. Therefore, they often rely on short-term reports from single institutions. Many authors have argued for a national/international donor registry to determine the impact living donor nephrectomy has on donor and graft health [50,59]. For instance, Shokeir recently reported a significant under-reporting and underestimation of complications from LDN. More surprising, no new series reporting open donor nephrectomy had been published since 1991, making the incidence of open donor nephrectomy complications and long-term outcomes in recent years unknown [59].

Summary

LDN has been a major advancement in the procurement of living kidneys for donation. The increase in living donors correlates with the advent of laparoscopic harvesting, as shown by the 11% increase in living donation from 2000 to 2001 [55]. Although many believe that the increased living donor pool is exclusively because of the application of LDN, it is difficult to definitely prove, and many other factors (such as extending the donor criteria) may play important roles [60]. Nonetheless, LDN is a known safe and effective alternative for living donor nephrectomy at centers with laparoscopic experience. Improvements continue to emerge in surgical techniques and perioperative management of the donors and recipients, which will continue to lead to the best possible outcomes for all parties involved.

Acknowledgment

The authors would like to acknowledge Dr. Henrique Melquiades, Professor, Recife, Brazil for his instrumental help in the preparation of the video.

References

[1] 2006 Annual report of the US Organ Procurement and Transplantation Network and the Scientific Registry of Transplant Recipients: transplant data 1996–2005. Department of Health and Human Services, Health Resources and Services Administration, Healthcare Systems Bureau, Division of Transplantation, Rockville (MD); United Network for Organ Sharing, Richmond, VA; University Renal Research and Education Association, Ann Arbor, MI.

[2] Ratner LE, Ciseck LJ, Moore RG, et al. Laparoscopic live donor nephrectomy. Transplantation 1995;60(9):1047–9.

[3] Clayman RV, Kavoussi LR, Soper NJ, et al. Laparoscopic nephrectomy: initial case report. J Urol 1991;146(2):278–82.

[4] Gill IS, Carbone JM, Clayman RV, et al. Laparoscopic live donor nephrectomy. J Endourol 1994; 8(2):143–8.

[5] Ratner LE, Montgomery RA, Kavoussi LR. Laparoscopic live donor nephrectomy: the four-year Johns Hopkins University experience. Nephrol Dial Transplant 1999;14(9):2090–3.

[6] Philosophe B, Kuo PC, Schweitzer EJ, et al. Laparoscopic versus open donor nephrectomy: comparing ureteral complications in the recipients and improving the laparoscopic technique. Transplantation 1999;68(4):497–502.

[7] Ratner LE, Montgomery RA, Kavoussi LR. Laparoscopic live donor nephrectomy. A review of the first 5 years. Urol Clin North Am 2001;28(4):709–19.

[8] Kasiske BL, Ravenscraft M, Ramos EL, et al. The evaluation of living renal transplant donors: clinical practice guidelines. Ad Hoc Clinical Practice Guidelines Subcommittee of the Patient care and Education Committee of the American Society of Transplant Physicians. J Am Soc Nephrol 1996; 7(11):2288–313.

[9] Live Organ Donor Consensus Group. Consensus statement on the live organ donor. JAMA 2000; 284:2919–26.

[10] Schlunt LB, Harper JD, Broome DR, et al. Improved detection of renal vascular anatomy using multidetector CT angiography: is 100% detection possible? J Endourol 2007;21(1):12–7.

[11] Kim J, Kim C, Jang M, et al. Can magnetic resonance angiogram be a reliable alternative for donor evaluation for laparoscopic nephrectomy? Clin Transplant 2007;21:126–35.

[12] Bhatti AA, Chugtai A, Haslam P, et al. Prospective study comparing three-dimensional computed tomography and magnetic resonance imaging for evaluating the renal vascular anatomy in potential living renal donors. BJU Int 2005;96:1105–8.

[13] Mandal A, Cohen C, Montgomery RA. Should the indications for laparoscopic live donor nephrectomy of the right kidney be the same for the open

procedure? Anomalous left renal vasculature is not a contraindication to laparoscopic left donor nephrectomy. Transplantation 2001;71(5):660–4.

[14] Troppmann C, Wiesmann K, McVicar JP, et al. Increased transplantation of kidneys with multiple renal arteries in the laparoscopic live donor nephrectomy era: surgical technique and surgical and nonsurgical donor and recipient outcomes. Arch Surg 2001;136(8):897–907.

[15] Lin CH, Steinberg AP, Ramani AP, et al. Laparoscopic live donor nephrectomy in the presence of circumaortic or retro-aortic left renal vein. J Urol 2004;171(1):44–6.

[16] Ratner LE, Kavoussi LR, Chavin KD, et al. Laparoscopic live donor nephrectomy: technical considerations and allograft vascular length. Transplantation 1998;65(12):1657–8.

[17] Buell JF, Edye M, Johnson M, et al. Are concerns over right laparoscopic donor nephrectomy unwarranted? Ann Surg 2001;233(5):645–51.

[18] Diner EK, Radolinski B, Murdock JD, et al. Right laparoscopic donor nephrectomy: the Washington Hospital experience. Urology 2006;68(6):1175–7.

[19] Buell JF, Abreu SC, Hanaway MJ, et al. Right donor nephrectomy: a comparison of hand-assisted transperitoneal and retroperitoneal laparoscopic approaches. Transplantation 2004;77(4):521–5.

[20] McDougal EM, Monk TG, Wolf JS, et al. The effect of prolonged pneumoperitoneum on renal function in an animal model. J Am Coll Surg 1996;182(4):317–28.

[21] Lind MY, Hazebroek EJ, Bajema IM, et al. Effect of prolonged warm ischemia and pneumoperitoneum on renal function in a rat syngeneic kidney transplantation model. Surg Endosc 2006;20(7):1113–8.

[22] Mertens zur Borg IR, Di Biase M, Verbrugge S, et al. Comparison of three perioperative fluid regimes for laparoscopic donor nephrectomy: a prospective randomized dose-finding study. Surg Endosc 2007 [epub ahead of print].

[23] Bergman S, Feldman LS, Carli F, et al. Intraoperative fluid management in laparoscopic live donor nephrectomy: challenging the dogma. Surg Endosc 2004;18(11):1625–30.

[24] Giessing M, Turk I, Roigas J, et al. Laparoscopy for living donor nephrectomy—particularities of the currently applied techniques. Transpl Int 2005;18(9):1019–27.

[25] Ruszat R, Sulser T, Dickenmann M, et al. Retroperitoneoscopic donor nephrectomy: donor outcome and complication rate in comparison with three different techniques. World J Urol 2006;24(1):113–7.

[26] Dunkin BJ, Johnson LB, Kuo PC. A technical modification eliminates early ureteral complications after laparoscopic donor nephrectomy. J Am Coll Surg 2000;190(1):96–7.

[27] Chan DY, Fabrizio MD, Ratner LE, et al. Complications of laparoscopic live donor nephrectomy: the first 175 cases. Transplant Proc 2000;32(4):778.

[28] Kerbl K, Chandhoke PS, Clayman RV, et al. Ligation of the renal pedicle during laparoscopic nephrectomy: a comparison of staples, clips, and sutures. J Laparoendosc Surg 1993;3(1):9–12.

[29] Baumert H, Ballaro A, Arroyo C, et al. The use of polymer (Hem-o-lok) clips for management of the renal hilum during laparoscopic nephrectomy. Eur Urol 2006;49(5):816–9.

[30] Meng MV, Freise CE, Kang SM, et al. Techniques to optimize vascular control during laparoscopic donor nephrectomy. Urology 2003;61(1):93–7.

[31] Winfield HN. Survey of endourology: laparoscopy. J Endourol 2006;20(11):852–4.

[32] Sundaram CP, Bargman V, Bernie JE. Methods of vascular control during laparoscopic donor nephrectomy. J Endourol 2006;20(7):467–9.

[33] Turk IA, Giessing M, Deger S, et al. Laparoscopic live donor right nephrectomy: a new technique with preservation of vascular length. Transplant Proc 2003;35(2):838–41.

[34] Deng DY, Meng MV, Nguyen HT, et al. Laparoscopic linear cutting stapler failure. Urology 2002;60(3):415–9.

[35] Friedman AI, Peters TG, Jones KW, et al. Fatal and nonfatal hemorrhagic complications of living kidney donation. Ann Surg 2006;243(1):126–30.

[36] Sulser T, Gurke L, Langer I, et al. Retroperitoneoscopic living donor nephrectomy: first clinical experiences in 19 operations. J Endourol 2004;18(3):257–62.

[37] Wolf JS, Tchetgan MB, Merion RM. Hand-assisted laparoscopic live donor nephrectomy. Urology 1998;52(5):885–7.

[38] Ruiz-Deya G, Cheng S, Palmer E, et al. Open donor, laparoscopic donor, and hand-assisted laparoscopic donor nephrectomy: a comparison of outcomes. J Urol 2001;166(4):1270–3.

[39] Velidedeoglu E, Williams N, Brayman KL, et al. Comparison of open, laparoscopic and hand-assisted approaches to live donor nephrectomy. Transplantation 2002;74(2):169–72.

[40] Horgan S, Galvani C, Gorodner MV, et al. Effect of robotic assistance on the learning curve for laparoscopic hand-assisted donor nephrectomy. Surg Endosc 2007;21(9):1512–7.

[41] Jacobs SC, Cho E, Dunkin BJ, et al. Laparoscopic live donor nephrectomy: the University of Maryland 3-year experience. J Urol 2000;164(5):1494–9.

[42] Shalhav AL, Siqueira TM, Gardner TA, et al. Manual specimen retrieval without a pneumoperitoneum-preserving device for laparoscopic live donor nephrectomy. J Urol 2002;168(3):941–4.

[43] Wolf JS, Merion RM, Leichtman AB, et al. Randomized controlled trial of hand-assisted laparoscopic versus open surgical, live donor nephrectomy. Transplantation 2001;72(2):284–90.

[44] Brook NR, Harper SJ, Bagul A, et al. Laparoscopic donor nephrectomy yields kidney with structure and function equivalent to those retrieved by open surgery. Transplant Proc 2005;37(2):625–6.

[45] Oyen O, Andersen M, Mathisen L, et al. Laparoscopic versus open living donor nephrectomy: experiences from a prospective, randomized, single-center study focusing on donor safety. Transplantation 2005;79(9):1236–40.

[46] Simforoosh N, Basiri A, Tabibi A, et al. Comparison of laparoscopic and open donor nephrectomy: a randomized controlled trial. BJU Int 2005;95(6):851–5.

[47] Andersen MH, Mathisen L, Oyen O, et al. Postoperative pain and convalescence in living kidney donors—laparoscopic versus open donor nephrectomy: a randomized study. Am J Transplant 2006; 6(6):1438–43.

[48] Kok NF, Lind MY, Hansson BM, et al. Comparison of laparoscopic and mini-incision open donor nephrectomy: single-blind, randomized controlled clinical trial. BMJ 2006;333(7561):221.

[49] Wilson CH, Bhatti AA, Rix DA, et al. Comparison of laparoscopic and open donor nephrectomy: UK experience. BJU Int 2005;95(1):131–5.

[50] Jacobs SC, Cho E, Foster C, et al. Laparoscopic donor nephrectomy: the University of Maryland 6-year experience. J Urol 2004;171(1):47–51.

[51] Breda A, Bui MH, Liao JC, et al. Association of bowel rest and ketorolac analgesia with short hospital stay after laparoscopic donor nephrectomy. Urology 2007;69(5):828–31.

[52] Lind MY, Liem YS, Bemelman WA, et al. Live donor nephrectomy and return to work: does the operative technique matter? Surg Endosc 2003;17(4):591–5.

[53] Leventhal JR, Deeik RK, Joehl RJ, et al. Laparoscopic live donor nephrectomy—is it safe? Transplantation 2000;70(4):602–6.

[54] Rawlins MC, Hefty TL, Brown SL, et al. Learning laparoscopic donor nephrectomy safely: a report on 100 cases. Arch Surg 2002;137(5):531–4.

[55] Sundaram CP, Martin GL, Guise A, et al. Complications after a 5-year experience with laparoscopic donor nephrectomy: the Indiana University Experience. Surg Endosc 2007;21(5):724–8.

[56] Abreu SC, Goldfarb DA, Derweesh I, et al. Factors related to delayed graft function after laparoscopic live donor nephrectomy. J Urol 2004; 171(1):52–7.

[57] Rizvi SA, Naqvi SA, Jawad F, et al. Living kidney donor follow-up in a dedicated clinic. Transplantation 2005;79(9):1247–51.

[58] Sansalone CV, Maione G, Aseni P, et al. Early and late residual renal function and surgical complications in living donors: a 15-year experience at a single institution. Transplant Proc 2006;38(4):994–5.

[59] Shokeir AA. Open versus laparoscopic live donor nephrectomy: a focus on the safety of donors and the need for a donor registry. J Urol 2007;178(5): 1860–6.

[60] Schweitzer EJ, Wilson J, Jacobs S, et al. Increased rates of donation with laparoscopic donor nephrectomy. Ann Surg 232(3):392–400.

[61] Breda A, Veale J, Liao J, et al. Complications of laparoscopic living donor nephrectomy and their management: the UCLA experience. Urology 2007; 69(1):49–52.

[62] Su L, Ratner LE, Montgomery RA, et al. Laparoscopic live donor nephrectomy: trends in donor and recipient morbidity following 381 consecutive cases. Ann Surg 2004;240(2):358–63.

ELSEVIER
SAUNDERS

Urol Clin N Am 35 (2008) 425–439

UROLOGIC
CLINICS
of North America

Minimally Invasive Approaches to Ureteropelvic Junction Obstruction

David Canes, MD[a], Andre Berger, MD[a],
Matthew T. Gettman, MD[b], Mihir M. Desai, MD[a],*

[a]Department of Urology, Center for Laparoscopic and Robotic Surgery, Glickman Urological and Kidney Institute,
Cleveland Clinic, 9500 Euclid Avenue, Cleveland, OH 44195, USA
[b]Department of Urology, Mayo Clinic, 200 First Street SW, Rochester, MN 55905, USA

Ureteropelvic junction obstruction (UPJO) is the most common congenital abnormality of the ureter, with an annual incidence of 5 per 100,000 population. For many years, open pyeloplasty remained the 'gold-standard' treatment, with success rates greater than 90%. During the last 2 decades, multiple minimally invasive methods have been used for the surgical management of UPJO, including endopyelotomy, endopyeloplasty, and laparoscopic and robotic pyeloplasty. The choice of initial surgical intervention is important because it is likely to influence the final outcome.

This review covers minimally invasive treatments for UPJO in the adult, including endopyelotomy (antegrade and retrograde), endopyeloplasty, laparoscopic pyeloplasty (LP), and robotic pyeloplasty. The relevant literature is summarized, and a rational algorithm for management is proposed.

Diagnostic workup

The goals of diagnostic evaluation in a patient suspected of having a UPJO are to confirm functional obstruction, determine differential renal function, and assess the anatomy at the uteropelvic junction (UPJ). Mercaptoacetyl-Tri-Glycine (MAG3) diuretic renal scan typically achieves the first two goals. A retrograde pyelogram (usually at the time of surgical procedure)

confirms the length of stricture and degree of hydronephrosis. A spiral CT angiogram may be useful in preoperative detection of a crossing vessel in a patient in whom endopyelotomy is being considered as a treatment option.

Endopyelotomy

In 1903, Albarran [1] first described full-thickness incision of a narrow ureteral segment followed by prolonged stenting. Endoscopic pyelolysis was first described by Wickham and Kellett [2] and popularized by Badlani and colleagues [3] as endopyelotomy. The key concept of endopyelotomy is based on the principle of intubated ureterostomy developed by Davis [4]: regeneration of the ureter over a stent for 6 weeks after a full-thickness incision, causing a durable increase in the caliber of the strictured segment. The exact mechanism of ureteral healing, however, remains unclear. A combination of wound contracture and smooth muscle regeneration likely contributes to healing of the endopyelotomy defect.

Many variables have been suggested as predictors of poor prognosis after endopyelotomy, including the presence of crossing vessels, severe hydronephrosis, long (> 1.5 cm) stricture length, poor ipsilateral renal function, and previous failed endopyelotomy. The discussion of the impact of crossing vessels on the outcome after endopyelotomy continues to be debated. Van Cangh and colleagues [5] reported 46% success in patients with crossing vessels and 86% without. Evaluating the Acucise technique, Nakada and colleagues

* Corresponding author.
    E-mail address: desaim1@ccf.org (M.M. Desai).

[6] reported lower success in patients with crossing vessels (96% versus 64%). One would expect a higher incidence of crossing vessels found at secondary pyeloplasty after failed endopyelotomy, but results are inconsistent. Knudsen and colleagues [7] and Van Cangh and colleagues [8] found crossing vessels in 83% and 87% of their cases, respectively. In contrast, Gupta and colleagues [9] attributed only 4% cases of endopyelotomy failure to crossing vessels.

Poor renal function and significant hydronephrosis seem to predict a higher failure rate after endopyelotomy. In patients with poor renal function, the success rate was 54% compared with 94% in patients with normal renal function [9]. Danuser and colleagues [10] described a success rate of 87% in patients with a pyelocalyceal volume less than 50 cm^3, 81% with a volume from 50 to 100 cm^3, and 69% with a volume greater than 100 cm^3.

Antegrade (percutaneous) endopyelotomy

Initially reported by Ramsay and colleagues [11] in 1984, the technique has several variations: cutting between two wires, cutting over a stent [12], invagination of the UPJ [13], and external incision of the UPJ through a transpelvic route [14]. Cold knife, electrocautery, and laser have each been reported, with none conclusively demonstrated to be superior over the others. Antegrade endopyelotomy is particularly suitable in patients who have concomitant large-volume stone disease. Success rates with antegrade endopyelotomy range between 67% and 88% (Table 1).

Retrograde endopyelotomy

Ureteroscopic approach

Ureteroscopic retrograde endopyelotomy was initially reported by Inglis and Tolley [18] in 1986. The most attractive feature of the ureteroscopic approach is the potentially reduced morbidity when compared with the percutaneous approach. The risk for subsequent ureteral stricture was historically higher with the use of large-diameter ureteroscopes and electrocautery [19]. Whereas preemptive stenting was previously necessary to achieve passive ureteral dilatation, current small profile semirigid ureteroscopes and flexible ureteroscopes have practically abolished this need and significantly reduced ureteral complications with this procedure. The incision is performed

using the holmium:yttrium-aluminum-garnet (YAG) laser at 10 W through a 200- to 365-μ laser fiber. Symptomatic and radiographic success range from 65% to 91% and from 73% to 85%, respectively [20–24]. Geavlete and colleagues [25] reported a success rate of 83.3% (18 months of follow-up) in 30 patients who had secondary UPJO (failed pyeloplasty [17 cases], failed endopyelotomy [13 cases]) (Table 2).

Acucise endopyelotomy

Acucise endopyelotomy consists of a balloon electrocautery incision performed under fluoroscopic control and was first proposed by Chandhoke and colleagues [26] in 1993. Drawbacks of cutting-wire endopyelotomy include difficulty in controlling the rate and depth of the incision and the risk for hemorrhage because of the lack of direct visual control. Bleeding complications have been reported in 3% to 10% of cases [27,28]. Results from select series of cutting-wire balloon endopyelotomy are summarized in Table 3.

El-Nahas and colleagues [35] compared Acucise with ureteroscopic endopyelotomy in 40 patients who had UPJO in a prospective randomized trial (follow-up of 30 months). Exclusion criteria included the presence of crossing vessels, renal function less than 20%, or hydronephrosis of grade 3 or greater. Success rates were 85% for the ureteroscopic group and 65% for the Acucise group. There was no difference in the complication rate.

Preference of the surgeon, anatomic factors, and concomitant calculi are the main factors considered in the choice between the percutaneous and ureteroscopic approaches for endopyelotomy. The main advantage of percutaneous approaches is the ability to treat concomitant calculi. Body habitus or anatomic issues that may have previously limited retrograde access have decreased with modern ureteroscope technology, and decreased morbidity makes retrograde endopyelotomy an attractive option for the appropriate short-segment stricture.

Stenting after endopyelotomy

Stenting after endopyelotomy is still debated. No consensus exists regarding optimal stent size or duration of stenting. The assumption that a larger stent would result in a larger final caliber if healing occurs around the stent has been analyzed. Danuser and colleagues [36] evaluated the influence of stent size in two consecutive series

Table 1
Antegrade endopyelotomy

First author	Senior author	Year	Cases	Technique	Primary UPJO (n)	Crossing vessels (%)	Open conversion (%)	OR time (minutes)	Hospital stay (days)	Follow-up (months)	Symptomatic success (%)	Radiographic success (%)	Complications (%)
Motola [15]	Smith	1993	212	Cold knife	110	79	1.5	119	4.1	25	85	86	16%
Van Cangh [5]	Lorge	1994	102	Cold knife	81	57	0	252	3.3	26	Not stated	73	Not stated
Kletscher [16]	Patterson	1995	50	Cold knife	49	42	5.4	185	4.5	14	92	88	Not stated
Gupta [9]	Smith	1997	401	Cold knife	235	42	5.5	164	2.6	19	Not stated	85	Not stated
Danuser [10]	Studer	1998	80	Cold knife	80	57	0	165	3.7	23	Not stated	81	13
Shalhav [17]	Clayman	1998	63	Electrocautery	40	16	6.4	179	4	12	89	85	27
Knudsen [7]	Denstedt	2004	80	Electrocautery (77), laser (3)	61	54	Not reported	246	3.1	24	Not stated	67	Not stated

Abbreviation: OR, operation.
Data from Desai MM, Hegarty N. Contemporary surgical management of adult ureteropelvic junction obstruction. AUA Update Series 2007;26.

Table 2
Retrograde endopyelotomy

First author	Senior author	Cases	Technique (n)	Primary UPJ (n)	Crossing vessels (%)	Follow-up (months)	Symptomatic success (%)	Radiographic success (%)
Conlin [23]	Bagley	21	Electrocautery (14), laser (6), cold knife (1)	15	57%	23	Not stated	81
Renner [24]	Rassweiler	34	Laser	27	Not stated	18	92	85
Giddens [20]	Grasso	23	Laser	18	17	10	Not stated	83
Gerber [21]	Kim	22	Electrocautery (16), laser (6)	18	Not stated	20.5	91	82
Matin [22]	Streem	45	Laser	40	Not stated	23.2	65	73

of patients who had UPJO managed by antegrade endopyelotomy. In group 1 (77 patients), a 14/8.2-French graduated stent was used. In group 2 (55 patients), a 27-French catheter was used for 3 weeks, followed by the same 14/8.2-French graduated stent for 3 weeks. The early success rates after 6 to 8 weeks in groups 1 and 2 were 83% and 94%, respectively. The long-term success rates after 2 years were 71% and 93%, respectively, suggesting that the benefit in the group with larger stents was durable. Similarly, Wolf and colleagues [37] evaluated 69 patients undergoing 77 endoureterotomies for ureteral strictures and found that for strictures longer than 1 cm, use of a stent sized 12 French or greater seems to be beneficial.

Series of retrospectives nonrandomized studies did not support any benefits from using larger stents. Comparing 14/7-French versus 8-French

stents after endopyelotomy, Kletscher and colleagues [16] found no statistically significant difference. Hwang and colleagues [38] evaluated 40 patients after percutaneous endopyelotomy, and the difference between 6-French and 14/7-French stents was not statistically significant.

What about duration of stenting? The classic study of Davis [4] still drives the empiric 6-week stenting time. In contrast, Mandhani and colleagues [39] compared 57 consecutive patients who had primary UPJO randomized to undergo 7/14-French internal endopyelotomy stent placement for 2 weeks (group 1) and 4 weeks (group 2), and no difference was found in drainage pattern stent-related symptoms, suggesting that 6 weeks may not be required. Properly conducted studies are required to establish evidence-based guidelines for stenting practice after endopyelotomy.

Table 3
Acucise endopyelotomy

First author	Senior author	Year	Cases (n)	Primary UPJO (n)	Follow-up (months)	Symptomatic success (%)	Radiographic success (%)	Complications
Nadler [29]	Clayman	1996	26	17	33	89	81	0
Preminger [28]	Smith	1997	66	52	8	Not stated	77	4.5
Faerber [30]	Ohl	1997	32	27	14	Not stated	81	15.6
Gelet [27]	Dubernard	1997	44	21	12	Not stated	78	4.6
Kim [31]	Albala	1998	77	61	12	Not stated	78	4
Lechevalier [32]	Coulange	1999	36	23	24	Not stated	75	Not stated
Biyani [33]	Hetherington	2002	42	34	27	64	52	10
Weikert [34]	Schrader	2005	24	24	32	58 (overall)	58 (overall)	12.5

Data from Desai MM, Hegarty N. Contemporary surgical management of adult ureteropelvic junction obstruction. AUA Update Series 2007;26.

Endopyelotomy for secondary ureteropelvic junction obstruction

Ng and colleagues [40] evaluated 42 patients (mean follow-up of 47.7 months) who underwent management of failed primary intervention for UPJO. Secondary intervention included open operative repair (n = 20) or percutaneous (n = 11), ureteroscopic (n = 5), or retrograde cautery wire balloon endopyelotomy (n = 6). Long-term success rate of endoscopic treatment of secondary UPJO was 59.1% overall, including a 71.4% success rate after a failed open operative procedure and a 37.5% success rate after a failed endourologic procedure. Success of open operative salvage was 95% overall, including 94.1% after failed endourologic intervention and 100% after failed open operative intervention. In summary, endopyelotomy may be the optimal initial intervention after failed pyeloplasty but has a poor outcome after failed endopyelotomy.

Endopyeloplasty

Endopyeloplasty consists of a Heineke-Mikulicz repair accomplished entirely through a percutaneous tract (Fig. 1). In 1996, Oshinsky and colleagues [41] reported percutaneous intrarenal suturing for the first time. Desai and colleagues [42] reported the use of a laparoscopic suturing device through a 26-French nephroscope to perform endopyeloplasty (Fenger) in a porcine model. Technical feasibility was established, with a wider caliber of the UPJ after endopyeloplasty compared with endopyelotomy. Presumably, healing by primary rather than secondary intention accounts for this finding.

In a clinical setting, Gill and colleagues [43] published the results of endopyeloplasty in 9 patients. Inclusion criteria were less than 1-cm segment stenosis, absence of crossing vessels on preoperative imaging, and absence of prior UPJ surgery. Success was defined as absence of pain and improvement of drainage on an excretory urogram or diuretic renal scan. Endopyeloplasty was completed in 53 patients. Mean operative time was 103 minutes, and suturing time was 27 minutes. Two cases of intraoperative complications were reported: suture cut-through and irrigation fluid extravasation. Prolonged ureteral stenting was required in five cases for pyrexia. Surgery relieved obstruction in 96.2% (n = 51) of the patients and failed in 3.8% (n = 2): one immediately after stent removal and the other

12 months after the procedure, in whom a crossing vessel was identified.

In 2004, Desai and colleagues [44] reported 1-year follow-up data retrospectively compared with matched cohorts undergoing endopyelotomy and LP in 44 patients who had primary UPJO. Resolution of symptoms and unobstructed drainage on intravenous urography or diuretic renography was noted in 100% and 100% of endopyeloplasties (n = 15, mean follow-up of 11.6 months), 93% and 88% of percutaneous endopyelotomies (n = 15, mean follow-up of 31.4 months), and 93% and 100% of LPs (n = 14, mean follow-up of 20 months). Using the same technique, however, Ost and colleagues [45] had only a 40% success rate (2 of 5 patients). This lower rate was explained by a previous balloon dilation of the UPJ, leading to a thinner ureteral wall, resulting in suture pull-through and fibrosis. Initial data suggest the feasibility and safety of percutaneous endopyeloplasty in selected patients who have primary UPJO. In general, indications are similar to those of endopyelotomy, and the results may be superior. Longer follow-up and multi-institutional experience are necessary to corroborate these promising findings.

Laparoscopic pyeloplasty

Initially reported by Schuessler and colleagues [46] in 1993, LP has now emerged as a standard approach to UPJO with results comparable to the gold-standard open pyeloplasty. LP allows correction of all anatomic variants of UPJO, transposition or displacement of crossing vessels when necessary, treatment of primary and secondary UPJO [47], extraction of concomitant renal calculi [48], and pelvic reduction when indicated. Indications have recently been carefully expanded to include pelvic and horseshoe kidneys [49] in addition to solitary kidneys [50].

Technique

The choice of trans- or retroperitoneal approaches is governed by surgeon preference and individual patient factors. Although either approach may be used in most patients who have primary UPJO, the retroperitoneal approach may be preferred in patients with obesity or a history of prior abdominal surgery. The transperitoneal approach is preferred in patients with prior retroperitoneal surgery on the ipsilateral kidney and in complex UPJ repairs in which salvage

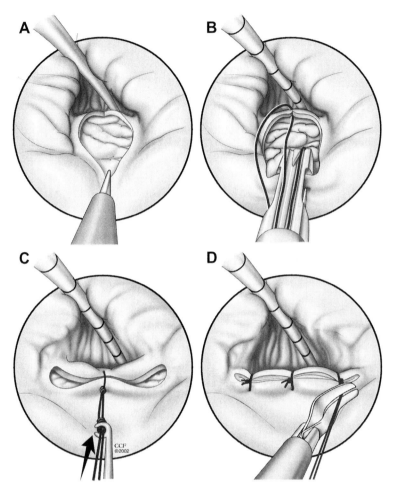

Fig. 1. Endopyeloplasty. Vertical incision is made down to peripelvic fat (*A*) and closed horizontally with an endoclose device (*B–D*). (*Courtesy of* the Cleveland Clinic Foundation, Cleveland, OH; with permission.)

procedures may be required. Most published series use the classic technique as described by Andersen and Hynes [51] in an attempt to duplicate established open surgical techniques. Nondismembered techniques, including Y-V plasty, Fengerplasty, and flap pyeloplasty, have all been described and are technically feasible but are indicated in few situations. Klingler and colleagues [52] noted higher success rates with dismembered pyeloplasty (96%) compared with nondismembered techniques (73%), suggesting superiority of the former, which the authors use in most cases.

A brief description of the authors' preferred technique is as follows (Figs. 2 and 3). They perform retrograde stenting before LP at the beginning of the case. In the authors' opinion, decompression of the renal pelvis by the stent

does not pose any significant disadvantage during mobilization of the pelvis and UPJ. The anesthetized patient is placed in the lithotomy position. A retrograde pyelogram is performed to confirm the level and extent of anatomic obstruction. The retrograde pyelogram alters management in the occasional patient in whom ureteral obstruction is revealed that was not apparent on preoperative imaging. A 4.7-French or similarly small-caliber ureteral stent is placed at the conclusion of the retrograde pyelogram. In the authors' experience, the 4.7-French stent easily admits dissecting scissors alongside it, facilitating spatulation and subsequent unhindered suturing compared with a standard 6-French stent. The patient is placed in a 45° flank position and a three- or four-port transperitoneal approach is

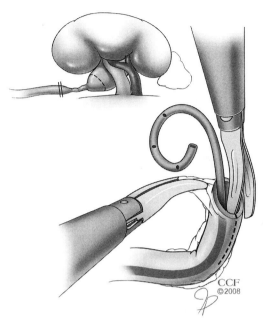

Fig. 2. Pyeloplasty. An oblique pyelotomy is made. The lateral edge of ureter is spatulated across the narrowed segment. A 4.7-French stent facilitates spatulation by leaving room for the scissors. (*Courtesy of* the Cleveland Clinic Foundation, Cleveland, OH; with permission.)

used. Anterior axillary line lateral retraction, when needed, is accomplished using a needlescopic grasper through a 2-mm Veres port.

The technique of dissection to expose the UPJ mimics open surgical principles. Aggressive distal ureteral dissection is avoided. An inflammatory rind, if present, is dissected sufficiently to expose the pelvic wall in the region of the UPJ. The UPJ is dismembered obliquely, and pelvic reduction and pyelolithotomy are performed when indicated. The lateral ureteral spatulation proceeds across the narrowed UPJ, and for a distance such that reapproximation accomplishes a dependent funneled configuration without undue tension but also without redundancy of the ureter. In patients with a crossing vessel, the decision to transpose depends on the surgeon's assessment of the obstructive nature of the crossing vessel and the relative position of the vessel in relation to the neo-UPJ. A 4-0 polyglactin suture on an RB-1 needle approximates the dependent portion of the pyelotomy to the caudal spatulated portion of ureter. This suture is run along the anterior wall as a forehand stitch. A separate 4-0 polyglactin running suture is then run along the posterior wall as a backhand stitch. Remaining open pelvis

is closed with 4-0 polyglactin if necessary. When tissue quality or tension is of some concern, kidney mobilization is performed and interrupted sutures are placed.

A closed-suction drain is placed in proximity to the repair. Free oral intake is commenced when the residua of anesthesia have passed, typically the evening of surgery or the following morning. The urethral catheter is removed after 1 to 2 days, followed by the drain, once output is low. The stent is removed at 4 weeks.

Results

Worldwide experience with LP is summarized in Table 4. Success rates of LP range from 88% to 100%, [53–58] depending on subjective (symptomatic) or objective (radiographic) measures. These results generally surpass those of endopyelotomy and match the established success rates (>90%) of open pyeloplasty [61]. Direct nonrandomized comparisons of open repairs with LP arrive at similar conclusions. Bauer and colleagues [62] compared 42 LPs with 35 open repairs. At 1 year of follow-up, symptomatic improvement was observed after 90% of LPs and 91% of open repairs. Radiographic improvement was present in 98% and 94%, respectively.

Crossing vessels

The routine transposition of crossing vessels continues to be the subject of some debate. Aron and colleagues [63] retrospectively compared 8 patients undergoing transposition with 23 not undergoing transposition. Obstruction was successfully treated in all patients, as evaluated by nuclear scintigraphy. More of the patients in the nontransposed group were operated on by means of a retroperitoneal approach, and vice versa. It seems clear that success has more to do with meticulous dismembered pyeloplasty than with the relation to overlying vessels, but the debate nevertheless continues.

Stern and colleagues [64] took a closer look at the impact of crossing vessels by performing intraoperative Whitaker tests in 10 patients at the time of LP. They measured differential pressures before any significant dissection and after mobilization of the vessels from the UPJ. In this small group, mere mobilization of the crossing vessels brought pressures down to unobstructed levels. This creative study has demonstrated that the vessels may be one of several contributing factors in UPJO. As others have shown [65], however, concomitant

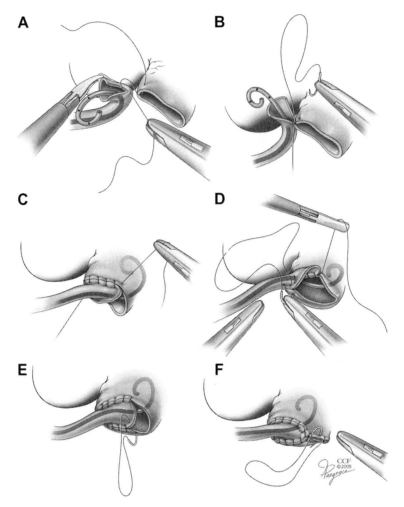

Fig. 3. (*A*) Corner is tied with a 4-0 Vicryl suture on an RB-1 needle. (*B–C*) This is run along the anterior wall as a forehand stitch (pelvis-ureter [*right*] or ureter-pelvis [*left*]). (*D*) With the assistant retracting the anterior wall suture, a backhand 4-0 Vicryl suture is placed. (*E*) Posterior wall is completed as a running backhand stitch. (*F*) U-stitch makes the transition onto the pelvis. A separate 3-0 or 4-0 running Vicryl suture from a cephalad-to-caudad direction closes the pyelotomy (varying size depending on need for pelvic reduction). (*Courtesy of* the Cleveland Clinic Foundation, Cleveland, OH; with permission.)

intrinsic obstruction is present in up to one third of patients with crossing vessels, necessitating pyeloplasty and not simple mobilization of the vessel. In addition, the findings still support the possibility that obstruction may resolve after nontransposed dismembered pyeloplasty.

Expanding indications

Patients requiring pyelolithotomy are excellent candidates for LP. In the authors' experience, most pelvic stones and many calyceal stones may be visualized and removed through the pyelotomy using standard laparoscopic grasping instruments. In the remainder, flexible nephroscopy can be performed through a laparoscopic trocar. In their report on 147 LPs, Inagaki and colleagues [58] included 22 renal units requiring simultaneous pyelolithotomy, with a 90% stone-free rate. Similarly, Ramakumar and colleagues [48] achieved a stone-free rate of 90% in 20 renal units requiring LP with pyelolithotomy.

Anatomic anomalies are generally no contraindication to LP. In fact, the anteriorly positioned

Table 4
Laparoscopic pyeloplasty

First author	Senior author	Year	Approach	Repair type (n)	Crossing vessels (%)	Open conversion (%)	Operative time (minutes)	Hospital stay (days)	Follow-up (months)	Symptomatic success (%)
Janetschek [53]	Bartsch	2000	Trans	Fengerplasty (67)	79	1.5	119	4.1	25	98
Soulie [54]	Plante	2001	Retro	Dismembered (48)	42	5.4	185	4.5	14	100[a]
Jarrett [55]	Kavoussi	2002	Trans	Dismembered (71)	57	0	252	3.3	26	98
Turk [56]	Loening	2002	Trans	Dismembered (49)	57	0	165	3.7	23	98
Mandhani [57]	Bhandari	2005	Trans	Dismembered (59), Fengerplasty (7), Y-V (20)	16	6.4	179	4	12	93
Inagaki [58]	Jarrett	2005	Trans	Dismembered (106), Fengerplasty (11), Y-V (28)	54	Not reported	246	3.1	24	95
Zhang [59]	Ye	2005	Retro	Dismembered (50)	12	0	81	7.6	22	98
Moon [60]	Eden	2006	Retro	Dismembered (170)	42	0.6	140	3	22	96

Abbreviations: Retro, Retroperitoneal; Trans, Transperitoneal.
[a] All patients pain free, with patent UPJ on intravenous pyelogram at 3 months; 88.9% had radiographic success, with decreased hydronephrosis at 3 months.
Data from Desai MM, Hegarty N. Contemporary surgical management of adult ureteropelvic junction obstruction. AUA Update Series 2007;26.

renal pelvis in horseshoe kidneys, for instance, may make laparoscopy the preferred approach. Bove and colleagues [66] reported on LP in five patients with horseshoe kidneys. The overall success rate of 91% included dismembered, Y-V, and Heineke-Mickulicz approaches. Three of these patients underwent concomitant pyelolithotomy. Similarly, Gupta and colleagues [67] reported two successful dismembered LPs in horseshoe kidneys. LP is also feasible in solitary kidneys. Wood and colleagues [68] reported 100% technical success in eight solitary kidneys undergoing LP, similar to results in a matched cohort undergoing open repair.

For secondary UPJO, LP has been reported with success. In general, LP is appropriate for failed endopyelotomy, and endopyelotomy is appropriate for failed LP. The first clinical report of LP for secondary UPJO in 1995 was updated in 2003 by Sundaram and colleagues [69]. This group of 36 patients had undergone a mean of 1.3 prior procedures. Radiographic patency was achieved in 89% of patients. Considering 2 patients with equivocal radiographic drainage but symptomatic resolution, the group reported a 94% overall success rate at 22 months. Other series of LP for secondary UPJO include those of Jarrett and colleagues [55] (88% success) and Siqueiria and colleagues [70] (88% success).

Robotic pyeloplasty

The steep learning curve for intracorporeal suturing that allows precise mucosal reapproximation has limited the widespread diffusion of LP. Just as robotic technology had an impact on prostatectomy, the application of robotics to pyeloplasty has found similar enthusiasm. Results from selected series of robotic-assisted LP are shown in Table 5. The robotic experience was built on the principles of LP, and, as expected, the results have similarly duplicated those of open repair, with success rates greater than 90%. The largest series by Schwentner and colleagues [76] includes 92 cases, with 96.7% radiographic success at 39 months and a mean operative time just shy of 2 hours. Although these investigators attribute these impressive results to the precision of robotic suturing, there is no firm reason to attribute this success to any factor other than surgeon experience and meticulous plastics closure of the UPJ, regardless of the method used. Experienced freehand laparoscopists can

and do place sutures with the same precision and have achieved similar results as shown previously.

Gettman and colleagues [77] reported on a comparison between robotic and laparoscopic approaches, with six patients in each group. Operative times were shorter for dismembered pyeloplasty in the robotic group (140 versus 235 minutes). This should not necessarily be taken to suggest that robotic pyeloplasty is a faster procedure in all hands or at all centers. Today, the choice between robotic and pure laparoscopic approaches has more to do with surgeon preference and availability of the robot. As a community, one hopes that the relative ease of robotic suturing may hasten the diffusion of minimally invasive approaches to UPJO in the future.

Single-port pyeloplasty

Desai and colleagues [78] published the first clinical case of laparoscopic single-port pyeloplasty. Whereas standard LP requires three to four ports, attempts to minimize morbidity further prompted exploration of single-port laparoscopy (SPL). A single trocar permitting passage of three instruments was deployed at the umbilicus. The three inlet valves contain a thermoplastic elastomer allowing the introduction of one 12-mm and two 5-mm instruments, with a separate dedicated insufflation channel. A combination of rigid and flexible or bent instruments limits external instrument crowding and accomplishes triangulation internally. For single-port pyeloplasty, a 2-mm needlescopic port was used as a left-handed instrument to aid intracorporeal suturing that did not require a formal skin incision. Operative time was 160 minutes, and the patient was discharged on the second postoperative day. The ultimate role of SPL remains to be determined. Theoretic advantages of improved cosmesis and decreased pain need to be evaluated in larger series with direct comparison to cohorts undergoing traditional laparoscopy. The same group has subsequently used the single umbilical approach for performing bilateral simultaneous pyeloplasty in two patients who had bilateral UPJO.

Approach to surgical treatment and summary

When Chen and colleagues [79] summarized LP for the *Urologic Clinics of North America* in 1998, they correctly stated, 'additional

Table 5
Robotic-assisted laparoscopic pyeloplasty

First author	Senior author	Year	N	Approach	Repair type (n)	Crossing vessels (%)	Operative time (minutes)	Hospital stay (days)	Follow-up (months)	Symptomatic success (%)	Radiographic success (%)	Complications (%)
Bentas [71]	Binder	2003	36	Trans	Dismembered	36	197	5.5	21	100[a]	100	9
Patel [72]	Same	2005	33	Trans	Dismembered	33	122	1.1	11.7	100	100	0
Palese [73]	Del Pizzo	2005	29	Trans	Dismembered	29	216	2.8	7.9	94	94	11
Siddiq [74]	Bird	2005	42	Trans	Dismembered (23), Y-V (3)	42	245	2	6	95	100	12
Mendez-Torres [75]	Thomas	2005	44	Trans	Dismembered (31), Fengerplasty (1)	44	300	1.1	10.3	94	94	3
Kaouk, (unpublished data, 2005)	—	—	30	Retro	Dismembered	30	157	2	15	100	100	0
Schwentner [76]	Peschel	2007	92	Trans	Dismembered	49	108	4.6	39	96.7	100	3

Abbreviations: Retro, Retroperitoneal; Trans, Transperitoneal.
[a] One patient who initially experienced flank pain and hydronephrosis after initial stent extraction responded to an additional 4 weeks of stenting.
Data from Desai MM, Hegarty N. Contemporary surgical management of adult ureteropelvic junction obstruction. AUA Update Series 2007;26.

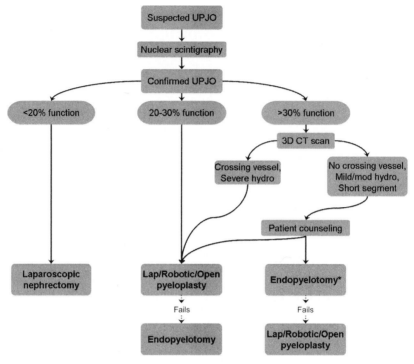

Fig. 4. Simplified algorithm for surgical management of UPJO. Endopyeloplasty can be used for select patients in place of endopyelotomy. Hydro, hydronephrosis; mod, moderate; lap, laparoscopic.

developments…may further simplify laparoscopic surgery, allowing laparoscopic reconstructive procedures to come into widespread use.' The dawn of robotics was imminent and has perhaps offered this 'simplification' to allow diffusion of this minimally invasive technique, albeit at a high cost. Over the past decade, we have seen LP established as a gold-standard procedure alongside open pyeloplasty, with commensurate results and lower morbidity. With the current minimally invasive treatments available in 2007 for the adult patient, only the rare patient now undergoes open pyeloplasty.

Fig. 4 provides a simplified rational approach to choosing the appropriate intervention. Key factors to consider include differential renal function, presence or absence of a crossing vessel, and stricture length. The reader is cautioned that the algorithm is not designed for the pediatric population, in which a different set of considerations are applied. As has been shown, the success rate for LP approaches 100% and addresses the spectrum of pathologic findings at the UPJ, including those patients who have failed other interventions. Indications have expanded to include concomitant

stone disease, solitary kidneys, and anatomically anomalous kidneys. Endopyelotomy should be avoided in patients with long-segment strictures, severe hydronephrosis, crossing vessels, or poor renal function ($<30\%$).

References

[1] Albarran JL. Operations plastiques et anastomosis dans la traitment des retention de vein. Theses, Paris 1903 [French].
[2] Wickham JE, Kellet MJ. Percutaneous pyelolysis. Eur Urol 1983;9(2):122–4.
[3] Badlani G, Eshghi M, Smith AD. Percutaneous surgery for ureteropelvic junction obstruction (endopyelotomy): technique and early results. J Urol 1986;135(1):26–8.
[4] Davis D. Intubated uterotomy: a new operation for ureteral and ureteropelvic stricture. Surg Gynecol Obstet 1943;76:513–23.
[5] Van Cangh PJ, Wilmart JF, Opsomer RJ, et al. Long-term results and late recurrence after endoureteropyelotomy: a critical analysis of prognostic factors. J Urol 1994;151(4):934–7.
[6] Nakada SY, Wolf JS Jr, Brink JA, et al. Retrospective analysis of the effect of crossing vessels on

successful retrograde endopyelotomy outcomes using spiral computerized tomography angiography. J Urol 1998;159(1):62–5.

[7] Knudsen BE, Cook AJ, Watterson JD, et al. Percutaneous antegrade endopyelotomy: long-term results from one institution. Urology 2004;63(2): 230–4.

[8] Van Cangh PJ, Nesa S, Galeon M, et al. Vessels around the ureteropelvic junction: significance and imaging by conventional radiology. J Endourol 1996;10(2):111–9.

[9] Gupta M, Tuncay OL, Smith AD. Open surgical exploration after failed endopyelotomy: a 12-year perspective. J Urol 1997;157(5):1613–8 [discussion: 1618–9].

[10] Danuser H, Ackermann DK, Böhlen D, et al. Endopyelotomy for primary ureteropelvic junction obstruction: risk factors determine the success rate. J Urol 1998;159(1):56–61.

[11] Ramsay JW, Miller RA, Kellett MJ, et al. Percutaneous pyelolysis: indications, complications and results. Br J Urol 1984;56(6):586–8.

[12] Savage SJ, Streem SB. Simplified approach to percutaneous endopyelotomy. Urology 2000;56(5): 848–50.

[13] Combe M, Gelet A, Abdelrahim AF, et al. Ureteropelvic invagination procedure for endopyelotomy (Gelet technique): review of 51 consecutive cases. J Endourol 1996;10(2):153–7.

[14] Ono Y, Ohshima S, Kinukawa T, et al. Endopyelouromy via a transpelvic extraurethral approach. J Urol 1992;147(2):352–5.

[15] Motola JA, Badlani GH, Smith AD. Results of 212 consecutive endopyelotomies: an 8-year followup. J Urol 1993;149(3):453–6.

[16] Kletscher BA, Segura JW, LeRoy AJ, et al. Percutaneous antegrade endopyelotomy: review of 50 consecutive cases. J Urol 1995;153(3 Pt 1):701–3.

[17] Shalhav AL, Giusti G, Elbahnasy AM, et al. Adult endopyelotomy: impact of etiology and antegrade versus retrograde approach on outcome. J Urol 1998;160(3 Pt 1):685–9.

[18] Inglis JA, Tolley DA. Ureteroscopic pyelolysis for pelviureteric junction obstruction. Br J Urol 1986; 58(3):250–2.

[19] Meretyk I, Meretyk S, Clayman RV. Endopyelotomy: comparison of ureteroscopic retrograde and antegrade percutaneous techniques. J Urol 1992;148(3): 775–82 [discussion: 782–3].

[20] Giddens JL, Grasso M. Retrograde ureteroscopic endopyelotomy using the holmium:YAG laser. J Urol 2000;164(5):1509–12.

[21] Gerber GS, Kim JC. Ureteroscopic endopyelotomy in the treatment of patients with ureteropelvic junction obstruction. Urology 2000;55(2):198–202 [discussion: 202–3].

[22] Matin SF, Yost A, Streem SB. Ureteroscopic laser endopyelotomy: a single-center experience. J Endourol 2003;17(6):401–4.

[23] Conlin MJ, Bagley DH. Ureteroscopic endopyelotomy at a single setting. J Urol 1998;159(3):727–31.

[24] Renner C, Frede T, Seemann O, et al. Laser endopyelotomy: minimally invasive therapy of ureteropelvic junction stenosis. J Endourol 1998;12(6): 537–44.

[25] Geavlete P, Georgescu D, Mirciulescu V, et al. Ureteroscopic laser approach in recurrent ureteropelvic junction stenosis. Eur Urol 2007;51(6):1542–8.

[26] Chandhoke PS, Clayman RV, Stone AM, et al. Endopyelotomy and endoureterotomy with the Acucise ureteral cutting balloon device: preliminary experience. J Endourol 1993;7(1):45–51.

[27] Gelet A, Combe M, Ramackers JM, et al. Endopyelotomy with the Acucise cutting balloon device. Early clinical experience. Eur Urol 1997;31(4): 389–93.

[28] Preminger GM, Clayman RV, Nakada SY, et al. A multicenter clinical trial investigating the use of a fluoroscopically controlled cutting balloon catheter for the management of ureteral and ureteropelvic junction obstruction. J Urol 1997;157(5):1625–9.

[29] Nadler RB, Rao GS, Pearle MS, et al. Acucise endopyelotomy: assessment of long-term durability. J Urol 1996;156(3):1094–7.

[30] Faerber GJ, Richardson TD, Farah N, et al. Retrograde treatment of ureteropelvic junction obstruction using the ureteral cutting balloon catheter. J Urol 1997;157(2):454–8.

[31] Kim FJ, Herrell SD, Jahoda AE, et al. Complications of Acucise endopyelotomy. J Endourol 1998; 12(5):433–6.

[32] Lechevallier E, Eghazarian C, Ortega JC, et al. Retrograde Acucise endopyelotomy: long-term results. J Endourol 1999;13(8):575–8.

[33] Biyani CS, Minhas S, el Cast J, et al. The role of Acucise endopyelotomy in the treatment of ureteropelvic junction obstruction. Eur Urol 2002;41(3):305–10 [discussion: 310–1].

[34] Weikert S, Christoph F, Müller M, et al. Acucise endopyelotomy: a technique with limited efficacy for primary ureteropelvic junction obstruction in adults. Int J Urol 2005;12(10):864–8.

[35] El-Nahas AR, Shoma AM, Eraky I, et al. Prospective, randomized comparison of ureteroscopic endopyelotomy using holmium:YAG laser and balloon catheter. J Urol 2006;175(2):614–8.

[36] Danuser H, Hochreiter WW, Ackermann DK, et al. Influence of stent size on the success of antegrade endopyelotomy for primary ureteropelvic junction obstruction: results of 2 consecutive series. J Urol 2001;166(3):902–9.

[37] Wolf JS Jr, Elashry OM, Clayman RV. Long-term results of endoureterotomy for benign ureteral and ureteroenteric strictures. J Urol 1997;158(3 Pt 1): 759–64.

[38] Hwang TK, Yoon JY, Ahn JH, et al. Percutaneous endoscopic management of upper ureteral stricture size of stent. J Urol 1996;155(3):8824.

[39] Mandhani A, Kapoor R, Zaman W, et al. Is a 2-week duration sufficient for stenting in endopyelotomy? J Urol 2003;169(3):886–9.

[40] Ng CS, Yost AJ, Streem SB. Management of failed primary intervention for ureteropelvic junction obstruction: 12-year, single-center experience. Urology 2003;61(2):291–6.

[41] Oshinsky GS, Jarrett TW, Smith AD. New technique in managing ureteropelvic junction obstruction: percutaneous endoscopic pyeloplasty. J Endourol 1996;10(2):147–51.

[42] Desai MM, Gill IS, Carvalhal EF, et al. Percutaneous endopyeloplasty: a novel technique. J Endourol 2002;16(7):431–43.

[43] Gill IS, Desai MM, Kaouk JH, et al. Percutaneous endopyeloplasty: description of new technique. J Urol 2002;168(5):2097–102.

[44] Desai MM, Desai MR, Gill IS. Endopyeloplasty versus endopyelotomy versus laparoscopic pyeloplasty for primary ureteropelvic junction obstruction. Urology 2004;64(1):16–21.

[45] Ost MC, Kaye JD, Guttman MJ, et al. Laparoscopic pyeloplasty versus antegrade endopyelotomy: comparison in 100 patients and a new algorithm for the minimally invasive treatment of ureteropelvic junction obstruction. Urology 2005;66(Suppl 5): 47–51.

[46] Schuessler WW, Grune MT, Tecuanhuey LV, et al. Laparoscopic dismembered pyeloplasty. J Urol 1993;150(6):1795–9.

[47] Eden C, Gianduzzo T, Chang C, et al. Extraperitoneal laparoscopic pyeloplasty for primary and secondary ureteropelvic junction obstruction. J Urol 2004;172(6 Pt 1):2308–11.

[48] Ramakumar S, Lancini V, Chan DY, et al. Laparoscopic pyeloplasty with concomitant pyelolithotomy. J Urol 2002;167(3):1378–80.

[49] Stein RJ, Desai MM. Management of urolithiasis in the congenitally abnormal kidney (horseshoe and ectopic). Curr Opin Urol 2007;17(2):125–31.

[50] Albani JM, Desai MM, Gill IS, et al. Repair of adult ureteropelvic junction obstruction in the solitary kidney: effect on renal function. Urology 2006; 68(4):718–22.

[51] Andersen JC, Hynes W. Retrocaval ureter. A case diagnosed pre-operatively and treated successfully by a plastic operation. Br J Urol 1949;21:209–14.

[52] Klingler HC, Remzi M, Janetschek G, et al. Comparison of open versus laparoscopic pyeloplasty techniques in treatment of uretero-pelvic junction obstruction. Eur Urol 2003;44(3):340–5.

[53] Janetschek G, Peschel R, Bartsch G. Laparoscopic Fenger plasty. J Endourol 2000;14(10):889–93.

[54] Soulié M, Salomon L, Patard JJ, et al. Extraperitoneal laparoscopic pyeloplasty: a multicenter study of 55 procedures. J Urol 2001;166(1):48–50.

[55] Jarrett TW, Chan DY, Charambura TC, et al. Laparoscopic pyeloplasty: the first 100 cases. J Urol 2002;167(3):1253–6.

[56] Türk IA, Davis JW, Winkelmann B, et al. Laparoscopic dismembered pyeloplasty—the method of choice in the presence of an enlarged renal pelvis and crossing vessels. Eur Urol 2002;42(3):268–75.

[57] Mandhani A, Kumar D, Kumar A, et al. Safety profile and complications of transperitoneal laparoscopic pyeloplasty: a critical analysis. J Endourol 2005;19(7):797–802.

[58] Inagaki T, Rha KH, Ong AM, et al. Laparoscopic pyeloplasty: current status. BJU Int 2005; 95(Suppl 2):102–5.

[59] Zhang X, Li HZ, Wang SG, et al. Retroperitoneal laparoscopic dismembered pyeloplasty: experience with 50 cases. Urology 2005;66(3):514–7.

[60] Moon DA, El-Shazly MA, Chang CM, et al. Laparoscopic pyeloplasty: evolution of a new gold standard. Urology 2006;67(5):932–6.

[61] O'Reilly PH, Brooman PJ, Mak S, et al. The long-term results of Anderson-Hynes pyeloplasty. BJU Int 2001;87(4):287–9.

[62] Bauer JJ, Bishoff JT, Moore RG, et al. Laparoscopic versus open pyeloplasty: assessment of objective and subjective outcome. J Urol 1999;162(3 Pt 1):692–5.

[63] Aron M, Desai MM, Rubinstein M, et al. Routine transposition of anterior crossing vessels during laparoscopic pyeloplasty: is it necessary? J Urol 2005; 173(Suppl):316 [abstract 1165].

[64] Stern JM, Park S, Anderson JK, et al. Functional assessment of crossing vessels as etiology of ureteropelvic junction obstruction. Urology 2007;69(6): 1022–4.

[65] Janetschek G, Peschel R, Frauscher F. Laparoscopic pyeloplasty. Urol Clin North Am 2000;27(4): 695–704.

[66] Bove P, Ong AM, Rha KH, et al. Laparoscopic management of ureteropelvic junction obstruction in patients with upper urinary tract anomalies. J Urol 2004;171(1):77–9.

[67] Gupta N, Mandhani A, Sharma D, et al. Is laparoscopic approach safe for ectopic pelvic kidneys? Urol Int 2006;77(2):118–21.

[68] Wood HM, Albani JM, Kaouk JH, et al. Laparoscopic versus open dismembered pyeloplasty in a solitary kidney. J Urol 2006;175(Suppl):20 [abstract 59].

[69] Sundaram CP, Grubb RL III, Rehman J, et al. Laparoscopic pyeloplasty for secondary ureteropelvic junction obstruction. J Urol 2003;169(6):2037–40.

[70] Siqueira TM Jr, Nadu A, Kuo RL, et al. Laparoscopic treatment for ureteropelvic junction obstruction. Urology 2002;60(6):973–8.

[71] Bentas W, Wolfram M, Bräutigam R, et al. Da Vinci robot assisted Anderson-Hynes dismembered pyeloplasty: technique and 1 year follow-up. World J Urol 2003;21(3):133–8.

[72] Patel V. Robotic-assisted laparoscopic dismembered pyeloplasty. Urology 2005;66(1):45–9.

[73] Palese MA, Stifelman MD, Munver R, et al. Robot-assisted laparoscopic dismembered

pyeloplasty: a combined experience. J Endourol 2005;19(3):382–6.

[74] Siddiq FM, Leveillee RJ, Villicana P, et al. Computer-assisted laparoscopic pyeloplasty: university of Miami experience with the daVinci surgical system. J Endourol 2005;19(3):387–92.

[75] Mendez-Torres F, Woods M, Thomas R. Technical modifications for robot-assisted laparoscopic pyeloplasty. J Endourol 2005;19(3):393–6.

[76] Schwentner C, Pelzer A, Neururer R, et al. Robotic Anderson-Hynes pyeloplasty: 5-year experience of one centre. BJU Int 2007;100(4):880–5.

[77] Gettman MT, Peschel R, Neururer R, et al. A comparison of laparoscopic pyeloplasty performed with the daVinci robotic system versus standard laparoscopic techniques: initial clinical results. Eur Urol 2002;42:453.

[78] Desai MM, Rao PP, Aron M, et al. Scar-less single-port transumbilical nephrectomy and pyeloplasty: a first clinical report. BJU Int 2008;101(1):83–8.

[79] Chen RN, Moore RG, Kavoussi LR. Laparoscopic pyeloplasty. Indications, technique, and long-term outcome. Urol Clin North Am 1998;25(2):323–30.

ELSEVIER
SAUNDERS

Urol Clin N Am 35 (2008) 441–454

UROLOGIC
CLINICS
of North America

Minimally Invasive Approaches to Upper Urinary Tract Urolithiasis

Geoffrey R. Wignall, MD[a], Benjamin K. Canales, MD, MPH[b],
John D. Denstedt, MD[c], Manoj Monga, MD[d],*

[a]*Division of Urology, University of Western Ontario, 268 Grosvenor Street, London, Ontario, Canada N6A 4V2*
[b]*University of Florida, 1600 SW Archer Rd, RM# N-213, Post Office BOX 100247, Gainesville, FL 32610, USA*
[c]*Department of Surgery, University of Western Ontario, 268 Grosvenor Street, London, Ontario, Canada N6A 4V2*
[d]*Department of Urologic Surgery, University of Minnesota, Mayo 394, 410 Delaware Street
Southeast, Minneapolis, MN 55455-0392, USA*

Since the first reported successful shock wave lithotripsy (SWL) treatment of a patient who had a renal stone in 1980 [1], urologists increasingly have employed minimally invasive techniques to treat patients who have ureteral or renal calculi. With over 25 years of experience in the techniques of SWL, percutaneous nephrolithotomy (PCNL), and ureteroscopy (URS), the amount of information available to objectively counsel a stone former on his/her treatment options can be overwhelming. This article reviews the recent literature that may affect surgical decision making for renal and ureteral calculi, including imaging and patient selection, and a step-by-step review of surgical minimally invasive approaches.

Factors influencing surgical stone-free rates

Hounsfield units—in vitro

Noncontrast, spiral CT has become the imaging modality of choice for assessing urinary stone disease, offering highly specific information such as stone location, size, number, density, and renal anatomy [2]. Because larger cystine, brushite, and calcium oxalate monohydrate stones are known to be more resistant to SWL fragmentation [3–5], CT attenuation values of urinary calculi in Hounsfield units (HU) have been used to differentiate stone composition with some degree of success. In vitro studies have demonstrated that uric acid stones consistently have attenuation levels below 1000 HU, whereas calcium oxalate and phosphate stones usually exceed 1000 HU [6–8]. Unfortunately, the range of HU values for calcium oxalate monohydrate and struvite stones overlap, suggesting that some stone compositions cannot be predicted reliably by CT [6,9]. In addition, several studies have shown that stone size plays a role in HU density calculations. In the early 1980s, Parienty and colleagues [10] found that stones of the same composition less than 5 mm in diameter had lower attenuation value than sized at 5 to 9 mm and proposed that the use of low-resolution beam collimation (5 mm) can yield artificially low attenuation values because of volume averaging [10]. More recently, Saw and colleagues [11] scanned 127 human calculi (ex vivo) and used a model, based on the physics of helical CT, to predict the effect of scan collimation width and stone size. As stone size decreased, HU for the same stone types also decreased, implying that smaller stones may decrease attenuation readings falsely and produce misleading results.

Hounsfield units—in vivo

Recently, correlating SWL success rates with in vivo CT HU attenuation levels has gained popularity. Joseph and associates studied 30 patients who had renal calculi undergoing SWL therapy using an electromagnetic lithotripter [12]. Patients who had calculi less than 500 HU (n = 12)

* Corresponding author.
E-mail address: endourol@yahoo.com (M. Monga).

had 100% stone clearance and required a median of 2500 shocks. Those who had calculi of 500 to 1000 HU (n = 7) had a clearance rate of 86% and required a median of 3390 shocks. Patients who had calculi HU greater than 1000 (n = 11) had a clearance rate of 56% and required a median of 7300 shocks [12]. Similarly, Gupta and colleagues [13] used high-resolution CT protocols to report a linear relationship between calculus density and number of SWL sessions in patients who had renal and proximal ureteral stones. For stones less than 1.1 cm with HU less than 750, they reported that 34 patients had three or fewer SWL sessions and a stone-free rate of 90%. In patients who had HU greater than 750 and stone size greater than 1.1 cm, almost 80% required three or more SWL treatments with stone-free rates of only 60% [13]. Two prospective trials have been published in this area. The first, Wang and colleagues [14] in 2005, described three important patient factors on SWL multivariate analysis: stone burden greater than 700 mm^3, stone density greater than 900 HU, and presence of nonoval (branched, irregular) stones. The second study, by El-Nahas and colleagues [15], found that stone density greater than 1000 HU and body mass index (BMI) were the only variables that predicted failure of renal stone disintegration using multivariate analysis. Leveraging the concept that stone morphology may be predictive of SWL fragility [16], this study is unique in that the authors use high-resolution bone windows to report stone size and narrow slide width protocols (1.2 mm versus 3.75 mm sections; stone HU calculated at lower, middle, and upper portion of stone versus one calculation) to predict a high-risk SWL failure group [15]. In contrast, Pareek and colleagues analyzed 64 patients who had lower pole renal calculi sized 5 to 15 mm undergoing SWL and did not find HU to be an independent risk factor for stone clearance. Because their stone-free group had significantly smaller lower pole stone sizes before SWL (P < .01), it is likely that stone size, stone density, and stone location, along with other patient factors are linked in the context of lower pole clearance rates. Further studies in the clinical area of HU and stone density, in particular lower pole stones, undoubtedly will aid in stratifying SWL outcomes.

Obesity—technical concerns

As the epidemic of obesity continues to grow in underdeveloped and developed countries, urologists increasingly will be presented with the therapeutic challenge of stone disease in patients who are obese and morbidly obese [17,18]. Technically speaking, each different minimally invasive approach in obese patients who have stone disease brings about its own unique set of nuances. SWL may be limited in these patients, as their weight may exceed gantry or table limits; their size may exceed lithotripter focal length, or body habitus may prevent adequate stone visualization at the time of SWL [19,20]. Proven to be just as safe and effective as in the nonobese population, PCNL in patients who are obese requires modifications in technique, specialized long equipment, and the ability of the patient to tolerate the prone position [21]. Although no new equipment or techniques are required for the ureteroscopic approach, the patient must be able to tolerate general anesthesia and must be able to fit on the operating table without interfering with fluoroscopy [22]. In addition, special attention to thromboembolic prophylaxis and prevention of pressure-induced iatrogenic injuries during prolonged dorsal lithotomy positioning may be warranted in the morbidly obese.

Obesity—shockwave lithotripsy concerns

Excluding positioning and technical concerns, the obese patient still may receive a suboptimal outcome after SWL. In 1994, Ackermann and colleagues [23] first described BMI as an independent predictor of SWL failure using a Dornier HM-3 lithotriptor (Dornier MedTech, Kennesaw, Georgia). Their data suggested that patients who had BMI less than or equal to 28 had the best chance at successful SWL and implied that SWL failure in obese patients may be because of hampered stone targeting or dampened shock wave blast path. In two more recent studies using second-generation electrohydraulic lithotriptors, Portis and colleagues and Pareek and colleagues [24,25] both reported a causal relationship between SWL failures and BMI. Because fat is distributed in different areas for different patients who have the same BMI, a quantitative measurement of the distance from the shockhead to the kidney was introduced in 2005, termed SSD or "skin to stone distance." SSD is calculated by measuring three distances from the renal stone to the skin at the 0°, 45°, and 90° using radiographic calipers or a computational measuring device [26]. The average of these values represents the SSD for a given stone. In a series of 64 lower pole stone patients undergoing SWL, Pareek and colleagues found that SSD greater than 10 cm was a more reliable predictor than either BMI or HU measurements alone for SWL failure. Conversely, El-Nahas and colleagues [15] published their series of 120 patients who underwent SWL for solitary renal stones 5 to 25 mm in size. Although it was shown to be predictive of SWL stone disintegration failure by univariate analysis ($P = .033$), SSD did not reach significance on multivariate analysis [15]. Interestingly, BMI predicted need for more than three SWL sessions and disintegration failure reliably. Overall, as both imaging technology and patients' abdominal girths expand, predicting SWL success by using surrogate markers, such as BMI, HU, or SSD, may lead to alternative stratification protocols.

Lower pole factors—shockwave lithotripsy

Although many different stone and patient factors play roles in the successful surgical management of upper tract urolithiasis, stones located in the lower pole of the kidney continue to be a challenge. In their meta-analysis, Lingeman and colleagues [27] noted that between 1984 and 1991, the incidence of lower pole stones treated with SWL increased from 2% to 48% of all SWL cases. The authors investigated the outcomes of SWL for lower pole calculi and found that stone-free rates ranged from 25% to 84.6%, with a mean stone-free rate of 59.2%. This falls well short of the expected stone-free rates for middle and upper pole stones, which are estimated to be 70% to 90% [28]. Outcomes were more favorable for patients who had stones less than 1 cm, with an overall stone-free rate of 74% for a single treatment as compared with patients who had stones 1 to 2 cm or greater than 2 cm (stone-free rates of 56% and 33%, respectively). These findings questioned the role of SWL in the management of larger, lower pole stones, and opened the door for numerous retrospective and prospective studies concerning the management of these calculi [29–34]. A summary of the most recent lower pole stone-free success rates stratified by procedure type and stone size is listed in Fig. 1. Where at all possible, stone-free rates are provided for single treatments, with the longest recorded follow-up based on strict CT criteria. Occasionally, mean stone size was used because of lack of individual stone size reporting. Multiple explanations have been offered for the poor stone-free rates in lower pole stones, including anatomic factors and the dependent position of the calculi limiting the passage of

fragments from the kidney. The explanation to this mystery, however, is likely multifactorial.

In 2001, the Lower Pole Study Group published a prospective, randomized trial comparing SWL and PCNL for treating lower pole stones [33]. One hundred twenty-eight patients who had symptomatic lower pole calculi were randomized to receive either PCNL or SWL. Overall, stone-free rates at 3 months were 95% for PCNL as opposed to only 37% for the SWL group ($P < .001$). When stratified by stone size, it became evident that SWL success rates declined as stone size increased. The stone-free rates following SWL for stones 11 to 20 mm and 21 to 30 mm were 23% and 14%, respectively, as compared with 93% and 86% for PCNL. Retreatment and the need for auxiliary procedures were more common in the SWL group, while hospital stay was significantly longer in the PCNL group. Overall morbidity was not significantly different between the two groups. The authors concluded that stones greater than 10 mm in diameter are managed better initially with PCNL because of the higher stone-free rates and acceptable rate of morbidity. An advantage of this multicenter trial was the fact that eight different lithotriptors were represented, minimizing the machine-specific effect on the success and complication rates.

In 2005, Pearle and colleagues conducted a multicenter trial comparing SWL and URS for treating lower pole calculi less than or equal to 1 cm in diameter [38]. There was no significant difference in stone-free rates for SWL and URS (35% versus 50%, $P = .92$). Additionally there was no difference in the number of patients requiring retreatment or ancillary treatments. Significant differences were found, however, regarding quality-of-life measures, with a more rapid return to driving, work, and overall shorter recovery time with SWL as compared with URS. In total, 90% of patients who underwent SWL would choose the procedure again as opposed to 63% in the URS group ($P < .05$). Complication rates were not significantly different between groups. The results of this study seem to support SWL treatment over URS for stones 1 cm or less in diameter because of superior patient acceptance; however, the authors point out that many of the symptoms encountered by the URS group could be accounted for by the ureteral stent.

In an effort to improve poor outcomes, Pace and associates investigated the effect of mechanical percussion inversion (MPI) and diuresis on residual lower pole fragments following SWL [50].

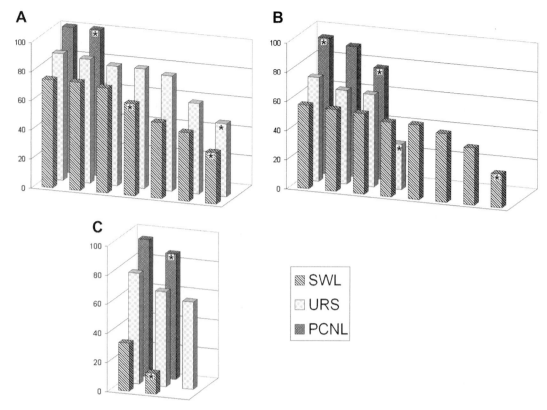

Fig. 1. Lower pole stone-free success rates stratified by procedure type and stone size. Prospective randomized controlled trials are marked by an asterisk. (*A*) Size <1 cm. Shock wave lithotripsy (SWL): 74% [27]; 74% [35]; 72% [36]; 63% [33]; 52% [37]; 47% [26]; 35% [38]. Ureteroscopy (URS): 87% [39]; 85% [40]; 82% [41]; 82% [42]; 79% [43]; 62% [37]; 50% [38]. Percutaneous nephrolithotomy (PCNL): 100% [27]; 100% [33]. (*B*) Size 1 to 2 cm. SWL: 57% [44]; 56% [27]; 55% [45]; 51% [46]; 51% [36]; 41% [35]; 39% [36]; 23% [33]. URS: 71% [41]; 64% [43]; 63% [42]; 31% [47]. PCNL: 93% [33]; 89% [27]; 76% [47]. (*C*) Size >2 cm. SWL: 33% [27]; 14% [33]; URS: 76% [48]; 65% [41]; 60% [49]. PCNL: 94% [27]; 86% [33].

In total, 69 patients who had residual lower pole fragments 3 months following SWL were randomized to receive either MPI or observation for 1 month. The group receiving MPI had a significantly better stone-free rate than the observed group (40% versus 3%) and a greater reduction in total stone area (−63.3% versus +2.7%) in patients who were not free of stones. The authors concluded that MPI is a safe and effective adjunct to SWL in patients who have lower pole calculi, significantly improving success rates and reducing stone burden in SWL failures.

Lower pole factors—ureteroscopy

As with SWL, ureteroscopic management of lower pole stones is frequently challenging, with lower success rates than for stones located elsewhere in the kidney. Grasso and Ficazzola reported overall stone-free rates of 82%, 71%, and 65% in patients with lower pole stones measuring 10 mm or less, 11 to 20 mm, and greater than 20 mm, respectively, managed with retrograde ureteropyeloscopy [41]. Several factors contribute to these poor success rates, including the difficulty of accessing the stone because of acute infundibular angles and reduced deflection in ureteroscopes associated with the passage of even small laser fibers. With the advent of small, flexible endoscopes and tipless nitinol stone baskets, many urologists have taken to relocating lower pole stones into a more favorable location before fragmentation. Kourambas and colleagues [40] described the use of either a 3.2F nitinol basket or 2.6F nitinol grasper in 10 cases where access to the lower pole was inhibited by decreased ureteroscopic deflection. Fragmentation was achieved in all 10 cases after stones were manipulated into a more favorable location. Schuster and colleagues reviewed their experience in 78 patients undergoing ureteroscopy for lower pole stones [43]. Success rates were significantly better in cases where stones were displaced into a more favorable location than in those where lithotripsy was performed in situ. This was statistically significant for stones measuring 1 to 2 cm, where only 29% of cases in the in situ group were successful compared with 100% success in the displacement group.

Although lower pole calculi continue to present challenges for the urologist, new technologies and improved techniques offer the promise of better success rates in these cases. As a general rule, lower pole calculi 1 cm or less are managed best initially with SWL when feasible, while most stones between 1 and 2 cm may be well managed with either URS or PCNL as primary therapy. Large calculi, especially those greater than 2 cm, have profoundly lower success rates in the lower pole and are managed best with PCNL when possible as this modality is influenced least by a lower calyceal location. As always, patient and stone factors, including comorbidities, anatomic factors, and stone composition, should be taken into account when choosing the treatment with the best chance of success.

Surgical management of ureteral calculi

Efficacy

The management of ureteral calculi has changed dramatically over the last 10 years because of an increased awareness and implementation of medical expulsive therapy (to facilitate ureteral stone passage) and advances in ureteroscope design and accessory instrumentation. In general, SWL remains the mainstay treatment for small (less than 1 cm) proximal stones. As stone size increases and as a stone moves distally, most authors agree that ureteroscopy is the more effective surgical approach. In early 2007, Nabi and colleagues [51] summarized results from six published prospective, randomized controlled trials

(PRCT) comparing URS head-to-head with SWL therapy for ureteral stones. Overall, stone-free rates were found to be lower in the SWL group (RR 0.84, 95% CI 0.73 to 0.96) with a trend toward lower retreatment rates in the ureteroscopy group (RR 3.34, 95% CI 0.82 to 13.62). Tables 1 and 2 summarize the results from the six PRCTs and several other recent publications in an attempt to stratify stone free rates (SWL and URS) based on stone size and ureteral stone location. If available, the stone-free rates are reported for single SWL or URS treatments. Retreatment rates and the time to complete stone clearance must be entertained when considering the value of SWL or URS.

Complications

Perhaps the more difficult consideration for patients and urologists is the spectrum of potential complications that may accompany a given ureteral stone treatment. The rate of reported complications in the six PRCTs was lower in the SWL group (RR 0.48, CI 0.26 to 0.91) with a significantly lower rate of hospital stay [51], but no specific details on the exact type of complications were given, except to say that most were minor. This review reported that pain symptoms were higher, but not significantly so, in the stented ureteroscopy group [51]. In a recent review of over 3000 procedures for ureteral stones (predominantly retrospective), significant complications for SWL and URS were 7% for each group [68]. Eighty-seven SWL complications were recognized (Fig. 2), with the most significant difference between URS coming in rates of acute ureteral obstruction (48% [42 oif 87] versus less than 1% 1 of 151]). Notably, the lack of ureteral obstruction in URS patients was likely because of stenting, but no objective measure of stent discomfort was included in this review. Within the URS group, 151 complications were recognized, with ureteral injury (63 of 151 complications, 41%) and ureteral stricture (7 151 complications) occurring exclusively in the URS (SWL group 0%, see Fig. 2) [68]. It comes as no surprise that ureteral injuries occur more frequently during

Table 1
Stone-free clearance rates for mid- and distal ureteral calculi, stratified by size and therapy

Therapy	<1 cm	>1 cm
Extracorporeal shockwave lithotripsy	51% [52]; 91% [34]; 78% [53]; 85% [54]; 79% [55]	95% [54]; 54% [55]
Ureteroscopy	99% [56]; 91% [52]; 91% [34]; 93% [53]; 100% [54]; 97% [57]; 98% [58]; 88% [55]	100% [54]; 94% [57]; 89% [58]; 89% [55]

Table 2
Stone-free clearance rates for proximal ureteral calculi, stratified by size and therapy

Therapy	<1 cm	>1 cm
Extracorporeal shockwave lithotripsy	78% [59]; 80% [60]; 60% [61]; 85% [62]; 70% [55]	32% [63]; 50% [60]; 45% [61]; 35% [62]; 43% [55]
Ureteroscopy	90% [59]; 100% [60]; 90% [61]; 91% [62]; 80% [57]; 91% [58]; 75% [55]	35% [63]; 93% [60]; 93% [61]; 77% [62]; 65% [57]; 71% [58]; 76% [55]
Percutaneous nephrolithotomy	N/A (Most studies examine large stone burden)	98% [64]; 86% [65]; 79% [66]; 94% [67];

ureteroscopy, and many of the previously mentioned studies were performed with older lithotripsy options (electrohydraulic, pneumatic), large semirigid ureteroscopes, and variability in evaluation for and definitions of complications. Overall, the potential for complications must be balanced with the surgeon's experience, type of anesthesia used, available equipment, efficacy, and potential for retreatment.

High-risk treatment groups—pregnancy and bleeding diathesis

Ureteral stones in pregnancy and in patients who have bleeding diathesis represent a high-risk group of stone patients in whom SWL or PCNL are absolutely contraindicated, leaving ureteroscopic lithotripsy as the only effective therapeutic alternative that treats the stone rather than temporizes the pain. Most calculi of pregnancy are eliminated with a combination of analgesia, rest, and hydration [69] or are managed temporarily with the insertion of a ureteral stent or

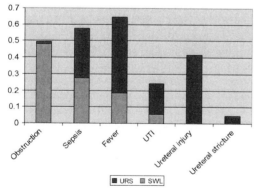

Fig. 2. Percent totals of selected complications for ureteral stones treated by SWL (n = 87) or ureteroscopy (n = 151). (*Data from* Wolf JS Jr. Treatment Selection and Outcomes: Ureteral Caculi. Urol Clin North Am 2007;34:421–30.)

nephrostomy tube [70]. When necessary, the ureteral dilation associated with pregnancy has been shown to facilitate passage of the ureteroscope [71], and several case reports of safe and effective ureteroscopy during pregnancy have been published [72,73]. Indeed, with improvement in ureteroscopic instrumentation and technique, primary definitive ureteroscopic stone extraction can supplant the need for frequent stent changes during pregnancy. Care should be taken to minimize fluoroscopy time and fetal exposure during the case. For patients with ureteral stones who cannot safely stop therapeutic anticoagulation therapy, ureteroscopy also has been shown to be safe and effective. In a retrospective series of 25 patients who had significant alterations in bleeding times and international normalized ratio (INR), Watterson and colleagues [74] successfully treated 18 of 19 (95%) ureteral stones with minimal morbidity.

Technique

Shockwave lithotripsy

SWL has evolved since its introduction in the early 1980s [1,75]. At present, SWL is the preferred first-line treatment in most patients who have renal calculi less than 2 cm in diameter [76]. Several patient and stone factors affecting success rates following SWL are described elsewhere in this article. This section focuses on ESWL technique at the authors' institution, although the authors recognize that there certainly will be variations, particularly given the large number of commercially available SWL units.

The authors generally reserve SWL for patients who have renal or ureteral calculi less than 2 cm in diameter with no evidence of distal ureteral obstruction. Patients who have a known history of cystine stones usually are treated with ureteroscopy or PCNL unless the stone is less than 1 cm.

A urine culture is obtained at the preadmission visit to document sterile urine. Any bacteriuria is treated with oral antibiotics, and urine culture is repeated before SWL to demonstrate resolution of the infection. Routine laboratory studies including coagulation studies are performed the week before the procedure. Contraindications to SWL include pregnancy, uncorrected coagulopathy, distal ureteral obstruction, and untreated urinary tract infection. The authors typically do not perform bilateral SWL in a single setting to avoid potential bilateral ureteral obstruction.

In patients who have a solitary functioning kidney, the authors routinely place a ureteral stent to assist with urine passage. Prophylactic antibiotics are not administered routinely if the preoperative urine culture is negative. Preoperative broad-spectrum antibiotics (ie, first-generation cephalosporin), however, are given to high-risk patients such as those who have indwelling ureteral stents, prostheses or artificial heart valves, and patients who have diabetes mellitus. The patient is counseled on the risk of bleeding requiring hospitalization (1 in 1000), the risk of residual stones or steinstrasse (tailored to the stone size and density), and the possible delayed increased risk of diabetes mellitus.

Following informed consent, the patient is placed in the supine position, and a foam bolster is placed under the knees to flatten the curve of the lumbar spine. Patients who have stones overlying the bony pelvis are placed in the prone position to allow the shockwave front to impact the stone. Short-acting narcotic sedative anesthesia is administered, and the stone is targeted with fluoroscopy in both the anteroposterior and oblique planes.

At this point, cystoscopy is performed if necessary with the patient supine using the flexible endoscope. This generally is required only if the patient requires a ureteral stent or if the stone is not visible and retrograde pyelography is necessary to identify the calculus. If contrast studies are required, the authors use a 5F open-ended ureteral catheter that is left in place throughout the case to allow for periodic injection of contrast as necessary to target the stone. Commonly, the patient has elected SWL because of concerns of transurethral instrumentation, in which case, intravenous contrast is used to delineate the collecting system.

The authors normally limit the total number of shocks to 3000 in a single setting with at least 4 weeks between SWL sessions. Stone position is monitored in the AP plane during the case, with additional targeting in the oblique plane reserved for instances where the patient has shifted during the procedure. The authors use a rate of 60 to 120 shocks per minute starting at a relatively low energy setting. Several in vitro studies suggest that slower rates of treatment improve stone fragmentation [77–79].

The patient is monitored continuously for dysrhythmia during the procedure. If a sustained abnormal heart rhythm is encountered, the lithotriptor is gated to the cardiac rate. The energy gradually is increased over the first 500 shocks to the full dose. This gradual increase is based on the theory of renal preconditioning, where a phase of lower energy SWL followed by a full treatment dose reduces renal injury. Willis and colleagues [80] studied the damage caused by SWL in a pig kidney model. It was noted that pretreatment of the same renal pole with 100 to 500 shocks before the treatment dose resulted in a significantly smaller lesion than in animals that had not received pretreatment. At present, clinical trials in people have yet to prove the utility of this approach in practice. In the setting of multiple calculi, the authors prefer to treat individual stones until there is radiographic evidence of good fragmentation, at which point remaining shockwaves are focused on additional stones.

Patients are discharged home on the day of surgery with a prescription for oral analgesia. The authors also suggest a short course of oral antibiotics in patients who have indwelling ureteral stents or those at high risk of infection (ie, diabetics, immunocompromised). Follow-up is arranged for 1 to 2 weeks following surgery with appropriate imaging, most commonly a plain film of the kidneys, ureters, and bladder (KUB). If a ureteral stent has been inserted, it is removed at this visit with a flexible cystoscope.

Ureteroscopy

Since its first description over 20 years ago, URS has progressed from an awkward diagnostic procedure with limited visualization to a precise, complex surgical intervention allowing access to the entire collecting system in more than 94% of cases [43]. A summary of some of the indications for a retrograde ureteroscopic approach to renal calculi can be found in Box 1. The expansion of these indications can be attributed primarily to the introduction of the 200 μm holmium laser fiber and to

Box 1. Accepted indications for ureteroscopic treatment of renal and ureteral calculi

Renal anatomic characteristics
Calyceal diverticulum
Infundibular stenosis
Skin-to-stone distance >10 cm
Horseshoe/ectopic kidney
Concomitant ureteral stricture, UPJ obstruction, or hydronephrosis
Lower pole anatomy
  Infundibular pelvic angle <70°
  Infundibular length >3 cm
  Infundibular width <5 mm

Patient characteristics
Obesity
Bleeding diathesis
Patient preference
Musculoskeletal deformities
Pregnancy
Unable to tolerate prone position
Requirement to be stone-free
  Airline pilots
  Astronauts

Stone characteristics
Failed previous SWL
Radiolucent
HU >1000
Size 5 to 30 mm
Ureteral location
Combined approach with PCNL
Composition
  Cysteine
  Brushite
  Calcium oxalate monohydrate

small-diameter flexible ureteroscopes with active primary and secondary deflection. As the role of URS continues to expand, a brief review of ureteroscopic technique is in order. Informed consent is obtained emphasizing the risk of minor ureteral perforation, major ureteral injury, bleeding, infection, residual stones, and stent discomfort.

For patients with ectopic kidneys in whom SWL is not feasible, URS is an excellent alternative with comparable stone-free rates. Many of the difficulties associated with accessing the pelvic kidney (ie, tortuous ureter, UPJ obstruction) have become less of an issue in recent years, with refinements in flexible, small-caliber endoscopes and associated technology such as ureteral access sheaths.

The patient is positioned in a lithotomy position with the ipsilateral leg slightly extended. One arm is tucked, for easy access by the fluoroscopy C-arm, while the C-arm monitor, video monitor, and holmium laser machine are positioned on the other side of the patient. Following cystoscopic inspection, the ureteral orifice is cannulated with a .035 in guide wire and advanced to the renal pelvis. If resistance is encountered, a 5F open-ended catheter is advanced to the level of resistance under fluoroscopic guidance, and the sensor guidewire is withdrawn and a retrograde pyelogram performed to delineate the ureteral anatomy. A .035 in hydrophilic wire then is placed through the open-ended catheter and advanced beyond the site of obstruction. The open-ended catheter is advanced to the renal pelvis and the hydrophilic wire replaced with a more secure wire. If the guidewire cannot be manipulated past the site of obstruction, a semi-rigid ureteroscope is gently advanced and wire advanced under direct vision. If all attempts to pass a guide wire are unsuccessful, then the URS is aborted.

The safety wire is secured to the drapes with a clamp. A semirigid ureteroscope is advanced into the bladder using a Microvasive single-action, hand-irrigation syringe (Boston Scientific, Natick, Massachusetts) as it allows easy intermittent manipulation of flow. The tip of the ureteroscope is used to tent the guidewire and open up the ureteral orifice. If difficulty is encountered in cannulating the ureteral orifice, a superstiff guidewire can be advanced through the working channel alongside the safety wire and used as a filiform to enter the ureter. After rotating the tip of the semirigid ureteroscope so it lies between the two wires, gently advance the scope into the ureter. It then may be used to clear the distal and middle ureter of any pathology before placement of a ureteral access sheath. In addition, the semirigid ureteroscope passively dilates the ureteral orifice, which the authors believe facilitates sheath placement. Lastly, the authors place the second working guide wire zz9superstiff .035 in through the working channel of the ureteroscope before removal.

A 12/14F ureteral access sheath then is advanced under fluoroscopic guidance up the ureter. It is important to liberally wet the sheath before placement to activate the hydrophilic coating. If the sheath cannot be advanced up the ureter, the inner dilator can be removed and a 6 mm × 4 cm balloon dilator advanced through the sheath to the site of obstruction and inflated with dilute contrast. The balloon then is removed and the inner dilator reintroduced. If the authors remain unable to advance the ureteral sheath, the ureteroscope is advanced over a superstiff guide wire. If the ureteroscope will not pass the site of obstruction, then a 6F ureteral stent is placed and URS reattempted after 2 weeks of passive dilation by the stent.

Once the sheath has been positioned adequately, the inner dilator and working guide wire are removed, leaving the safety wire outside of the sheath lumen. A flexible ureteroscope is advanced through the sheath into the proximal ureter and renal pelvis. The authors inspect the collecting system starting with the upper pole calyx and working systematically down to the lower pole calyx. If laser lithotripsy is required, the authors use a 200 μm laser fiber with a 20 W laser set at 8 Hz and 0.8 J. It is important to pass the laser fiber with the flexible ureteroscope in a neutral position, as passage while deflected may damage the working channel. In the event that the stone cannot be visualized once the laser fiber is passed, the authors remove the fiber and reposition the stone in an upper pole calyx with a tipless stone basket.

If there are stone fragments adherent to the renal papilla, the authors prefer to use a 2.2F tipless nitinol basket, as the wires are more pliable and can be distorted with gentle pressure until they surround and grasp the adherent stone. Gentle partial opening and closing of the basket can help disengage the stone. Forceful irrigation may be needed to wash a difficult-to-access stone into the basket. At the end of the procedure, the ureter is inspected as the ureteral access sheath is removed.

Percutaneous nephrolithotomy

Technological advancements have improved the ability to manage renal calculi dramatically. Unfortunately, stone-free rates for URS and SWL decrease significantly with factors such as increasing stone size, lower pole stones, and unfavorable stone composition (ie, cystine, brushier, calcium oxalate monohydrate). For this reason, percutaneous stone removal remains the standard of care for patients who have large renal stone burdens. In 1941, Rupel and Brown [81] first described the removal of a renal calculus through a surgically established nephrostomy tract. Since that time, PCNL has virtually eliminated the need for open stone surgery in patients who have calculi not amenable to less-invasive therapies. The authors

acquire their own percutaneous access, as they feel this provides optimal control with the greatest chance of entry into the desired calyx, and the ability to obtain additional access points as required during the procedure.

The authors generally reserve PCNL for managing upper tract stones in patients who have a body habitus not suitable for SWL, failed SWL not amenable to ureteroscopy, cystine stones, and large or complicated stones such as staghorn calculi. Contraindications to PCNL include uncorrected coagulopathy and pregnancy. It is imperative to adequately treat any urinary tract infection, and sterile urine should be documented before surgery. Informed consent is obtained after the risks and benefits of the procedure have been explained, including bleeding, infection, and associated organ injury. Preoperative broad-spectrum antibiotics are administered on the day of surgery. The transfusion rate at the authors' institution is less than 1%, and the authors do not routinely cross-match patients for blood products before surgery.

Under general anesthesia, the patient is placed in the prone position, and all pressure points are checked carefully and padded. The authors typically place a pillow under the chest as a support to allow optimal ventilation. If there is a significant curvature of the lumbar spine, a 1 L irrigation bag may be placed beneath the lower abdomen for support. The flank and genitals are prepared widely and draped to allow exposure for cystoscopy and percutaneous renal access. Flexible cystoscopy is performed, and the ipsilateral ureteral orifice is visualized. The orifice is cannulated with a .038 in Bentson guide wire (Cook Urological, Spencer, Indiana). The wire is advanced in a cephalad direction under fluoroscopic guidance to the level of the collecting system. The cystoscope is removed, and a 5F open-ended ureteral catheter is advanced over the wire, taking care to avoid curling in the bladder. A 16F Foley catheter (Bard Medical, Covington, Georgia) is placed in the bladder, and the guide wire is removed, leaving the ureteral catheter in place. The authors then secure a contrast-filled syringe to the ureteral catheter and cover the area with a sterile towel. At this point, the authors change for clean surgical gloves and begin the percutaneous access portion of the procedure.

Contrast is injected through the ureteral catheter under fluoroscopy to define the calyceal anatomy. The authors prefer to enter by means of a posterior calyx, as this gives the most direct route to the renal pelvis and ureter and helps to minimize unnecessary torquing of the nephroscope during the procedure. A subcostal access is ideal. Certain situations, however, require access to be placed above the 11th or 12th ribs, and this may be accomplished with a slight increase in lung-related complications such as hydrothorax. Situations where intercostal access might be required include large, branched calculi and those cases where access to the ureteropelvic junction is necessary. In the setting of an isolated calyceal or diverticular stone, access is best acquired directly into the stone-bearing calyx or diverticulum. A small volume of air injected through the ureteral catheter may assist in identifying posterior calyces, as these will preferentially fill with air in the prone position. With the C-arm in the AP plane, an 18G Chiba needle (Cook Urological, Spencer, Indiana) is positioned over the tip of the desired entry calyx. The needle is advanced along the AP plane in a controlled fashion until the tip of the needle begins to deflect with the respiratory movement of the kidney. The C-arm is rotated 30° laterally, and the needle is advanced carefully until the tip penetrates the entry calyx. The stylet of the needle is removed, and further insertion of the needle should be avoided at this point. Urine may be seen flowing from the hub of the needle; however, the absence of urine does not indicate that the needle is positioned incorrectly. The authors generally confirm positioning in the collecting system by the gentle passage of a .035 in hydrophilic guide wire that should pass easily and follow the contour of the calyx. In the event that calyceal puncture is unsuccessful, the needle should be withdrawn and access reattempted.

Once correct placement of the needle has been confirmed, the .035 in hydrophilic wire is advanced into the collecting system. Ideally, the wire is passed into the ureter and down to the bladder. The authors routinely employ a 5F Kumpe angled catheter to assist in the passage of the wire down the ureter. They then advance the Kumpe catheter down the ureter and exchange the hydrophilic wire for a .038 in superstiff guide wire with the distal end curled in the bladder. Occasionally, when it is not possible to pass the hydrophilic wire into the ureter, the authors will curl a Bentson wire in the renal pelvis and proceed with tract dilation. Once the nephrostomy tract has been established, a wire usually can be passed down the ureter under direct vision. After the stiff guide wire has been passed, the authors make a 2 cm skin incision and advance a one-step balloon dilator with the radio-opaque marker positioned

in the renal pelvis. The tract is dilated, and a 30F working sheath is advanced under fluoroscopy. It is important to avoid advancing either the balloon dilator or the working sheath beyond the renal pelvis and into the UPJ or proximal ureter. At this point, the guide wire is secured to the drapes, and rigid nephroscopy is performed.

Calculi up to 1 cm in diameter often may be removed through the nephrostomy sheath without fragmentation. Stones may be removed using various baskets, forceps, and graspers. Larger stones are fragmented using an appropriate intracorporeal lithotriptor such as pneumatic, laser, or ultrasonic devices. The authors' preference is to use ultrasonic lithotripsy, as this offers excellent stone fragmentation combined with suction to simultaneously evacuate stone debris. Stones in the entry calyx and renal pelvis should be cleared initially to increase the working space. Once these are clear, attention may be turned to stones in other calyces. Often the nephroscope may be maneuvered gently to allow access to opposing calyces; however, excess torque should be avoided. Once all accessible calculi have been fragmented and removed, the authors carry out flexible nephroscopy to assess the remaining calyces for further stones. In the event that stones remain that cannot be reached safely with the rigid nephroscope, the authors place a second tract into the calyx containing the stone(s), or use the flexible nephroscope with either the holmium laser or electrohydraulic lithotripsy (EHL).

The authors do not routinely place a ureteral stent following PCNL; however in situations where the UPJ or proximal ureter have been manipulated, they will consider passing a stent in an antegrade fashion before exiting the kidney. Once lithotripsy is complete, the authors remove the sheath under direct vision with the rigid nephroscope, as calculi may be concealed alongside the sheath. The authors then place a nephrostomy tube under fluoroscopic guidance. For this purpose, the authors most commonly employ a 16F Council tipped urethral catheter (Bard Medical, Covington, Georgia) with 2 to 3 cc of contrast in the balloon to confirm position in the renal pelvis. Other types of nephrostomy drainage (ie, 8F pigtail) may be used as per surgeon preference. Although other investigators have reported the successful performance of tubeless PCNL, recent studies suggest a lack of benefit and higher complication rate [82], and as such, the authors prefer to maintain drainage and access in the immediate postoperative period. The nephrostomy is secured at the skin with a silk suture, and the wound is cleaned and dressed. Active hemorrhage from the nephrostomy site often may be controlled by passage of a larger caliber nephrostomy tube over a guide wire. In the event that this is not successful, it may be necessary to use a Kaye tamponade catheter to control bleeding. Finally, if bleeding persists or the patient becomes hemodynamically unstable, selective embolization may be required.

The authors' patients routinely are admitted for 24 to 48 hours postoperatively, and a plain radiograph of the KUB is obtained on the first postoperative day. If there is no further evidence of residual calculi, the nephrostomy is clamped, and the patient is observed for flank pain or fever. The authors do not typically obtain an antegrade nephrostogram unless there is a strong clinical suspicion of distal obstruction. Provided the patient tolerates the trial of tube clamping, the nephrostomy may be removed and the patient discharged. In the event that postoperative imaging suggests small residual calculi, the authors often will take a second look with the flexible nephroscope in the clinic and basket remaining stones through the tract. More extensive residual stone burden might require a second PCNL under general anesthesia to render the patient stone-free. If a stent has been placed, the authors will see the patient in the clinic the week after surgery and remove the stent with flexible cystoscopy. All patients are seen in the clinic 4 to 6 weeks postoperatively to be assessed and to arrange further follow-up as required.

While the authors have described their technique for PCNL, there are many variations, from the access technique to the surgical devices used during the case. Hosking and Reid [83] described their experience with over 200 cases of retrograde nephrostomy. The authors reported successful establishment of a nephrostomy tract in 98% of cases, with a mean time of 27.9 minutes to establish the tract. As with any technique of percutaneous access, retrograde access should not be attempted without a suitable period of mentoring under a urologist skilled in the technique. As mentioned previously, the authors' preferred tool for dilation of the nephrostomy tract is a one-step balloon dilator. Other options for tract dilation include introduction of progressively larger serial fascial dilators such as Amplatz renal dilators (Cook Urological, Spencer, Indiana) or Alken metal coaxial dilators (Karl Storz, Tuttlingen, Germany). The authors occasionally will advance a single 8/10F Amplatz coaxial dilator over the guide wire if resistance is met while passing the balloon dilator. This maneuver usually will allow for smooth passage of the balloon into the kidney. There are many other technical nuances and equipment types that urologists may find useful in performing PCNL, and surgeons should experiment with various equipment to find what works best for them.

Laparoscopic

Although uncommonly performed, laparoscopic pyelolithotomy can be an effective treatment modality for stone extraction, especially in the setting of UPJ repair or renal ectopia. A retrospective case series of 19 patients who underwent concomitant laparoscopic pyelolithotomy during pyeloplasty demonstrated stone-free rates of 90% and 80% at 3 and 12 months respectively [84]. In a more contemporary series, transperitoneal laparoscopy was shown to be safe and 100% effective in four patients who had large stone burdens (mean size 2280 mm^2) within either a pelvic or horseshoe kidney [85]. In both reports, pancalicoscopy was achieved by guiding a flexible cystoscope into the renal pelvis through a lap port site. Indwelling stents and peritoneal drains were placed in all patients. Conversely, although ureterolithotomy has been described for ureteral stone removal, most consider this a salvage treatment for the rare case of endoscopic failure.

Summary

The past several decades have seen profound advancements in the management of upper urinary tract urolithiasis. SWL, URS, and PCNL have rendered open stone surgery virtually obsolete. Although factors such as obesity, stone fragility, and unfavorable stone location present challenges to the urologist, new instruments such as smaller caliber ureteroscopes and laser fibers allow increasing numbers of stones to managed with high success rates and minimal patient morbidity. It is imperative for surgeons to keep apprised of new technology and techniques to provide individualized treatments for each patient with the greatest chance of success.

References

[1] Chaussy C, Brendel W, Schmiedt E. Extracorporeally induced destruction of kidney stones by shock waves. Lancet 1980;2:1265–8.
[2] Smith RC, Rosenfield AT, Choe KA, et al. Acute flank pain: comparison of noncontrast-enhanced

CT and intravenous urography. Radiology 1995;
194:789–94.

[3] Dretler SP. Stone fragility—a new therapeutic distinction. J Urol 1988;139:1124–7.

[4] Klee LW, Brito CG, Lingeman JE. The clinical implications of brushite calculi. J Urol 1991;145:715–8.

[5] Zhong P, Preminger GM. Mechanisms of differing stone fragility in extracorporeal shockwave lithotripsy. J Endourol 1994;8:263–8.

[6] Mostafavi MR, Ernst RD, Saltzman B. Accurate determination of chemical composition of urinary calculi by spiral computerized tomography. J Urol 1998;159:673–5.

[7] Nakada SY, Hoff DG, Attai S, et al. Determination of stone composition by noncontrast spiral computed tomography in the clinical setting. Urology 2000;55:816–9.

[8] Zarse CA, McAteer JA, Tann M, et al. Helical computed tomography accurately reports urinary stone composition using attenuation values: in vitro verification using high-resolution microcomputed tomography calibrated to fourier transform infrared microspectroscopy. Urology 2004;63:828–33.

[9] Motley G, Dalrymple N, Keesling C, et al. Hounsfield unit density in the determination of urinary stone composition. Urology 2001;58:170–3.

[10] Parienty RA, Ducellier R, Pradel J, et al. Diagnostic value of CT numbers in pelvocalyceal filling defects. Radiology 1982;145:743–7.

[11] Saw KC, McAteer JA, Monga AG, et al. Helical CT of urinary calculi: effect of stone composition, stone size, and scan collimation. AJR Am J Roentgenol 2000;175:329–32.

[12] Joseph P, Mandal AK, Singh SK, et al. Computerized tomography attenuation value of renal calculus: can it predict successful fragmentation of the calculus by extracorporeal shock wave lithotripsy? A preliminary study. J Urol 2002;167:1968–71.

[13] Gupta NP, Ansari MS, Kesarvani P, et al. Role of computed tomography with no contrast medium enhancement in predicting the outcome of extracorporeal shock wave lithotripsy for urinary calculi. BJU Int 2005;95:1285–8.

[14] Wang LJ, Wong YC, Chuang CK, et al. Predictions of outcomes of renal stones after extracorporeal shock wave lithotripsy from stone characteristics determined by unenhanced helical computed tomography: a multivariate analysis. Eur Radiol 2005;15: 2238–43.

[15] El-Nahas AR, El-Assmy AM, Mansour O, et al. A prospective multivariate analysis of factors predicting stone disintegration by extracorporeal shock wave lithotripsy: the value of high-resolution non-contrast computed tomography. Eur Urol 2007;51: 1688–93 [discussion: 1693–4].

[16] Williams JC Jr, Paterson RF, Kopecky KK, et al. High-resolution detection of internal structure of renal calculi by helical computerized tomography. J Urol 2002;167:322–6.

[17] Koo BC, Burtt G, Burgess NA. Percutaneous stone surgery in the obese: outcome stratified according to body mass index. BJU Int 2004;93:1296–9.

[18] Rigby N, Baillie K. Challenging the future: the Global Prevention Alliance. Lancet 2006;368: 1629–31.

[19] Cass AS. Equivalence of mobile and fixed lithotriptors for upper tract stones. J Urol 1991;146:290–3.

[20] Busby JE, Low RK. Ureteroscopic treatment of renal calculi. Urol Clin North Am 2004;31:89–98.

[21] Pearle MS, Nakada SY, Womack JS, et al. Outcomes of contemporary percutaneous nephrostolithotomy in morbidly obese patients. J Urol 1998; 160:669–73.

[22] Dash A, Schuster TG, Hollenbeck BK, et al. Ureteroscopic treatment of renal calculi in morbidly obese patients: a stone-matched comparison. Urology 2002;60:393–7 [discussion: 397].

[23] Ackermann DK, Fuhrimann R, Pfluger D, et al. Prognosis after extracorporeal shock wave lithotripsy of radiopaque renal calculi: a multivariate analysis. Eur Urol 1994;25:105–9.

[24] Portis AJ, Yan Y, Pattaras JG, et al. Matched pair analysis of shock wave lithotripsy effectiveness for comparison of lithotriptors. J Urol 2003;169: 58–62.

[25] Pareek G, Armenakas NA, Panagopoulos G, et al. Extracorporeal shock wave lithotripsy success based on body mass index and Hounsfield units. Urology 2005;65:33–6.

[26] Pareek G, Hedican SP, Lee FT Jr, et al. Shock wave lithotripsy success determined by skin-to-stone distance on computed tomography. Urology 2005;66: 941–4.

[27] Lingeman JE, Siegel YI, Steele B, et al. Management of lower pole nephrolithiasis: a critical analysis. J Urol 1994;151:663–7.

[28] Renner C, Rassweiler J. Treatment of renal stones by extracorporeal shock wave lithotripsy. Nephron 1999;81(Suppl 1):71–81.

[29] Obek C, Onal B, Kantay K, et al. The efficacy of extracorporeal shock wave lithotripsy for isolated lower pole calculi compared with isolated middle and upper caliceal calculi. J Urol 2001;166:2081–4 [discussion: 2085].

[30] Havel D, Saussine C, Fath C, et al. Single stones of the lower pole of the kidney. Comparative results of extracorporeal shock wave lithotripsy and percutaneous nephrolithotomy. Eur Urol 1998;33:396–400.

[31] Chen RN, Streem SB. Extracorporeal shock wave lithotripsy for lower pole calculi: long-term radiographic and clinical outcome. J Urol 1996;156: 1572–5.

[32] May DJ, Chandhoke PS. Efficacy and cost-effectiveness of extracorporeal shock wave lithotripsy for solitary lower pole renal calculi. J Urol 1998;159:24–7.

[33] Albala DM, Assimos DG, Clayman RV, et al. Lower pole I: a prospective randomized trial of

extracorporeal shock wave lithotripsy and percutaneous nephrostolithotomy for lower pole nephrolithiasis—initial results. J Urol 2001;166:2072–80.

[34] Pearle MS, Nadler R, Bercowsky E, et al. Prospective randomized trial comparing shock wave lithotripsy and ureteroscopy for management of distal ureteral calculi. J Urol 2001;166:1255–60.

[35] Sorensen CM, Chandhoke PS. Is lower pole caliceal anatomy predictive of extracorporeal shock wave lithotripsy success for primary lower pole kidney stones? J Urol 2002;168:2377–82 [discussion: 2382].

[36] Gupta NP, Singh DV, Hemal AK, et al. Infundibulopelvic anatomy and clearance of inferior caliceal calculi with shock wave lithotripsy. J Urol 2000; 163:24–7.

[37] Elbahnasy AM, Shalhav AL, Hoenig DM, et al. Lower caliceal stone clearance after shock wave lithotripsy or ureteroscopy: the impact of lower pole radiographic anatomy. J Urol 1998;159:676–82.

[38] Pearle MS, Lingeman JE, Leveillee R, et al. Prospective, randomized trial comparing shock wave lithotripsy and ureteroscopy for lower pole caliceal calculi 1 cm or less. J Urol 2005;173:2005–9.

[39] Elashry OM, DiMeglio RB, Nakada SY, et al. Intracorporeal electrohydraulic lithotripsy of ureteral and renal calculi using small caliber (1.9F) electrohydraulic lithotripsy probes. J Urol 1996;156:1581–5.

[40] Kourambas J, Delvecchio FC, Munver R, et al. Nitinol stone retrieval-assisted ureteroscopic management of lower pole renal calculi. Urology 2000; 56:935–9.

[41] Grasso M, Ficazzola M. Retrograde ureteropyeloscopy for lower pole caliceal calculi. J Urol 1999; 162:1904–8.

[42] Hollenbeck BK, Schuster TG, Faerber GJ, et al. Flexible ureteroscopy in conjunction with in situ lithotripsy for lower pole calculi. Urology 2001;58: 859–63.

[43] Schuster TG, Hollenbeck BK, Faerber GJ, et al. Ureteroscopic treatment of lower pole calculi: comparison of lithotripsy in situ and after displacement. J Urol 2002;168:43–5.

[44] Madbouly K, Sheir KZ, Elsobky E. Impact of lower pole renal anatomy on stone clearance after shock wave lithotripsy: fact or fiction? J Urol 2001;165: 1415–8.

[45] Saw KC, Lingeman JE. Management of calyceal stones. AUA Update Series 1999;20:154–9.

[46] Sumino Y, Mimata H, Tasaki Y, et al. Predictors of lower pole renal stone clearance after extracorporeal shock wave lithotripsy. J Urol 2002;168:1344–7.

[47] Kuo RL, Lingeman JE, Leveillee RJ, et al. A randomized clinical trial of ureteroscopy and percutaneous nephrolithotomy for lower pole stones between 11 and 25 mm. J Endourol 2003;17:A31.

[48] Grasso M, Conlin M, Bagley D. Retrograde ureteropyeloscopic treatment of 2 cm or greater upper urinary tract and minor Staghorn calculi. J Urol 1998; 160:346–51.

[49] El-Anany FG, Hammouda HM, Maghraby HA, et al. Retrograde ureteropyeloscopic holmium laser lithotripsy for large renal calculi. BJU Int 2001;88: 850–3.

[50] Pace KT, Tariq N, Dyer SJ, et al. Mechanical percussion, inversion, and diuresis for residual lower pole fragments after shock wave lithotripsy: a prospective, single-blind, randomized controlled trial. J Urol 2001;166:2065–71.

[51] Nabi G, Downey P, Keeley F, et al. Extracorporeal shock wave lithotripsy (ESWL) versus ureteroscopic management for ureteric calculi. Cochrane Database Syst Rev 2007 Jan 24;(1):CD006029.

[52] Hendrikx AJ, Strijbos WE, de Knijff DW, et al. Treatment for extended-mid and distal ureteral stones: SWL or ureteroscopy? Results of a multicenter study. J Endourol 1999;13:727–33.

[53] Zeng GQ, Zhong WD, Cai YB, et al. Extracorporeal shock wave versus pneumatic ureteroscopic lithotripsy in treatment of lower ureteral calculi. Asian J Androl 2002;4:303–5.

[54] Peschel R, Janetschek G, Bartsch G. Extracorporeal shock wave lithotripsy versus ureteroscopy for distal ureteral calculi: a prospective randomized study. J Urol 1999;162:1909–12.

[55] Park H, Park M, Park T. Two-year experience with ureteral stones: extracorporeal shockwave lithotripsy v ureteroscopic manipulation. J Endourol 1998;12:501–4.

[56] Sofer M, Watterson JD, Wollin TA, et al. Holmium: YAG laser lithotripsy for upper urinary tract calculi in 598 patients. J Urol 2002;167:31–4.

[57] Aghamir SK, Mohseni MG, Ardestani A. Treatment of ureteral calculi with ballistic lithotripsy. J Endourol 2003;17:887–90.

[58] Sozen S, Kupeli B, Tunc L, et al. Management of ureteral stones with pneumatic lithotripsy: report of 500 patients. J Endourol 2003;17:721–4.

[59] Fong YK, Ho SH, Peh OH, et al. Extracorporeal shockwave lithotripsy and intracorporeal lithotripsy for proximal ureteric calculi—a comparative assessment of efficacy and safety. Ann Acad Med Singapore 2004;33:80–3.

[60] Lam JS, Greene TD, Gupta M. Treatment of proximal ureteral calculi: holmium:YAG laser ureterolithotripsy versus extracorporeal shock wave lithotripsy. J Urol 2002;167:1972–6.

[61] Parker BD, Frederick RW, Reilly TP, et al. Efficiency and cost of treating proximal ureteral stones: shock wave lithotripsy versus ureteroscopy plus holmium:yttrium-aluminum-garnet laser. Urology 2004;64:1102–6 [discussion: 1106].

[62] Wu CF, Chen CS, Lin WY, et al. Therapeutic options for proximal ureter stone: extracorporeal shock wave lithotripsy versus semirigid ureterorenoscope with holmium:yttrium-aluminum-garnet laser lithotripsy. Urology 2005;65:1075–9.

[63] Lee YH, Tsai JY, Jiaan BP, et al. Prospective randomized trial comparing shock wave lithotripsy

and ureteroscopic lithotripsy for management of large upper third ureteral stones. Urology 2006;67: 480–4 [discussion: 484].

[64] Toth CS, Varga A, Flasko T, et al. Percutaneous ureterolithotomy: direct method for removal of impacted ureteral stones. J Endourol 2001;15:285–90.

[65] Kumar V, Ahlawat R, Banjeree GK, et al. Percutaneous ureterolitholapaxy: the best bet to clear large bulk-impacted upper ureteral calculi. Arch Esp Urol 1996;49:86–91.

[66] Srivastava A, Ahlawat R, Kumar A, et al. Management of impacted upper ureteric calculi: results of lithotripsy and percutaneous litholapaxy. Br J Urol 1992;70:252–7.

[67] Anselmo G, Bassi E, Fandella A, et al. Antegrade ureterolitholapaxy in the treatment of obstructing or incarcerated proximal ureteric stones. Br J Urol 1990;65:137–40.

[68] Wolf JS Jr. Treatment selection and outcomes: ureteral calculi. Urol Clin North Am 2007;34:421–30.

[69] Stothers L, Lee LM. Renal colic in pregnancy. J Urol 1992;148:1383–7.

[70] Delakas D, Karyotis I, Loumbakis P, et al. Ureteral drainage by double-J catheters during pregnancy. Clin Exp Obstet Gynecol 2000;27:200–2.

[71] Scarpa RM, De Lisa A, Usai E. Diagnosis and treatment of ureteral calculi during pregnancy with rigid ureteroscopes. J Urol 1996;155:875–7.

[72] Lemos GC, El Hayek OR, Apezzato M. Rigid ureteroscopy for diagnosis and treatment of ureteral calculi during pregnancy. Int Braz J Urol 2002;28: 311–5 [discussion: 316].

[73] Akpinar H, Tufek I, Alici B, et al. Ureteroscopy and holmium laser lithotripsy in pregnancy: stents must be used postoperatively. J Endourol 2006;20: 107–10.

[74] Watterson JD, Girvan AR, Cook AJ, et al. Safety and efficacy of holmium:YAG laser lithotripsy in patients with bleeding diatheses. J Urol 2002;168: 442–5.

[75] Chaussy C, Schmiedt E, Jocham D, et al. First clinical experience with extracorporeally induced destruction of kidney stones by shock waves. J Urol 1982;127:417–20.

[76] Kerbl K, Rehman J, Landman J, et al. Current management of urolithiasis: progress or regress? J Endourol 2002;16:281–8.

[77] Greenstein A, Matzkin H. Does the rate of extracorporeal shock wave delivery affect stone fragmentation? Urology 1999;54:430–2.

[78] Weir MJ, Tariq N, Honey RJ. Shockwave frequency affects fragmentation in a kidney stone model. J Endourol 2000;14:547–50.

[79] Paterson RF, Lifshitz DA, Lingeman JE, et al. Stone fragmentation during shock wave lithotripsy is improved by slowing the shock wave rate: studies with a new animal model. J Urol 2002;168:2211–5.

[80] Willis LR, Evan AP, Connors BA, et al. Prevention of lithotripsy-induced renal injury by pretreating kidneys with low-energy shock waves. J Am Soc Nephrol 2006;17:663–73.

[81] Rupel E, Brown R. Nephroscopy with removal of stone following nephrostomy for obstructive calculous anuria. J Urol 1941;46:177–82.

[82] Choi M, Brusky J, Weaver J, et al. Randomized trial comparing modified tubeless percutaneous nephrolithotomy with tailed stent with percutaneous nephrostomy with small-bore tube. J Endourol 2006; 20(10):766–70.

[83] Hosking D, Reid R. The evaluation of retrograde nephrostomy in over 200 procedures. In: Walker V, Sutton R, Cameron E, editors. Urolithiasis: proceedings of the Sixth International Symposium on Urolithiasis. New York: Plenium Press; 1989.

[84] Ramakumar S, Lancini V, Chan DY, et al. Laparoscopic pyeloplasty with concomitant pyelolithotomy. J Urol 2002;167:1378–80.

[85] Kramer BA, Hammond L, Schwartz BF. Laparoscopic pyelolithotomy: indications and technique. J Endourol 2007;21:860–1.

ELSEVIER
SAUNDERS

Urol Clin N Am 35 (2008) 455–466

UROLOGIC
CLINICS
of North America

Laparoscopic Radical Cystectomy

Amr F. Fergany, MD[a,b,]*,
Inderbir S. Gill, MD[a,b]

[a]*Center for Laparoscopy and Robotics, and Comprehensive Center for Urologic Oncology,
Department of Urology, Glickman Urological and Kidney Institute, Cleveland Clinic,
Cleveland, OH, USA*
[b]*Cleveland Clinic Lerner School of Medicine at Case Western University,
Cleveland, OH, USA*

Bladder cancer accounts for more than 63,000 new cases and 13,000 deaths annually. Radical surgery remains the mainstay of treatment in cases of muscle-invasive disease and some cases of refractory or high-risk superficial bladder cancer, even with the modern concepts of integrating neoadjuvant or adjuvant chemotherapy into treatment strategies. A high-quality cystectomy, with the main objectives of negative surgical margins and an adequate lymphadenectomy, has been shown to have significant impact upon patient survival [1].

The application of laparoscopic techniques to radical cystectomy has been a recent and natural evolution of successful laparoscopic applications in renal surgery and prostatectomy. Initial case reports and small series of laparoscopic radical cystectomy (LRC) were reported in the early 1990s [2,3], soon yielding to larger series with varying techniques and dependable results. The authors' ongoing international registry comprises over 700 cases from 14 countries. Most LRC operations are performed using standard laparoscopic technique, with a minority of hand-assisted or robotic-assisted procedures. This article attempts to provide an overview of the current status of LRC, with technical details, modifications, and results of various techniques as reported by the authors' group and other groups.

The current standard: open radical cystectomy

Open radical cystectomy (ORC) remains the gold standard treatment for invasive bladder cancer, setting the bar for other treatment approaches to be measured against. Nevertheless, wide variations in the quality of ORC exist among academic and community settings, with the experience of the individual surgeon being a highly significant variable as regards nodal yield and positive surgical margins, both factors impacting on oncologic outcomes of ORC. At centers of excellence, a contemporary quality ORC is a technically efficient procedure with positive margin rates in the 0% to 2% range for organ-confined disease and less than 10% overall. A critical component of ORC is an extended lymphadenectomy up to the common iliac and presacral nodes, and recently, even para-caval, interaorto–caval, and para-aortic nodes, providing nodal yields greater than or equal to 20. Cancer-specific survival correlates with lymph node counts, even among node-negative patients.

ORC, however, does confer substantial morbidity, even at experienced centers. Major complication rates are 10% to 12%; overall complication rates are 30% to 60%, and perioperative mortality ranges from 2% to 5%. Factors impacting upon complications of ORC include surgeon experience, hospital volume, and patient factors such as advanced age and medical comorbidities.

* Corresponding author. Center for Laparoscopy and Robotics, and Comprehensive Center for Urologic Oncology, Department of Urology, Glickman Urological and Kidney Institute, Cleveland Clinic, 9500 Euclid Avenue, A-100, Cleveland, OH 44195.

E-mail address: fergana@ccf.org (A.F. Fergany).

The rationale for laparoscopic radical cystectomy

Fundamentally, LRC must deliver a high-quality, technically superb loco–regional onco-logic clearance comparable to ORC, thereby guaranteeing equivalent oncologic outcomes. Additionally, LRC potentially can reduce morbidity and shorten convalescence, thereby leading to improved postoperative quality of life over the short term. Similar to other laparoscopic onco-logic procedures (renal, prostate), the excellent visualization and decreased blood loss during laparoscopy allows for a highly precise technical operation. Smaller skin/fascial incisions decrease pain and convalescence, with the potential for decreasing certain perioperative complications. By minimizing bowel manipulation and its exposure to the atmosphere, postoperative ileus may be reduced. Partly because of patient demand, the application of minimally invasive surgery continues to rapidly increase not only in urologic oncology, but also across the entire surgical spectrum. Risks of port site recurrence and peritoneal seeding are exceedingly rare. LRC data require careful scrutiny to ensure that soft tissue margins, nodal yields, local recurrences, and cancer-specific survival meet the standards established by ORC. Such data are accruing. For LRC to become a widely accepted viable treatment option for aggressive bladder cancer, considerable work lies ahead.

Patient selection for laparoscopic radical cystectomy

Careful selection of patients for LRC is paramount for good outcomes. Invasive bladder cancer is an aggressive tumor; there will be no second opportunity for surgical cure, given a positive margin confers a death sentence. Adjuvant treatments (chemotherapy, radiotherapy) cannot salvage patients who have had a surgically sub-optimal excision. Tumor, patient, and surgeon factors should be taken into account when selecting the optimal approach, laparoscopic or open, for radical cystectomy.

At this time, the authors offer LRC to select patients who have clinically low volume, organ-confined tumors without lymphadenopathy. Patients who have locally advanced or bulky tumors or gross lymphadenopathy (before or after chemotherapy) are handled best with an open surgical approach. In these cases, wide excision

with possible adjacent organ resection may be necessary, which may require adequate intraoper-ative palpation to determine local tumor exten-sion. Also, it is difficult to manipulate bladders with heavy tumors laparoscopically; these tumors leave little working space in the pelvis, compro-mising proper laparoscopic visualization.

Patient factors play a significant role in selec-tion for LRC. General contraindications to lapa-roscopy (uncorrected bleeding tendency, active intra-abdominal infection, ascites) typically will contraindicate an open surgical cystectomy also. Other specific factors like previous pelvic radia-tion, multiple abdominal surgery, or previous pelvic surgery would favor selection of an open radical cystectomy. LRC has been reported after neoadjuvant chemotherapy, without mention of any added difficulty in such cases. Obese patients present a particular challenge to laparoscopy, with difficulty in obtaining access, identifying planes and landmarks, inability to reach ade-quately into the pelvis, and operator fatigue from difficult manipulation. Although robotic assistance can alleviate some of these difficulties, open surgery may be a more reasonable (although still challenging) option.

Finally, LRC should be limited to laparoscopic surgeons who have adequate experience and skills. These procedures are long, complicated, and require detailed knowledge of pelvic anatomy and bladder cancer pathology. Experience with laparoscopic pelvic surgery is vital to an oncolog-ically adequate procedure for the patient. Open surgical experience is also essential for transfer of surgical experience to the laparoscopic setting, possible open conversion if needed, and perform-ing open urinary diversion. The presence of an experienced surgical team in a tertiary care setting is the optimal situation, necessary to cover the laparoscopic, anesthetic, and postoperative care of such patients.

Techniques of laparoscopic radical cystectomy

Male

Bladder cancer is more common in males, and as a result 75% to 80% of all radical cystectomies are performed in male patients. A similar tech-nique of LRC with minor modifications has been reported in various initial series [4–7]. LRC is per-formed transperitoneally, with four to five ports placed in a peri-umbilical fan arrangement across the lower abdomen, with a possible sixth port in the suprapubic area (Fig. 1). The camera port is placed two fingerbreadths above the umbilicus, but may be moved to just below the umbilicus in large patients; this supra-umbilical camera position facilitates performance of the high-extended lymphadenectomy up to the inferior mesenteric artery. Although surgery can be performed in the supine position, a low lithotomy is preferred to allow access to the rectum and allow perineal pressure as needed during the urethral anastomosis in an orthotopic reconstruction. A steep Trendelenburg position is essential to keep the bowel out of the pelvis during surgery.

Surgery usually starts by visualizing the pelvis and releasing adhesions of the sigmoid colon to the pelvic side wall, which are present in almost all cases. This mobilization of the sigmoid allows retraction out of the pelvis and identification of the left ureter, and assists in the subsequent lymphadenectomy. If the sigmoid continues to fall into the pelvis, it can be held in place by a suture placed through an appendix epiploica and held to the abdominal wall. At this time, the major landmarks in the pelvis should be visualized; these are the ureters, medial umbilical ligaments, vasa deferentia, and the urachus. The

tip of the urethral catheter frequently is seen in the bladder dome also.

Important planes of dissection for radical cystectomy are the posterior plane between the seminal vesicles and prostate anteriorly, and the rectal wall posteriorly, as well as the lateral plane, between the bladder within the perivesical fat and the pelvic side wall including the iliac vessels, obturator fossa, and pelvic floor muscles. These planes are generally avascular; understanding and meticulously developing and following them are essential for a technically and oncologically sound operation.

The posterior plane usually is developed first, keeping the bladder attached to the anterior abdominal wall to allow exposure (Fig. 2). The ureters can be dissected and mobilized distally towards the bladder before or after opening the posterior plane. This plane is entered by dividing the peritoneum of the recto–vesical pouch a little higher than its lowest point. Following the vas deferens medially can facilitate identifying this

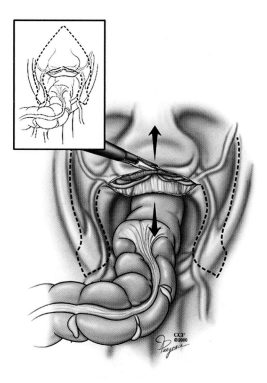

Fig. 2. Pelvic peritoneotomy incision. The initial peritoneotomy incision is made posteriorly, deep in the cul-de-sac, staying posterior to the seminal vesicles and vas. Dotted line indicates the ultimate peritoneotomy required as the operation proceeds. (*Courtesy of* the Cleveland Clinic Foundation, Cleveland, Ohio; with permission.)

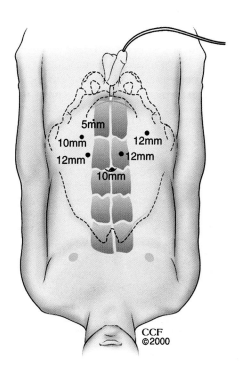

Fig. 1. Port placement. (*Courtesy of* the Cleveland Clinic Foundation, Cleveland, Ohio; with permission.)

plane in difficult cases. The tips of the seminal vesicles are visualized easily, and keeping the seminal vesicles anterior, the plane is developed distally towards the prostate (Fig. 3). Denonvillier's fascia is encountered at the level of the prostate–vesicular junction posteriorly. This fascia needs to be divided sharply, allowing the posterior plane to be developed further distally between the prostate and the anterior rectal surface (Fig. 4). Extreme care should be exercised at this time to avoid injuring the rectum, which lies in an oblique, rather than transverse plane in this area.

If the ureters have not been mobilized previously, they should be at this time. Proximal dissection to a level above the iliac vessels greatly facilitates the subsequent lymphadenectomy and the urinary diversion. The ureters are divided distally close to the bladder between clips, and the distal ureter margin is sent for frozen section pathological examination.

The lateral planes then are developed. This is done easiest by dividing the peritoneum over the obliterated medial umbilical ligaments until the anterior abdominal wall. The vas deferens is encountered commonly at this time and can be divided also. The lateral plane is identified readily lateral to the ligament, which is retracted medially. This plane is developed distally into the pelvis until the pelvic floor muscle and the endopelvic fascia is reached. The reflection of the endopelvic fascia over the prostate can be divided at this time or left for a later stage in the operation.

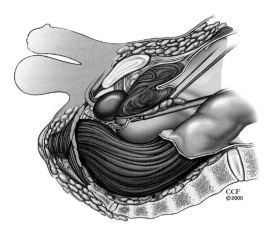

Fig. 4. Incising Denonvillier's fascia. (*Courtesy of* the Cleveland Clinic Foundation, Cleveland, Ohio; with permission.)

The posterolateral bladder pedicles thus are exposed between the posterior and lateral planes. These pedicles are sometimes separable into a lateral and posterior portion (with the ureter between the two), or in some thin patients may be one posterolateral attachment. The superior and inferior vesical vessels course with the lateral portion of the pedicle, and accordingly, the pedicles usually are divided with a laparoscopic linear stapler (Fig. 5). Other energy-based coagulating instruments or clips can be used also. These pedicles are followed to the level of the pelvic floor, or if the endopelvic fascia has been opened, along the side of the prostate as distally as the apex of the prostate.

After the posterior and lateral bladder attachments are freed, the bladder is mobilized from the

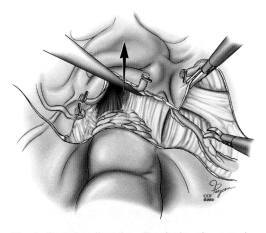

Fig. 3. Posterior dissection. Developing the posterior plane and the right postero–lateral vesicle pedicle. (*Courtesy of* the Cleveland Clinic Foundation, Cleveland, Ohio; with permission.)

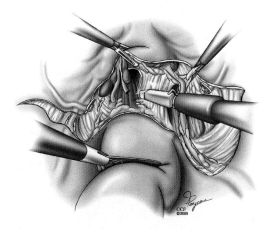

Fig. 5. Transecting the right posterior pedicle using the endo-GIA stapler. (*Courtesy of* the Cleveland Clinic Foundation, Cleveland, Ohio; with permission.)

anterior abdominal wall, including a triangle of peritoneum with the urachus to the umbilicus (Fig. 6). The pubic bones are exposed, the space of Retzius developed, and the puboprostatic ligaments exposed. The superficial branch of the dorsal vein is coagulated and divided. The endopelvic fascia is opened on both sides of the prostate at this time if not previously opened; the pelvic floor muscles are swept off the sides of the prostate, exposing the apex, urethra, and sides of the dorsal vein complex. The dorsal vein can be controlled by various techniques (Fig. 7). The authors commonly utilize a laparoscopic GIA stapler to control the well-mobilized complex, although a controlling stitch can be placed across the dorsal vein. Coagulating instruments like bipolar electrocautery also can be used, although they are less reliable. After the puboprostatic ligaments and the dorsal vein complex are divided, the urethra comes into view. The attachments of the prostatic apex to the pelvic floor are released, and the urethral catheter can be removed at this time. A locking clip or a suture should be placed at the proximal urethra to prevent tumor spillage from the bladder, and the urethra is divided. Proximal traction on the prostatic apex allows the final attachments of the prostate to the anterior rectal surface (rectourethralis muscle) to come into view; these are divided carefully, and the specimen is placed in an impermeable laparoscopic retrieval sac, which is placed out of the pelvis to allow subsequent inspection, hemostasis, and lymphadenectomy.

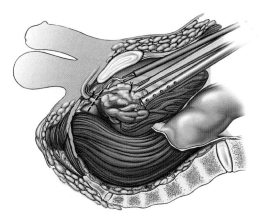

Fig. 7. Completing the prostate apical dissection. Transection of the dorsal vein complex and urethra. The specimen side of the transected prostate apex is secured with a stitch or clip to eliminate local spillage of urine from the bladder. (*Courtesy of* the Cleveland Clinic Foundation, Cleveland, Ohio; with permission.)

Female

LRC in the female usually involves an anterior exenteration with en bloc resection of the bladder, uterus, fallopian tubes, and ovaries. The authors' technique in females [8] starts similar to a laparoscopic cystectomy in the male, with identification of the ureters and dissection into the pelvis. The ovarian vessels are divided in the infundibulopelvic ligaments, allowing the ovaries to be mobilized into the pelvis. The bladder is mobilized laterally in the same manner as in males, using the obliterated medial umbilical ligament as a guide, and dividing the round ligament of the uterus in the process. The endopelvic fascia is visualized, although it does not need to be divided in the female. Anterior retraction of the uterus is very helpful, and facilitates identification of the posterior and posterolateral structures. This can be accomplished with a laparoscopic instrument held by an assistant, or by various instruments that can be placed vaginally and used to manipulate the uterine cervix. A good example is the RUMI uterine manipulator with the Koch colpotomizer system (Cooper Surgical, Trumbull, Connecticut). The posterolateral bladder pedicles are identified; these include the uterine vessels and are controlled with a linear stapler.

The posterior fornix is identified with a sponge stick placed in the vagina, and the vagina is opened close to the cervix. The vaginal incision is continued around the cervix, and distally along the anterior vaginal wall. The vaginal wall is

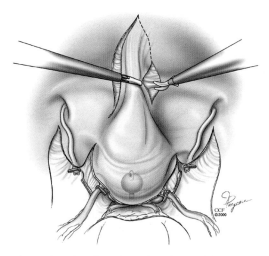

Fig. 6. Anterior dissection. The triangular inverted V peritoneotomy is created and space of Retzius entered. (*Courtesy of* the Cleveland Clinic Foundation, Cleveland, Ohio; with permission.)

well-vascularized, and various cutting/coagulating instruments (eg, Harmonic scalpel, Ligasure) are especially useful for this part of the procedure. As the bladder neck area is reached, this dissection can proceed closer to the urethra, which is removed in its entirety. If an orthotopic neobladder is planned, the dissection ends at the bladder neck; the urethra is transected at the bladder neck, and the bladder neck is sutured closed immediately to prevent spillage. The distal dissection of the bladder neck and urethra can be performed vaginally, and the specimen can be removed from the vaginal incision (useful in cases where intracorporeal diversion is planned). The vagina then is closed with a continuous Vicryl suture. The distal part of this closure also can be performed vaginally according to surgical preference.

Laparoscopic extended pelvic lymphadenectomy for bladder cancer

Pelvic lymphadenectomy is an integral part of radical cystectomy, and has been proven to have a significant impact on patient survival in addition to accurately staging the tumor. Numerous publications recently have advocated extension of the standard pelvic lymph node dissection to a more extensive template [9,10]. Within the pelvis, the anatomical limits of the lymphadenectomy are the genitofemoral nerve (laterally), the obturator vessels (medially), and the node of Cloquet (distally). The proximal extent of the dissection has become an area of significant debate recently, with most oncologists advocating a common iliac lymphadenectomy, and a few extending that to the level of the inferior mesenteric origin from the aorta. The presacral nodes also should be removed. The number of lymph nodes correlates well with the extent of the lymphadenectomy. Difficulty in standardizing a specific number arises from different surgical practices as far as the number of packets sent, the pathologist's diligence in counting the lymph nodes, and to a certain extent, interpatient variability.

Keeping all these principles in mind, a laparoscopic lymphadenectomy for bladder cancer has to cover the same template as an open lymphadenectomy. Standard lymphadenectomy (to the bifurcation of the common iliac artery) has been performed by urologists for decades, being one of the earliest laparoscopic procedures integrated into urological practice. The authors prefer to perform the lymphadenectomy after the bladder is removed, with the pelvis empty and landmarks readily visible. An extended lymphadenectomy can be adequately performed laparoscopically [11]. Generous mobilization of the sigmoid helps to achieve exposure of the iliac vessels, especially on the left side, and vessel loop retraction of the common iliac arteries may facilitate exposure in the area just distal to the aortic bifurcation. Intermittent decrease of pneumoperitoneum to 5 mm Hg is helpful in identifying the veins, which are typically empty and flat at standard pressure. To avoid difficulty with the most proximal part of the dissection, it is advisable to place the main operating ports slightly more cephalad at the start of the procedure. The authors routinely perform extended lymphadenectomy after cystectomy, with removal of the common iliac and presacral lymph nodes, with a pathological yield similar to open surgical extended templates. An average yield of 21 lymph nodes is the result of this technique, with an increase of about 1 hour of operating time [11]. The authors recently performed extended lymphadenectomy to the inferior mesenteric artery in five patients (A.F. Fergany and I.S. Gill, unpublished data), demonstrating that a laparoscopic lymphadenectomy can cover the same templates as an open procedure (Fig. 8). Long-term oncological results are awaited.

Numerous modifications to the standard technique of radical cystectomy in males and females have been suggested as a means to minimize the functional impact of surgery on sexual function and urinary continence. All of these modifications have been incorporated readily into the laparoscopic technique, mainly nerve-sparing, female reproductive organ-sparing, and prostate-sparing techniques.

Modified techniques of laparoscopic radical cystectomy

Nerve-sparing techniques

Nerve-sparing techniques similar to those performed during prostatectomy have been advocated and applied in select cystectomy situations with low-stage disease, where tumor control is not compromised by this modification. Such nerve-sparing presents patients, especially younger ones, with the option of retaining erectile activity, and may improve urinary continence. Laparoscopic nerve-sparing radical cystectomy has been performed along the same principles as the open procedure [12] and is a fairly straightforward

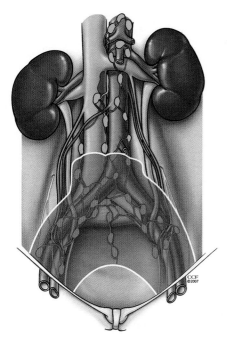

Fig. 8. High extended lymphadenectomy template. This template excises level I, II, and III nodal tissue. Level I: bilateral external iliac, internal iliac, obturator, perivesical packets. Level II: bilateral common iliac, internal iliac, presacral packets. Level III: aortic bifurcation and the pericaval, interaorto–caval, and peri-aortic packets up to the inferior mesenteric artery. (*Courtesy of* the Cleveland Clinic Foundation, Cleveland, Ohio; with permission.)

modification of the standard technique. The autonomic nerves run in the posterior bladder pedicles, close to the tip and sides of the seminal vesicles. At the prostate–vesicular junction, they are somewhat further away from the bladder; then they become closely applied to the posterolateral aspect of the prostate, with some neural fibers running more posterior or more lateral than the main bundles.

Preserving these nerve fibers requires a careful dissection of the posterior bladder pedicles— applying individual clips rather than a stapler— very close to the lateral sides of the seminal vesicles, to preserve as much of the pedicle as possible. Any energy-producing coagulation devices should be avoided, as they result in some degree of thermal damage to the nerves. Only cold scissors should be used to divide between the clips. When the inferior bladder pedicle is divided, the neurovascular bundles should be separated from the sides of the prostate similar to a radical prostatectomy, opening the lateral prostatic fascia

and gently dissecting the bundles aside, again with cold scissors, all the way until the urethra is reached. The bundles should be separated from the urethra before it is divided, to avoid injury to the bundles during division of the urethra or the subsequent neobladder–urethral anastomosis. Using the described technique, two of four patients maintained postoperative potency; 75% and 100% achieved day and night time continence, respectively [12].

Female nerve sparing is performed, with the primary objective of maintaining urethral innervation and urinary continence, although an added advantage is better preservation of vaginal lubrication and sensation. This also is performed laparoscopically similar to the open surgical technique. The surgical goal is avoiding any dissection on the lateral walls of the vagina, and avoiding any dissection distal to the bladder neck, leaving the urethra and distal vagina intact with the endopelvic fascial covering. In this way, the nerve fibers coursing along the lateral vaginal walls, as well as those innervating the urethra from the pelvic floor, remain undisturbed.

Female reproductive organ sparing

Although bladder cancer is less common in females, clinicians often are faced with female patients who are sexually active, premenopausal, or even within childbearing age. The sexual and hormonal effects of an anterior exenteration in such patients are not realistically acceptable; in addition to loss of hormonal function, most females will report a decrease or absence of sexual activity after radical cystectomy. A significant number of such patients will report dyspareunia from vaginal stenosis, decreased lubrication, or shortening of the vagina. At the same time, very low rates of direct cancer spread to female organs, especially in patients who have low-stage disease, warrant a relaxation of the oncologic principle of wide excision of all female organs in patients who have bladder cancer.

For premenopausal patients in whom preservation of hormonal function is desirable, sparing one or both ovaries can be accomplished by dividing the ovarian ligament (between the ovary and the uterus) and mobilizing the ovary on its blood supply cephalad into the abdomen. The ovary then can be pexed outside of the pelvis to avoid interfering with the subsequent cystectomy.

For female patients who are sexually active, (possibly all female patients if tumor control is not compromised), a vaginal-sparing approach should be used. If the uterus is in place, the posterior and lateral vaginal fornices should be opened as close to the cervix as possible. The anterior vaginal wall is divided close to the cervix, and with the bladder retracted anteriorly, the anterior vaginal wall is retracted posteriorly with a laparoscopic Allis clamp. This exposes the plane between the anterior vaginal wall and the base of the bladder. This plane is followed carefully to the bladder neck (if a neobladder reconstruction is planned), or to the distal urethra if a urethrectomy is planned. Avoiding entry into the bladder is critical. After the specimen is removed, a running closure of the vaginal vault is performed, leaving a vagina of normal length and capacity.

This type of dissection is oncologically safe only in low-stage (Ta, T1) tumors and tumors away from the posterior bladder wall. In higher-stage posterior wall tumors, resection of the anterior vaginal wall is safer. In these cases, the authors try to minimize the extent of vagina resected, avoiding excision of any part of the lateral walls. In all cases, the authors attempt to separate the urethra from the anterior vaginal wall distal to the tumor-bearing area, preserving the anterior vaginal wall below the urethra only. This preserves a full ring of intact vaginal skin at the introitus, avoiding any scarring in this area. This rim of vaginal skin also facilitates closure of the vaginal vault, which always is performed transversely to avoid vaginal stenosis.

In younger female patients within childbearing age who desire to preserve the uterus, a full reproductive organ-sparing cystectomy can be performed [8]. This occasionally can be performed in the older female patient who has low-stage disease as a simpler option to an anterior exenteration. With this technique, the ureters are dissected distal to the crossing of the uterine arteries; the peritoneum of the vesicouterine fold is opened, and the plane between the cervix and the bladder base is developed and followed distally between the anterior vaginal wall and the urethra for the desired distance. The distal clipped ends of the ureters can be used for anterior traction to facilitate following this plane distally.

Prostate-sparing cystectomy

Prostate-sparing cystectomy recently was introduced as an alternative to a standard radical cystectomy in male patients. This is an attractive option, as it maintains potency and urinary continence in a much larger percentage of patients, by removing the bladder above the level of the seminal vesicles and prostate. In this manner, the neural pathways for erection, the drainage pathway for semen, and the continence mechanism around the prostate are undisturbed. A flurry of debate surrounds the surgical principles of this technique, because of concerns about oncological adequacy. This debate is beyond the scope of this article, although the authors mention that advocates of the technique recommend careful selection of patients with low-stage disease, and careful exclusion of prostatic involvement with urothelial carcinoma or prostate cancer prior to surgery.

To perform a prostate sparing laparoscopic cystectomy, the plane between the bladder base anteriorly and the seminal vesicles posteriorly is developed and followed to the level of the bladder neck. At this point, a prostatic enucleation (adenomectomy) can be performed, leaving the outside capsule of the prostate. Alternatively, some authors prefer performing a transurethral resection of the prostatic adenoma prior to cystectomy, at which time the bladder is divided off the capsule of the prostate just distal to the bladder neck. After a neobladder is formed, it is sutured to the cut edge of the prostatic capsule.

Only one study of adequate sample size in the literature describes the results of laparoscopic prostate-sparing cystectomy [13]. The study comprised 25 patients in whom a laparoscopic technique was used, based on experience from about 100 cases of open surgery. The average operative time was 285 minutes; blood loss was 640 cc, and the complication rate was 16%. One patient had a local recurrence; two developed metastatic disease, and one died of progressive cancer. All patients were continent without pads; no patient had urinary retention, and 84% of patients maintained preoperative potency. Although this study clearly shows the functional benefit of the technique, widespread acceptance remains lacking because of the perceived risk of local tumor recurrence. The long-term utility of the technique remains to be seen.

Urinary diversion techniques: intra- or extracorporeal

A current area of debate in the field of LRC is whether to perform the urinary diversion intracorporeally using laparoscopic technique, or extracorporeally through a minilaparotomy that is required for specimen extraction (at least in males).

Early reports of LRC used intracorporeal technique [4,6,14] for ileal conduit, orthotopic neobladder, and rectal sigmoid pouch, and proved conclusively that such an endeavor is technically feasible. Prolonged operative time and significant complications from the urinary diversion and bowel reconstruction portions of the operation have led to a shift favoring extracorporeal bowel work, with intracorporeal suturing of the pouch–urethral anastomosis for orthotopic neobladders. Lack of enthusiasm for rectal urinary diversion (ureterosigmoidostomy, rectal pouches) within the United States has decreased the utility of intracorporeal diversion using these techniques. Within the robotic assisted literature, the same situation has prevailed, with reports of totally intracorporeal diversion [15,16] giving way to an overwhelming majority of extracorporeal urinary diversions.

The authors' experience with both techniques is representative of the current status on this topic [17]. The authors compared their initial 17 cases where intracorporeal urinary diversion was formed with the subsequent 37 cases where an extracorporeal diversion was formed. The second group had decreased operative time, blood loss, time to ambulation, time to oral diet, and significantly fewer complications. Re-exploration for anastomotic leak, bowel obstruction, or sepsis was required in 29% of the first group versus 11% of the second group. With this clearly safer and shorter approach, the authors have abandoned intracorporeal urinary diversion altogether. This experience also has been that of other major operators in this field [18].

Robotic radical cystectomy

Robotic-assisted laparoscopy has become prevalent, especially in regards to radical prostatectomy. With increasing robotic experience, it was natural for surgeons to attempt the more complex, closely related pelvic surgery, cystoprostatectomy. Proponents claim the benefits of improved three-dimensional visualization, freedom of movement offered by robotic instruments, and ergonomic comfort. The surgical steps are similar to the laparoscopic technique. The initial report in the literature described the nerve-sparing technique in 17 patients, 14 of whom were males [19]. The same group described the technique for female cystoprostatectomy, with and without uterus and vagina sparing, similar to that previously described in this article [20]. Mean operating

time for the cystectomy and lymphadenectomy portion was 140 minutes; mean blood loss was 150 cc. Urinary diversion was performed through a laparotomy. All surgical margins were negative; one reoperation for bleeding was required. The complication rate was not reported. The same group subsequently reported a port site recurrence (the only one for LRC in the literature) within this patient group [21]. A more recent study compared 20 patients undergoing robotic cystectomy with extracorporeal urinary diversion with 24 patients undergoing ORC [22]. Operating time was longer (6.1 versus 3.8 hours); blood loss was less (313 versus 588), and a total complication rate of 30% was reported. Mean lymph node yield was 19 nodes, and no positive margins were encountered. Similar results were obtained in a larger study comparing 21 ORCs with 33 robotic-assisted LRCs [23].

As widespread experience and availability of robotic systems increases, there no doubt will be an increase in the overall published experience with robotic cystoprostatectomy. Reconstruction and intracorporeal suturing are where the robotic assistance is most helpful, and single case reports have performed intracorporeal ileal conduits and neobladders. Whether a significant advantage is achieved through robotic assistance in LRC will remain to be seen, as the operation remains an extirpative procedure, with the reconstructive urinary diversion portion being performed through open surgery in most cases.

Hand-assisted laparoscopic radical cystectomy

Hand-assisted laparoscopic technique has been used extensively for renal surgery, but has been significantly slower to permeate into the field of pelvic laparoscopic procedures. Possible reasons for lack of widespread use for LRC may be the inherent length of operative time, making hand assistance ergonomically more difficult. LRC is also technically quite challenging, being undertaken by laparoscopic surgeons with extensive experience with pure laparoscopic technique, who do not feel a distinct advantage for hand assistance.

Hand-assisted laparoscopic technique (HALRC) first was reported in 2002 [24], with two small case series appearing in the literature since then. McGinnis and colleagues [25] reported seven cases of HALRC with mean operative time of 7.6 hours, blood loss of 420 mL, and hospital stay of 4.6 days without reporting oncologic results. One open conversion was necessary for unresectable lymph nodes, and surgical margins were all negative. Taylor and colleagues [26] compared eight patients undergoing ORC with eight patients undergoing HALRC; all patients had ileal conduit urinary diversion. Patients in the HALRC group had less blood loss (637 versus 957 cc), less parenteral analgesia requirement, faster return of bowel function, and shorter hospital stay (6.4 versus 9 days). Operative time was not different. One rectal injury and one positive surgical margin were reported. All these studies taken together do not show a distinct advantage for HALRC over pure LRC.

Outcomes of laparoscopic radical cystectomy

LRC is a fairly new development in the field of surgery for bladder cancer, a field where long-term patient survival and tumor recurrence are the ultimate measures. As such, long-term studies of patient survival, let alone randomized studies comparing laparoscopic with open surgical cystectomy, are not available, although the authors are starting such a prospective randomized study. The literature contains retrospective series of laparoscopic cystectomy, mainly describing operative, perioperative, and pathological results. Of these, the authors present the results of the more mature experiences, disregarding initial experiences and case reports. The perioperative outcomes of these studies are detailed in Table 1.

Few studies compare LRC with ORC. A prospective nonrandomized study from Italy [28] compared 22 ORC patients with 20 LRC patients. One open conversion in the laparoscopic group was necessary, and mean lymph node count was 18.4 in the ORC group and 19.5 in the LRC group; there were no positive surgical margins in either group. Significantly decreased postoperative narcotics and shorter time to oral diet were noted. All other parameters including operative time, blood loss, transfusion rate, and hospital stay were equivalent.

A retrospective comparison of LRC (13 patients) versus ORC (11 patients) reported no difference in operating time, blood loss, or complication rates between the two procedures [27]. A surprising finding in this study was the mean blood loss of 1 L in the laparoscopic cases, much higher than most of the studies in the literature. Two of the LRC patients underwent elective open conversion because of large tumor size and previous pelvic surgery. LRC patients had a significantly less postoperative

Table 1
Operative results of laparoscopic radical cystectomy

Study	Number of patients	Diversion	Operating time (min)	Blood loss (mL)	Transfusion	Hospital stay	Complications
Basillote and colleagues [27]	13	15 cm Pfannenstiel; all ileal neobladder	480 + 77	1000 + 414	62%	5.1 + 1.2	Major 30%; minor 15%
Porpiglia and colleagues [28]	20	Extra	284	520	10%	18.1[a]	30%
Deger and colleagues [29]	20	Intra (Mainz II)	485	200	5%	15[a]	10% reoperation
Cathelineau and colleagues [30]	84 (40 prostate sparing)	Extra	280[b]	550[b]	5%	12[a]	18%
Castillo and colleagues [31]	59	Extra	337	488	20%	—	42%; 3.3% reoperation
Gerullis and colleagues [32]	34	Extra	244	325	5.9%	—	—
Huang and colleagues [33]	33	Extra	390	460	—	—	18%
Rassweiler and colleagues [34]	48	Intra and extra	352–649	—	—	13[a]	25%; 1 conversion
Sighinolfi and colleagues [35]	83	Extra	520	376	6%		2 open conversion

[a] European discharge times.
[b] Median not mean value.

narcotic requirement, earlier resumption of oral diet (2.8 versus 5 days), and shorter hospital stay (5.1 versus 8.4 days).

A single report described intermediate-term (less than 5 years) oncological outcomes [36]. Of 37 patients who had a median follow-up interval of 31 months, extending to 5 years, two patients had positive surgical margins and a mean lymph node count of 6 in early cases (11 patients), and 21 in later cases (26 patients). Surgical pathology showed tumor stage to be T1, T2a, T2b, T3a, T3b, and T4a in 29%, 11%, 22%, 11%, 16%, and 11% of patients, respectively. Although 11 patients (30% of the study) died of various noncancer-related causes (five unknown cases of death), no patient in the study had a local recurrence or a port site metastasis. Two patients developed distant metastatic disease and subsequently died. Ignoring the five unknown deaths resulted in a 5-year actuarial overall and cancer specific survival of 63% and 92%, assuming those five deaths were from cancer yielded 58% and 68% survival, respectively.

In two other studies with all margin-negative patients reporting oncological follow- up, 3 of 20 patients (15%) developed metastatic disease without local recurrence within a median follow-up period of 2.7 years [29]. A smaller study of 10 patients reported a 40% rate of distant metastases without local recurrence over a mean follow-up period of 5 years [37], although this was an initial experience study. It is also noteworthy that 70% of patients in this study had pT2b or higher disease, much higher than contemporary series (open or laparoscopic).

Summary

At experienced centers, LRC is emerging as a minimally invasive alternative to ORC, offering reduced blood loss, postoperative pain, and possibly recovery time. With careful patient selection, LRC achieves the surgical goals of wide excision, negative margins, and extended lymphadenectomy. Long-term oncologic data are awaited.

References

[1] Herr HW, Faulkner JR, Grossman HB, et al. Surgical factors influence bladder cancer outcomes: a cooperative group report. J Clin Oncol 2004; 22(14):2781–9.

[2] Puppo P, Perachino M, Ricciotti G, et al. Laparoscopically assisted transvaginal radical cystectomy. Eur Urol 1995;27(1):80–4.

[3] Parra RO, Andrus CH, Jones JP, et al. Laparoscopic cystectomy: initial report on a new treatment for the retained bladder. J Urol 1992;148(4):1140–4.

[4] Gill IS, Fergany A, Klein EA, et al. Laparoscopic radical cystoprostatectomy with ileal conduit performed completely intracorporeally: the initial 2 cases. Urology 2000;56(1):26–9.

[5] Denewer A, Kotb S, Hussein O, et al. Laparoscopic assisted cystectomy and lymphadenectomy for bladder cancer: initial experience. World J Surg 1999; 23(6):608–11.

[6] Turk I, Deger S, Winkelmann B, et al. Laparoscopic radical cystectomy with continent urinary diversion (rectal sigmoid pouch) performed completely intracorporeally: the initial 5 cases. J Urol 2001; 165(6 Pt 1):1863–6.

[7] Abdel-Hakim AM, Bassiouny F, Abdel Azim MS, et al. Laparoscopic radical cystectomy with orthotopic neobladder. J Endourol 2002;16(6):377–81.

[8] Moinzadeh A, Gill IS, Desai M, et al. Laparoscopic radical cystectomy in the female. J Urol 2005;173(6): 1912–7.

[9] Poulsen AL, Horn T, Steven K. Radical cystectomy: extending the limits of pelvic lymph node dissection improves survival for patients with bladder cancer confined to the bladder wall. J Urol 1998;160(6 Pt 1): 2015–9 [discussion: 2020].

[10] Herr HW, Bochner BH, Dalbagni G, et al. Impact of the number of lymph nodes retrieved on outcome in patients with muscle invasive bladder cancer. J Urol 2002;167(3):1295–8.

[11] Finelli A, Gill IS, Desai MM, et al. Laparoscopic extended pelvic lymphadenectomy for bladder cancer: technique and initial outcomes. J Urol 2004; 172(5 Pt 1):1809–12.

[12] Lane BR, Finelli A, Moinzadeh A, et al. Nerve-sparing laparoscopic radical cystectomy: technique and initial outcomes. Urology 2006;68(4):778–83.

[13] Arroyo C, Andrews H, Rozet F, et al. Laparoscopic prostate-sparing radical cystectomy: the Montsouris technique and preliminary results. J Endourol 2005; 19(3):424–8.

[14] Gill IS, Kaouk JH, Meraney AM, et al. Laparoscopic radical cystectomy and continent orthotopic ileal neobladder performed completely intracorporeally: the initial experience. J Urol 2002;168(1):13–8.

[15] Beecken WD, Wolfram M, Engl T, et al. Robotic-assisted laparoscopic radical cystectomy and intra-abdominal formation of an orthotopic ileal neobladder. Eur Urol 2003;44(3):337–9.

[16] Balaji KC, Yohannes P, McBride CL, et al. Feasibility of robot-assisted totally intracorporeal laparoscopic ileal conduit urinary diversion: initial results of a single institutional pilot study. Urology 2004;63(1):51–5.

[17] Haber G, Campbell S, Colombo J Jr, et al. Perioperative outcomes with laparoscopic radical cystectomy: pure laparoscopic and open assisted laparoscopic techniques 2007;70(5):910–5.

[18] Cathelineau X, Jaffe J. Laparoscopic radical cystectomy with urinary diversion: what is the optimal technique? Curr Opin Urol 2007;17(2):93–7.

[19] Menon M, Hemal AK, Tewari A, et al. Nerve-sparing robot-assisted radical cystoprostatectomy and urinary diversion. BJU Int 2003;92(3):232–6.

[20] Menon M, Hemal AK, Tewari A, et al. Robot-assisted radical cystectomy and urinary diversion in female patients: technique with preservation of the uterus and vagina. J Am Coll Surg 2004;198(3):386–93.

[21] El-Tabey NA, Shoma AM. Port site metastases after robot-assisted laparoscopic radical cystectomy. Urology 2005;66(5):1110.

[22] Pruthi RS, Wallen EM. Robotic-assisted laparoscopic radical cystoprostatectomy: operative and pathological outcomes. J Urol 2007;178(3 Pt 1): 814–8.

[23] Wang GJ, Barocas DA, Raman JD, et al. Robotic vs open radical cystectomy: prospective comparison of perioperative outcomes and pathological measures of early oncological efficacy. BJU Int 2008;101(1): 89–93.

[24] Peterson AC, Lance RS, Ahuja S. Laparoscopic hand-assisted radical cystectomy with ileal conduit urinary diversion. J Urol 2002;168(5): 2103–5 [discussion: 2105].

[25] McGinnis DE, Hubosky SG, Bergmann LS. Hand-assisted laparoscopic cystoprostatectomy and urinary diversion. J Endourol 2004;18(4):383–6.

[26] Taylor GD, Duchene DA, Koeneman KS. Hand-assisted laparoscopic cystectomy with minilaparotomy ileal conduit: series report and comparison with open cystectomy. J Urol 2004; 172(4 Pt 1):1291–6.

[27] Basillote JB, Abdelshehid C, Ahlering TE, et al. Laparoscopic-assisted radical cystectomy with ileal neobladder: a comparison with the open approach. J Urol 2004;172(2):489–93.

[28] Porpiglia F, Renard J, Billia M, et al. Open versus laparoscopy-assisted radical cystectomy: results of a prospective study. J Endourol 2007;21(3):325–9.

[29] DeGer S, Peters R, Roigas J, et al. Laparoscopic radical cystectomy with continent urinary diversion (rectosigmoid pouch) performed completely intracorporeally: an intermediate functional and oncologic analysis. Urology 2004;64(5):935–9.

[30] Cathelineau X, Arroyo C, Rozet F, et al. Laparoscopic-assisted radical cystectomy: the Montsouris experience after 84 cases. Eur Urol 2005;47(6): 780–4 [Epub 2005 Apr 11].

[31] Castillo OA, Abreu SC, Mariano MB, et al. Complications in laparoscopic radical cystectomy. The South American experience with 59 cases. Int Braz J Urol 2006;32(3):300–5.

[32] Gerullis H, Kuemmel C, Popken G. Laparoscopic cystectomy with extracorporeal-assisted urinary diversion: experience with 34 patients. Eur Urol 2007;51(1):193–8.

[33] Huang J, Xu KW, Yao YS, et al. Laparoscopic radical cystectomy with orthotopic ileal neobladder: report of 33 cases. Chin Med J (Engl) 2005;118(1):27–33.

[34] Rassweiler J, Frede T, Teber D, et al. Laparoscopic radical cystectomy with and without orthotopic bladder replacement. Minim Invasive Ther Allied Technol 2005;14(2):78–95.

[35] Sighinolfi MC, Micali S, Celia A, et al. Laparoscopic radical cystectomy: an Italian survey. Surg Endosc 2007;21(8):1308–11.

[36] Haber GP, Gill IS. Laparoscopic radical cystectomy for cancer: oncological outcomes at up to 5 years. BJU Int 2007;100(1):137–42.

[37] Simonato A, Gregori A, Lissiani A, et al. Laparoscopic radical cystoprostatectomy: our experience in a consecutive series of 10 patients with a 3 years follow-up. Eur Urol 2005;47(6):785–90 [discussion: 790–2].

ELSEVIER
SAUNDERS

Urol Clin N Am 35 (2008) 467–476

UROLOGIC
CLINICS
of North America

Minimally Invasive Treatment of Stress Urinary Incontinence and Vaginal Prolapse

Elizabeth B. Takacs, MD[a],*, Kathleen C. Kobashi, MD[b]

[a]Department of Urology, University of Iowa, 200 Hawkins Drive, 3 RCP, Iowa City, IA 52242–1089, USA
[b]Section of Urology and Renal Transplantation, Virginia Mason Medical Center,
1100 Ninth Avenue, Seattle, WA 98111, USA

Disorders of the female pelvic floor, specifically stress urinary incontinence (SUI) and pelvic organ prolapse (POP), are prevalent among women of all ages. Numerous challenges await those who evaluate and treat these particular disorders, however. First, the risk factors for prolapse and incontinence are poorly understood, making it difficult to implement preventive measures. Second, there is no clear definition or agreement on what defines clinically significant prolapse. Objective measures of treatment are variable, and the definitions of success or failure of treatment options are vague. It has also been well established that discrepancies between subjective and objective outcome measures are not uncommon. Finally, we are hindered by the fact that much of the available literature is limited in length of follow-up and cohort size. These are important issues to recognize as we review the current literature.

The estimated lifetime risk for undergoing corrective surgery for POP is 11% [1,2]. This estimate is based on hospital admission and surgical codes data and likely underestimates the overall prevalence of SUI and POP in the general population. Two studies examined data on POP from the large multi-institutional Women's Health Initiative Hormone Replacement Therapy Clinical Trial. Hendrix and colleagues [3] presented the baseline data from the 27,342 patients enrolled. On visual inspection alone during the Valsalva maneuver, 41.1% of patients with an intact uterus had some degree of descent versus 38% of patients who had undergone a hysterectomy. In an ancillary study, Nygaard and colleagues [4] examined the rate of prolapse in women with an intact uterus. The mean age of the 270 participants was 68.3 years, and 65.5% were found to have stage 2 (leading edge within 1 cm proximal to hymen) or greater prolapse based on the standardized pelvic organ position quantification description (POP-Q [5]) examination. If the definition of prolapse was further narrowed to the leading edge at or beyond the hymen, 25.2% were defined as having prolapse.

In the past 10 years there has been significant evolution in the treatment of SUI and POP. The laparoscopic retropubic urethropexy was first introduced in 1991 [6] but was abandoned because of several small studies reporting lower cure rates. The next major stride in minimally invasive treatment of SUI occurred in 1996 with the introduction of the tension-free vaginal tape (TVT) [7]. This sling has been a significant impetus for the development of the vaginal mesh "kits" that are now available for treatment of SUI and POP. Attributable in great part to the simplicity of these techniques, the number of pelvic reconstructive cases performed per annum has increased significantly over the past decade.

In an effort to incorporate minimally invasive techniques in POP treatment, laparoscopic and robotic approaches have been applied to several transabdominal surgical techniques. The often-cited advantages of laparoscopic and robotic surgery include improved visualization because of magnification and insufflation, better cosmesis and hemostasis, shorter hospital stay and less postoperative pain with an overall more rapid

---

* Corresponding author.
  E-mail address: elizabeth-takacs@uiowa.edu
(E.B. Takacs).

recovery relative to corresponding open approaches. The disadvantages of minimally invasive techniques are the long "learning curve," the potentially increased difficulty of the retroperitoneal dissection, and the potential increase in hospital costs. It is likely that with the increased application of robotics and laparoscopy, the learning curve is eventually likely to become a less significant barrier.

Only recently have well-designed trials with longer term and appropriate minimum follow-up (1–2 years) begun to appear in the literature. The aim of this article is to review the laparoscopic and robotic techniques that have been described for treatment of POP and SUI and to present the longer term results available to date. Although considered by many to be "minimally invasive," the transvaginal techniques are not covered in this article.

Operative indications and anatomy

The indications for a laparoscopic or robotic approach to surgery for POP or SUI are identical to those for the open abdominal and vaginal routes. Repairs are reserved for those patients who are symptomatic from the prolapse. Symptoms may vary from patient to patient. The obvious bulge protruding from the vagina creating significant discomfort for the patient provides a clear indication for repair. More subtle findings of lower degrees of prolapse with variable associated voiding symptoms may require more contemplation.

The decision between a vaginal, abdominal, or laparoscopic or robotic approach depends on surgeon experience and patient preference. Other factors, such as prior prolapse repairs or anti-incontinence surgery, prior abdominal procedures, vaginal caliber and length in addition to age, weight, comorbidities, and ability to tolerate general anesthetic, are all important considerations for a laparoscopic or robotic approach.

The endopelvic fascia contributes to the integrity of the vaginal wall—anteriorly, the endopelvic fascia is referred to as the pubocervical fascia, and, posteriorly, the rectovaginal fascia. DeLancey [8] described three levels of support to the vagina and pelvic structures based on suspension, attachment, and fusion of the pelvic tissues at the corresponding levels (Fig. 1; Table 1). POP represents a break in the continuity of the endopelvic fascia or loss of the corresponding

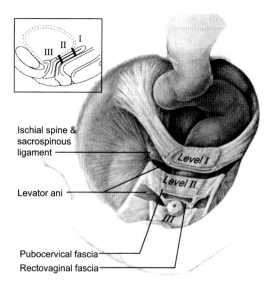

Fig. 1. Three levels of support to the vagina and pelvic structures based on suspension, attachment, and fusion of the pelvic tissues at the corresponding levels described by DeLancey.

suspension, attachment, or fusion. Pelvic reconstructive surgery aims to re-establish and correct the defects to restore normal anatomy and visceral (bowel and bladder) and sexual function.

With any surgical procedure (open, laparoscopic, or robotic), there are important anatomic landmarks with which the surgeon must be familiar. Pertinent landmarks are discussed as the various approaches to pelvic floor reconstruction are reviewed.

Laparoscopic surgery for stress urinary incontinence: procedure and results

In 2004, the Third International Consultation on Incontinence reported that level 1 evidence to support the use of open Burch colpopexy for the treatment of SUI exists; however, data for laparoscopic colposuspension were insufficient, and no recommendations could be made regarding its use [9]. Conversely, the 2005 Cochrane review reported that laparoscopic colposuspension provided benefits, such as more rapid recovery, but that long-term efficacy is unknown [10].

In 2006, two randomized trials of open versus laparoscopic Burch colposuspension with a minimum follow-up of 24 months suggested similar outcomes between the two procedures. Kitchener and colleagues [11] reported a 2-year objective

Table 1
Supportive structures of the vaginal levels as described after hysterectomy by DeLancey and resulting POP when the support fails or is deficient

	Technique	Support mechanism	Supported structure	Result of support failure
Level I	Suspension	Cardinal/uterosacral complex	Uterus Proximal one fourth of the vagina (vault/apex)	Uterine descensus Vaginal vault (apical) prolapse
Level II	Attachment	Lateral attachment of the pubocervical and rectovaginal endopelvic fascia to the ATFP	Middle half of vagina Bladder, bladder neck Proximal rectum	Cystocele Urethral hypermobility Rectocele
Level III	Fusion	Fusion to the perineal body	Distal one fourth of the vagina	Distal rectocele Perineal descent

Abbreviation: ATFP, arcus tendineus fasciae pelvis.
Data from DeLancey JO. Anatomic aspects of vaginal eversion after hysterectomy. Am J Obstet Gynecol 1992;166:1717–24.

cure rate (<1 g on pad test) of 79.7% in the laparoscopic group versus 70.1% for the open group. Similar subjective data (never or <1 incontinent episode per month) of 55.4% versus 53.1%, respectively, were also demonstrated. Carey and colleagues [12] reported subjective (no incontinence) results at 24 months of follow-up for all subjects of 63% and 70% for laparoscopic versus open approaches, respectively. With an intent-to-treat analysis, the success rates decreased to 61% and 50%, respectively, but this did not represent a statistically significantly difference. Neither study commented on the development of POP after surgery.

These data suggest that when performed in a fashion similar to the open procedure, the laparoscopic Burch colposuspension may be comparable to open surgery. Together with the data supporting the use of the laparoscopic Burch colposuspension at the time of sacrocolpopexy for patients without symptoms of SUI [13], there may still be a role for the laparoscopic Burch colposuspension in conjunction with other laparoscopic or robotic procedures.

Laparoscopic and robotic procedures for treatment of pelvic organ prolapse: anatomy and procedures

Anterior prolapse

The fact that a single surgical technique has not been readily accepted for treating cystoceles suggests a complexity of the condition beyond current understanding. Anterior colporrhaphy has long been the primary approach to correction of cystoceles despite reported failure rates of 40% to 70% [14,15]. This emphasizes the fact that several different defects can result in a cystocele, and, accordingly, the defect specific to a given patient needs to be identified and corrected.

In 1909, White [16] described the lateral detachment of the endopelvic fascia from the arcus tendineus fasciae pelvis (ATFP) as a cause for anterior compartment prolapse and a transvaginal approach for repair. A corresponding abdominal paravaginal repair was described in 1976 [17] and has been replicated laparoscopically [18].

The anatomic landmarks for a paravaginal repair are similar to those used for a Burch retropubic urethropexy. The space of Retzius is developed to identify the lateral detachment of the endopelvic fascia from the ATFP. Key structures include Cooper's ligaments, accessory or aberrant obturator veins, obturator neurovascular bundles that lie 3 to 4 cm anterior to the ATFP, the bladder neck, the ATFP itself, and the arcus tendineus levator ani.

In a laparoscopic transperitoneal approach, the bladder must first be mobilized. After filling the bladder for identification, a transverse incision 2 cm cephalad to the bladder reflection is made between the medial umbilical folds. Dissection is performed through the loose areolar tissue in an infralateral direction, moving toward the posterior-superior aspect of the pubic symphysis until Cooper's ligaments, the bladder neck, the obturator internus muscle and foramen, and the ATFP are identified. A vaginal manipulator (finger) helps to identify the torn edges of the pubocervical fascia from the ATFP. This paravaginal defect is closed with a series of nonabsorbable sutures starting distally, alternating sides. The most distal sutures (generally three sutures) incorporate vaginal tissue and the obturator internus and iliopectineal ligaments, whereas the most proximal suture only incorporates vaginal tissue and the iliopectineal ligament. The sutures are then tied without tension. If there is concern that significant urethral hypermobility is contributing to the SUI, the sutures may be tied more tightly [19]. Further level I defects require correction with hysteropexy or colpopexy. Cystoscopy is performed to confirm ureteral patency.

Posterior prolapse

Most surgeons prefer a transvaginal route for rectocele repair [20]; however, a laparoscopic approach has been described. The important landmarks for the abdominal approach include the rectovaginal septum, its lateral attachments to the medial aspect of the levator ani muscles, and the perineal body. During the procedure, the rectovaginal space is developed to the level of the rectovaginal septum. The perineal body is secured to the rectovaginal septum, and the rectovaginal fascial defects are closed with nonabsorbable sutures. In addition, the iliococcygeus and rectovaginal fascia can be reapproximated, and a levator ani placation can be performed if needed.

Apical prolapse

Identification and treatment of apical descent is fundamental to the success of pelvic floor reconstruction. Apical repair involves obliteration of the defect responsible for re-establishment of apical support.

Culdoplasty

Laparoscopic Moschowitz and Halban procedures are performed in a manner identical to the open abdominal repairs using nonabsorbable sutures to obliterate the cul-de-sac. In the Moschowitz procedure, the suture is placed in a purse-string fashion circumferentially around the cul-de-sac, whereas the Halban procedure uses sutures placed longitudinally incorporating the sigmoid serosa, the peritoneum of the cul-de-sac, and the posterior vagina. Cystoscopy should be performed after intravenous administration of indigo carmine or methylene blue to confirm ureteral integrity,

keeping in mind that the risk for ureteral kinking is reportedly greater with the Moschowitz procedure [21]. Cadeddu and colleagues [22] described a modified Moschowitz procedure in which the posterior vaginal fascia is reapproximated with the anterior wall of the rectum.

Enterocele excision and closure

During a laparoscopic enterocele repair, the enterocele sac is dissected laparoscopically or vaginally with identification of defects of the endopelvic fascia, pubocervical fascia, and rectovaginal fascia. For large enteroceles, a transvaginal approach is used to excise the redundant peritoneum and vagina, with care taken to avoid foreshortening or narrowing of the vagina. The vaginal apex and rectum can be delineated during laparoscopic dissection by intravaginal placement of an obturator, sponge-stick, or equivalent vaginal manipulator. A nonabsorbable suture placed in an interrupted fashion is then used to reapproximate the pubocervical and rectovaginal fascial edges until the defect is closed. Koninckx and colleagues [23] described vaporization of the enterocele sac with the carbon dioxide laser. Enterocele closure and excision performed concomitantly with uterosacral ligament suspension re-establishes support of the vaginal apex.

Uterosacral ligament suspension

The uterosacral ligaments have been used as supporting structures to re-establish level I support to the vaginal apex or uterus. Important anatomic landmarks in the laparoscopic uterosacral ligament vaginal vault suspension (LUSVS) or laparoscopic uterosacral ligament uterine vault suspension suspension (LUSUS) include the pubocervical and rectovaginal fascias, the uterosacral ligament, and the ureters. The ureters are in close proximity (1–1.5 cm lateral) to the uterosacral ligament as it courses beneath the uterine artery.

For the LUSVS, the uterosacral ligament at the proximal portion of its break is sutured with a nonabsorbable suture to the vaginal apex. The apical stitch is placed through the full thickness of the uterosacral and cardinal ligament complex and the rectovaginal fascia, excluding the vaginal epithelium. Additional sutures are placed more proximally on the uterosacral ligaments for support of the rectovaginal fascia. If a concomitant enterocele repair is planned, the uterosacral ligaments are identified and tagged before dissection of the posterior vagina [24]. Ross [25] described an apical repair that brought the rectovaginal septum and uterosacral and cardinal ligaments together with the use of purse-string sutures and plication of the uterosacral ligaments. In that procedure, the peritoneum is dissected free from the vaginal apex and pubocervical fascia. A series of nonabsorbable sutures are placed in a purse-string fashion incorporating the left and right uterosacral and cardinal ligaments, the rectovaginal septum, and the posterior vaginal wall. The first sutures are placed in the uterosacral ligament 3 to 4 cm proximal to the vaginal apex; subsequent sutures are placed until the vaginal apex is reached, with the final suture incorporating the pubocervical fascia.

Several researchers have described the LUSUS with minor differences in techniques. The basic principle involves placement of a nonabsorbable suture full thickness through the uterosacral ligament at the level of the ischial spine and then again at its insertion at the lower uterine segment to create shortening of the ligament [26,27].

Sacrocolpopexy

(Movie 1: Robotic assisted laparoscopic sacrocolpopexy*) Laparoscopic and robotic sacrocolpopexy (L/RSCP) procedures have been described with the goal of replicating the open surgical technique. Important anatomic landmarks at the sacrum include the middle sacral artery and vein and the anterior longitudinal ligament on the sacral promontory. The aortic bifurcation and vena cava lie superiorly at L4 to L5. Along the lateral margins of the presacral space are the iliac vessels and ureters bilaterally and the sigmoid colon, which is reflected to the left.

Final port placement configuration between the laparoscopic and robotic approaches is similar. For the laparoscopic approach, primary ports include an intraumbilical port and then a 10- to 12-mm port in each lower quadrant. One to two ancillary 5-mm ports may be placed at the level of the umbilicus lateral to the rectus muscle. For the robotic approach, the primary 12-mm port is placed at the inferior umbilical crease and two lateral 8-mm ports are then placed just below the level of the umbilicus and lateral to the rectus muscle. Two additional assistant ports are then placed in the lower quadrants.

Once port placement is complete and the robot, when employed, is docked, a vaginal

obturator is used to delineate the vaginal apex. The peritoneum overlying the apex is dissected off the vagina, and the incision of the posterior peritoneum is extended cephalad toward the sacral promontory.

Exposure of the presacral space and sacral promontory can be facilitated by "airplaning" the patient to the left and using a "snake" retractor. For improved exposure, retraction of the sigmoid can be facilitated using a figure-of-eight silk suture placed through the tenia coli and exiting percutaneously. The incision in the peritoneum overlying the sacral promontory is continued longitudinally extending through the cul-de-sac, and the presacral fat is cleared to expose the sacral periosteum. Hemostasis can be achieved by coagulation or clip placement. A Y-shaped synthetic mesh or biologic graft is secured to the vagina with nonabsorbable sutures placed through the full thickness of the vaginal wall. The mesh is secured to the sacral promontory with two nonabsorbable sutures preplaced into the anterior spinous ligament or by means of sutures attached to titanium bone anchors. The mesh should be placed without tension to support the vagina in an anatomic position. Redundant mesh is excised, and the posterior peritoneum is reapproximated over the mesh. If the mesh cannot be completely retroperitonealized, sigmoid epiploic fat can be used to cover it.

In the presence of a uterus, sacrohysteropexy can be performed for uterine preservation. This involves dissecting the rectovaginal space for approximately one third of the length of the posterior vaginal wall. The mesh or biologic graft is secured in several rows along the rectovaginal fascia and posterior cervix to the level of the internal os. Peritoneal closure is then performed.

Surgeon preference and anatomic detail should dictate the use of concomitant procedures. In the presence of a deep cul-de-sac, a Halban or Moschcowitz "culdeplasty" may be used. Urethral hypermobility is addressed with laparoscopic Burch or paravaginal repair. In the presence of rectal prolapse, rectopexy with or without the assistance of a colorectal surgeon can be performed.

Laparoscopic and robotic procedures for treatment of pelvic organ prolapse: results

Assessment of pelvic floor reconstructive techniques is challenging. As mentioned previously, objective measures of surgical treatment options are variable, the definition of success or failure is vague, and discrepancies between subjective and

---

* Videos for this article can be accessed by visiting www.urologic.theclinics.com. In the online table of contents for this issue, click on "add-ons."

objective outcome measures are frequently encountered. Long-term pelvic floor reconstructive data are also limited, and correction of pelvic floor defects often entails a combination of procedures, making assessment of any single procedure more challenging. With these limitations in mind, the data that are available with emphasis on series with a minimum follow-up of 12 months are reviewed.

Anterior repairs

Ostrzenski [28] prospectively evaluated the effectiveness of an isolated laparoscopic paravaginal repair for SUI and found an objective and subjective cure rate of 93%. Mean operative time was 165 minutes with no major perioperative complications reported.

Behnia-Willison and colleagues [19] reported on 212 patients who had POP and were treated with bilateral laparoscopic paravaginal repair with or without concomitant level I or posterior repair at a mean follow-up of 14.2 months. Of the 212 patients, 84 (39.6%) had a concomitant central defect that was not repaired at the initial surgery. Based on the presence of paravaginal sulci, only 3 patients had failure. Objective cure, defined as stage 0 or 1 on POP-Q examination, was achieved in 76.4% of patients. Twenty-three of the 40 failures occurred in the anterior compartment of patients with combined central and lateral defects. This article provides evidence that the laparoscopic paravaginal repair can recreate the lateral vaginal sulcus and, in some patients with a combined anterior defect, provide adequate support for improvement in stage. Operative time varied from 55 to 255 minutes but included concomitant procedures. These investigators reported a major complication rate (bowel, ureter, or bladder injury; anesthetic complication; unintended laparotomy; or blood loss >1 L) of 4.2%.

Posterior repairs

The vaginal approach to rectocele repair is often the preferred route of correction. with reported success rates of 76% to 96% and, importantly, low rates of complications [29]. There are limited reports on the success of isolated laparoscopic posterior repair. Lyons and Winer [30] reported that in 20 patients undergoing laparoscopic rectocele repair with polyglactin mesh with or without concomitant hysterectomy, 80% had resolution of symptoms at 1 year of follow-up.

Apical repairs

Three recent series have examined the results of LUSUS or LUVSV for apical repair. Diwan and colleagues [26] reported the results of LUSUS versus total vaginal hysterectomy (TVH) for correction of uterine prolapse with less than 1 year of follow-up. Patients who had a TVH had a concomitant McCall's culdoplasty, sacrospinous ligament suspension, or laparoscopic uterosacral ligament suspension. POP quantification of the apical data points revealed the LUSUS point D (−9 cm) compared with the TVH point C (−7.6 cm). Overall, one apical recurrence was reported in the LUSUS group compared with five in the TVH cohort. Schwartz and colleagues [24] reported statistically significant improvement in the sum of POP-Q values in 72 patients who had undergone LUSUS or LUSVS at less than 1 year of follow-up. The only series to report a mean follow-up greater than 12 months was that of Medina and Takacs [27]. In this series with a mean follow-up of 15.9 months (range: 6–40 months), LUSUS resulted in statistically significant improvement in points C and D. No major intraoperative complications were reported. These studies support LUSUS or LUVSV as a viable option for recreating level I support; however, longer follow-up is pending.

In a comprehensive review of the abdominal sacrocolpopexy, a 78% to 100% success rate was achieved when defined as no apical recurrence, and this decreased to 58% to 100% when success was defined as no postoperative prolapse [31]. The Third International Consultation on Incontinence (ICI) issued a grade A recommendation that sacrocolpopexy-based abdominal POP surgery is likely to result in a better and possibly more durable anatomic outcome than sacrospinous-based vaginal approaches but is limited by the increase in short-term morbidity [32]. This has naturally encouraged progression of laparoscopic and robotic approaches. The question is whether or not the long-term success of the open procedures transfers to the minimally invasive techniques in terms of efficacy, comparable operative time, decreased hospital stay, and no increase in complications.

Operative outcomes

Paraiso and colleagues [33] published a comparison of the first 56 laparoscopic sacrocolpopexies (LSCPs) to 61 open sacrocolpopexies (SCPs) completed during the same period with mean follow-ups of 14 and 16 months, respectively. Mean operative time was significantly longer for the LSCP (269 versus 218 minutes), but the hospital stay was significantly shorter (1.8 versus 4 days). There were no differences in clinical outcomes and reoperation rates. This is the only report available that compares open and laparoscopic techniques.

Other long-term reports continue to support the feasibility and efficacy of the LSCP (Table 2). Higgs and colleagues [34] evaluated 103 of 140 patients who had undergone LSCP. Sixty-six patients underwent repeat physical examination, and 103 responded to questionnaires. Median follow-up was 66 months, but all follow-ups were at least 36 months from surgery. Median surgery duration for all procedures was 145 minutes; surgical time was 107 minutes for those who underwent LSCP alone. Of the 103 patients evaluated, 4 had intraoperative complications (two bladder injuries, two bowel injuries). Mesh erosion rates were reported as 20% when placed through a transvaginal route and as 6% when placed laparoscopically. Subjectively, 71% of patients were very or quite satisfied with the procedure. The reoperation rate was 16% for all prolapses. On physical examination, 62% had stage 0 or 1 prolapse, 32% had stage 2 (10% apical), and 6% had stage 3. During a follow-up period of 5 years, Ross and Preston [35] analyzed 51 cases of LSCP for grade III and IV apical prolapse and reported a 93% cure rate.

With increasing documentation of the technical feasibility of LSCP and its comparable outcomes to open SCP, more attention is being drawn to the surgical techniques of LSCP and concomitant procedures. Antiphon and colleagues [36] sought to answer the question of whether the posterior limb of support is necessary when there is no evidence of posterior prolapse. A single anterior mesh (SAM) was placed in 31 patients and a double-mesh (DM), with mesh placed both anteriorly and posteriorly, was placed in 71 patients. Mean follow-up times were 16 and 17 months, respectively. A global failure rate of a Baden-Walker grade II or greater prolapse for any compartment was 25%, with 43.8% versus 16.2%, respectively, in the SAM versus DM groups. Furthermore, these investigators found that in patients who had undergone a prior or concomitant Burch procedure, the failure rate was statistically significantly higher in the patients in whom mesh was placed anteriorly (SAM [55%]) versus those in whom the mesh was placed anteriorly and posteriorly (DM [12.5%]). The final conclusion was that posterior mesh should be reserved for patients who have a documented rectocele or enterocele, or when associated with a Burch procedure.

In a second study, DM was placed uniformly in all patients with variability of the anti-incontinence procedure performed [37]. Overall, LSCP was completed successfully in 41 (86%) of 46 patients; 32% had LSCP alone, 36% had a concomitant laparoscopic Burch procedure, and 32% had concomitant TVT. The median follow-up was 24 months, with a 12-month minimum. The mean operative time was 206 minutes overall and 171 minutes for LSCP alone. The mean postoperative stay was 4 days overall and 3.1 days for LSCP alone. There were three intraoperative bladder injuries and one postoperative fever. Objective cure of Baden-Walker grade 0 or 1 was achieved in 83% of patients; 5 patients had recurrence of rectocele, all of whom had had a concomitant laparoscopic Burch procedure. In this study, despite placement of a posterior limb, Burch urethropexy was a risk for recurrent rectocele formation. Both studies together raise the question of whether a concomitant Burch urethropexy should be performed.

The overall complication rate for LSCP is low according to the available studies. The incidence of small bowel obstruction was 1%, and the rate of mesh erosion was 3.7% (see Table 2). Both rates are similar to those reported for open sacrocolpopexy at 1.1% and 3.4%, respectively [31].

Recently, initial reports on robotic sacrocolpopexy (RSCP) have begun to appear. In 2005, Ayav and colleagues [38] published a small case series of 18 consecutive patients who underwent RSCP (n = 12) or rectopexy (n = 6). Mean setup time (wrapping and positioning the robot and ports) was 30 minutes, and mean operative time was 170 minutes. All procedures were successfully completed, and the only reported complication was in the rectopexy group, in which one patient had a rectal tear. At 12 months of follow-up, no patient had evidence of POP. A case series from the Cleveland Clinic evaluated the use of robotic abdominal sacrocolpopexy or sacrouteropexy for stage III and IV POP [39]. The follow-up is short, with a mean of 3.1 months, but all POP-Q points demonstrated improvement. The surgery was completed successfully in 12 of the 15 patients, with a mean estimated blood loss (EBL) of 81 mL, hospital stay of 2.4 days, and operative time of 317 minutes. Elliott and colleagues [40] evaluated 21 patients who had undergone RSCP with a minimum of 12 months of follow-up and

Table 2
Summary of the perioperative and complication data for laparoscopic sacrocolpopexy and robotic sacrocolpopexy available in the literature

Authors	Procedure	N	Follow-up (months)	OR time (minutes)	EBL (cm³)	Hospital stay (days)	Conversion to open	Complications
Paraiso et al [33]	LSCP	56	13.5 (1–46)	269 ± 65 (150–467)	172 ± 166 (0–1100)	1.8 ± 1.0 (1–6)	1 (1.7%) Excessive bleeding during rectopexy	Bladder injury/suture, 6 (10.7%) Enterotomy, 1 (1.8%) SBO, 1 (1.8%) Mesh erosion, 2 (3.6%)
Higgs et al [34]	LSCP	140	66 (37–124) Median	145 (95–265)	—	3.8 (2–12)	1 (0.7%) Bladder perforation	Cystotomy, 2 (1.4%) Enterotomy, 2 (1.4%) Mesh erosion, 9 (9%)
Ross and Preston [35]	LSCP portion	—	—	107 (62–170)	—	—	—	No intraoperative complications
	LSCP	51	5 years	—	—	—	—	SBO, 2 (4%)
Antiphon et al [36]	LSCP portion	—	—	96 ± 42	100 ± 20	—	—	Mesh erosion, 4 (8%)
	LSCP	108	17 ± 16 (1–68)	261 ± 79 (120–450)	—	7 ± 4 (2–32)	3 (2.8%) Obesity factor	Bladder injury, 3 (2.8%) Reoperation, 4 (7.4%)
	SAM	33	16 ± 18	261 ± 120 (120–450)	—	—	—	1: SB injury
	DM	71	17 ± 19	261 ± 69 (130–430)	—	—	—	1: SB ischemia 1: SBO 1: Intervertebral disc infection
Gadonneix et al [37]	LSCP	46	24 (12–60) Median	206 ± 56 (105–360)	—	4.0 ± 2.1	5 (11%) 1: Hypercapnia 4: Difficult promontory	Bladder injury, 3 (7%)
Ayav [38]	LCSP portion	—	—	171 ± 37 (105–225)	—	—	—	—
	RSCP	12	—	170 (74–280)	—	7 (4–13)	0	—
Dangeshgari et al [39]	RSCP	15	3.1 (3–8)	317 (258–363)	81 (50–150)	2.4 (1–7)	3 (20%)	Serosal injury, 1 (6.6%) Wound infection, 0 (0%)
Elliott et al [40]	RSCP	30	—	186 (2.15–4.75 hours)	—	—	1 (3.3%) Bladder adhesions	Mesh erosion, 2 (6.6%)

Abbreviations: EBL, estimated blood loss; OR, operating room; RSCP, robotic sacrocolpopexy; SB, small bowel; SBO, small bowel obstruction.

a mean of 24 months. In this study, all patients had a preoperative Baden-Walker grade 4 apical prolapse. Mean total operative time was 186 minutes; however, with experience, these investigators report routinely completing the procedure in 150 minutes. All but 1 patient were discharged on the first postoperative day. Complications included one conversion to an open procedure for anatomic reasons, port site infections, and one postoperative vaginal bleed related to the anti-incontinence procedure. Two patients (10%) developed a small vaginal extrusion of the mesh at the vaginal cuff. Overall, 18 of 20 patients in whom the RSCP was successfully completed had no evidence of recurrent prolapse: 1 patient had recurrent vault prolapse, and 1 patient developed a grade 3/4 rectocele.

Summary

POP and SUI are prevalent conditions that have been approached using a variety of surgical techniques, with more than 40 procedures described for correction of POP alone [20]. There remain many unanswered questions regarding the optimal management of POP. Whether or not a graft should be used, whether that graft should be a biograft or synthetic mesh, and whether minimally invasive techniques can achieve outcomes similar to those of open approaches remain topics of debate and discussion. How to measure anatomic outcome most accurately and what other parameters should be assessed remain active considerations within the subspecialty as well.

In 2005, the World Health Organization (WHO) Third ICI Committee on Surgery for POP reported three conclusions based on level 1 evidence: (1) overall outcomes indicate that abdominal and vaginal surgery are relatively equivalent; (2) sacrospinous-based vaginal procedures have a higher anterior and apical anatomic recurrence rate than SCP-based abdominal repairs; and (3) abdominal surgery has greater morbidity, at least in the short-term [32]. Many clinicians have started to apply laparoscopy and robotics to pelvic floor reconstruction in the hopes of capitalizing on the advantages of minimally invasive surgery. Properly conducted randomized prospective studies are needed to definitively establish the advantages of minimally invasive pelvic floor surgery.

References

[1] Olsen A, Smith VA, Bergstrom JO, et al. Epidemiology of surgically managed pelvic organ prolapse and urinary incontinence. Obstet Gynecol 1997;89: 501–6.

[2] Fialkow MF, Newton KM, Lentz GM, et al. Lifetime risk of surgical management for pelvic organ prolapse or urinary incontinence. Int Urogynecol J Pelvic Floor Dysfunct 2008;19:437–40.

[3] Hendrix SL, Clark AC, Nygaard I, et al. Pelvic organ prolapse in the women's health initiative: gravity and gravidity. Am J Obstet Gynecol 2002;186: 1160–6.

[4] Nygaard I, Bradley C, Brandt D. Pelvic organ prolapse in older women: prevalence and risk factors. Obstet Gynecol 2004;104:489–97.

[5] Bump RC, Mattiasson A, Bøo K, et al. The standardization of terminology of female pelvic organ prolapse and pelvic floor dysfunction. Am J Obstet Gynecol 1996;175:10–7.

[6] Vancaillie TG, Schuessler W. Laparoscopic bladderneck suspension. J Laparoendosc Surg 1991;1:169–73.

[7] Ulmsten U, Henriksson L, Johnson P, et al. An ambulatory surgical procedure under local anesthesia for treatment of female urinary incontinence. Int Urogynecol J Pelvic Floor Dysfunct 1996;7:81–6.

[8] DeLancey JO. Anatomic aspects of vaginal eversion after hysterectomy. Am J Obstet Gynecol 1992;166: 1717–24.

[9] Smith ARB, Daneshgari F, Dmochowski R, et al. Surgery for urinary incontinence in women. In: Abrams P, Cardozo L, Khoury S, et al, editors. Incontinence, Management. Third International Consultation on Incontinence. vol. 2, Monaco: International Continence Society; 2005. p. 1297–370, chap 20.

[10] Lapitan MC, Cody DJ, Grant AM. Open retropubic colposuspension for urinary incontinence in women. Cochrane Database Syst Rev 2005 Jul 20;(3): CD002912.

[11] Kitchener HC, Dunn G, Lawton V, et al. Laparoscopic versus open colposuspension—results of a prospective randomised controlled trial. BJOG 2006;113:1007–13.

[12] Carey MP, Goh JT, Rosamilia A, et al. Laparoscopic versus open Burch colposuspension: a randomised controlled trial. BJOG 2006;113:999–1006.

[13] Brubaker L, Cundiff GW, Fine P, et al. Abdominal sacrocolpopexy with Burch colposuspension to reduce urinary stress incontinence. N Engl J Med 2006;354:1557–66.

[14] Sand PK, Koduri S, Lobel RW, et al. Prospective randomized trial of polyglactin 910 mesh to prevent recurrence of cystoceles and rectoceles. Am J Obstet Gynecol 2001;184:1357–64.

[15] Weber AM, Walters MD, Piedmonte MR, et al. Anterior colporrhaphy: a randomized trial of three surgical techniques. Am J Obstet Gynecol 2001; 185:1299–306.

[16] White GR. Cystocele: a radical cure by suturing lateral sulci of vagina to white line of fascia. J Am Med Assoc 1909;53:1707–10.

[17] Richardson AC, Saye WB, Miklos JR. Repairing paravaginal defects laparoscopically. Contemp Ob Gyn 1997;42:125–31.

[18] Margossian H, Walters MD, Falcone T. Laparoscopic management of pelvic organ prolapse. Eur J Obstet Gynecol 1999;85:57–62.

[19] Behnia-Willison F, Seman EI, Cook JR, et al. Laparoscopic paravaginal repair of anterior compartment prolapse. J Minim Invasive Gynecol 2007;14:475–80.

[20] Daneshgari F, Paraiso MF, Kaouk J, et al. Robotic and laparoscopic female pelvic floor reconstruction. BJU Int 2006;98(Suppl 1):62–8.

[21] Paraiso MFR, et al. Laparoscopic abdominal sacral colpopexy. In: Vasavada SP, Appell RA, Sand PK, et al, editors. Female urology, urogynecology, and voiding dysfunction. London: Informa Healthcare; 2004. p. 691–700, chapter 49.

[22] Cadeddu JA, Micali S, Moore RG, et al. Laparoscopic repair of enterocele. J Endourol 1996;10:367–9.

[23] Koninckx PR, Poppe W, Deprest J. Carbon dioxide laser for laparoscopic enterocele repair. J Am Assoc Gynecol Laparosc 1995;2:181–5.

[24] Schwartz M, Abbott KR, Glazerman L, et al. Positive symptom improvement with laparoscopic uterosacral ligament repair for uterine or vaginal vault prolapse: interim results from an active multicenter trial. J Minim Invasive Gynecol 2007;14:570–6.

[25] Ross JW. Apical vault repair, the cornerstone of pelvic vault reconstruction. Int Urogynecol J Pelvic Floor Dysfunct 1997;8:146–52.

[26] Diwan A, Rardin CR, Strohsnitter WC, et al. Laparoscopic uterosacral ligament uterine suspension compared with vaginal hysterectomy with vaginal vault suspension for uterovaginal prolapse. Int Urogynecol J Pelvic Floor Dysfunct 2005;17:79–83.

[27] Medina C, Takacs P. Laparoscopic uterosacral uterine suspension: a minimally invasive technique for treating pelvic organ prolapse. J Minim Invasive Gynecol 2006;13:472–5.

[28] Ostrzenski A. Genuine stress urinary incontinence in women. New laparoscopic paravaginal reconstruction. J Reprod Med 1998;43:477–82.

[29] Cundiff GW, Fenner D. Evaluation and treatment of women with rectocele: focus on associated defecatory and sexual dysfunction. Obstet Gynecol 2004;104:1403–21.

[30] Lyons TL, Winer WK. Laparoscopic rectocele repair using polyglactin mesh. J Am Assoc Gynecol Laparosc 1997;4:381–4.

[31] Nygaard IE, McCreery R, Brubaker L, et al. Abdominal sacrocolpopexy: a comprehensive review. Am J Obstet Gynecol 2004;104:805–23.

[32] Brubaker L, Bump R, Fynes M, et al. Surgery for pelvic organ prolapse. In: Abrams P, Cardozo L, Khoury S, et al, editors. Incontinence, Management. Third International Consultation on Incontinence. vol. 2, Monaco: International Continence Society; 2005. p. 1371–402, chapter 21.

[33] Paraiso MFR, Walters MD, Rackley RR, et al. Laparoscopic and abdominal sacral colpopexies: a comparative cohort study. Am J Obstet Gynecol 2005;192:1752–8.

[34] Higgs PJ, Chua H-L, Smith ARB. Long term review of laparoscopic sacrocolpopexy. BJOG 2005;112:1134–8.

[35] Ross JW, Preston M. Laparoscopic sacrocolpopexy for severe vaginal vault prolapse: five-year outcome. J Minim Invasive Gynecol 2005;12:221–6.

[36] Antiphon P, Elard S, Benyoussef A, et al. Laparoscopic promontory sacral colpopexy: is the posterior, recto-vaginal, mesh mandatory? Eur Urol 2004;45:655–61.

[37] Gadonneix P, Ercoli A, Salet-Lizée D, et al. Laparoscopic sacrocolpopexy with two separate meshes along the anterior and posterior vaginal walls for multicompartment pelvic organ prolapse. J Am Assoc Gynecol Laparosc 2004;11:29–35.

[38] Ayav A, Bresler L, Hubert J, et al. Robotic-assisted pelvic organ prolapse surgery. Surg Endosc 2005;19:1200–3.

[39] Daneshgari F, Kefer JC, Moore C, et al. Robotic abdominal sacrocolpopexy/sacrouteropexy repair of advanced female pelvic organ prolapse (POP): utilizing POP-quantification-based staging and outcomes. BJU Int 2007;100:875–9.

[40] Elliott DS, Krambeck AE, Chow GK. Long-term results of robotic assisted laparoscopic sacrocolpopexy for the treatment of high grade vaginal vault prolapse. J Urol 2006;176:655–9.

ELSEVIER
SAUNDERS

Urol Clin N Am 35 (2008) 477–488

**UROLOGIC
CLINICS
of North America**

Minimally Invasive Treatment
of Vesicoureteral Reflux

Matthew H. Hayn, MD*, Marc C. Smaldone, MD, Michael C. Ost, MD,
Steven G. Docimo, MD

*Department of Urology, University of Pittsburgh Medical Center, Kaufmann Medical Building,
Suite 700, 3471 Fifth Avenue, Pittsburgh, PA 15213, USA*

Vesicoureteral reflux (VUR) is a common problem in childhood, affecting approximately 1% to 2% of the pediatric population [1]. Mild cases of VUR are likely to resolve spontaneously, but high-grade VUR may require surgical correction. Pediatric urologists are familiar with open antireflux operations, which can be accomplished with minimal operative morbidity. Minimally invasive endoscopic and laparoscopic techniques now exist that may serve to reduce morbidity further. This article reviews the endoscopic materials, techniques, and outcomes in the treatment of VUR in addition to the techniques and outcomes of laparoscopic and robotic ureteroneocystotomy.

Endoscopic correction of vesicoureteral reflux

Materials used

Many injectable biomaterials have been produced as bulking agents for use in the endoscopic correction of VUR. For an injectable biomaterial to be ideal, it must be nontoxic and stable without migration to vital organs and cause minimal local inflammation while being well encapsulated by normal fibrous tissue and fibrocytes. It should be easy to inject through a rigid or flexible needle that passes easily through standard pediatric endoscopic equipment.

Polytetrafluoroethylene paste

Polytetrafluoroethylene (PTFE) paste is one of the most commonly used biomaterials in medicine. It is considered to be relatively inert chemically and biologically and has not been found to cause malignancy in humans. PTFE paste has been used as an injectable agent for the embolization of blood vessels [2] and injection of vocal cords [3], and as a bulking agent for stress urinary incontinence (SUI) [4–6].

PTFE paste was first reported as a bulking agent for treatment of VUR in 1981 by Matouschek [7]. This technique was popularized as the STING (subureteric transurethral injection) procedure by O'Donnell and Puri [8]. Puri [9] later reported on a large series of patients treated for VUR who demonstrated a 76% overall success rate after a single injection, which subsequently increased to 84.9% with repeat injection. PTFE paste was also used in a large European multicenter survey reporting on 6216 ureters in 4166 children with 10 years of follow-up. This survey reported a cure rate of 86% after one to four injections [10].

Despite its clinical effectiveness and widespread use in Europe, PTFE paste has never gained US Food and Drug Administration (FDA) approval because of concerns of distant particle migration. The rigid PTFE spheres have been found to migrate into the lymph nodes, lungs, liver, spleen, and brain in experimental studies [11]. Subsequent clinical reports confirming particle migration have been reported, including a case with clinically significant particle migration to the lungs [12] and another with

* Corresponding author.
E-mail address: haynm2@upmc.edu (M.H. Hayn).

doi:10.1016/j.ucl.2008.05.006

migration to the lungs and brain [13]. Because of these concerns and the availability of other injectable agents, the use of PTFE has been largely abandoned.

Polydimethylsiloxane

Polydimethylsiloxane (PDS) is a solid, silicone, elastomer, soft tissue bulking agent that has been incorporated into a patented medical device. It is made of 40% solid-textured highly cross-linked PDS elastomer spheres suspended in a 60% low-molecular-weight polyvinylpyrrolidone gel. It has been used clinically in treating SUI in women [14] and men [15]. The efficacy of this device for the correction of VUR has been well documented. Dodat and colleagues [16] reported a success rate of 79.4% at 5 years of follow-up in 590 refluxing ureters in 389 patients. Herz and colleagues [17] reported a success rate of 81% after a single injection and 90% after a repeat injection in 112 refluxing ureters. In a similar fashion, van Capelle and colleagues [18] showed an 82.3% success rate in 311 ureters over a 10-year period from two European centers. Oswald and colleagues [19]compared this PDS device versus dextranomer and hyaluronic acid copolymer and found similar results after a single endoscopic injection. Although the PDS device has demonstrated good long-term results, it has not received FDA approval for correction of VUR because of concerns about the potential for particulate migration, which has been demonstrated in one animal model study [20].

Collagen

Medical collagen is made of bovine collagen, which is a natural matrix protein commonly found in bone and connective tissue. It is commercially available in the injectable form as a solution of 95% type I collagen mixed with 5% type III collagen. Frey and colleagues [21] reported a success rate of 63% after one injection in 204 ureters of 100 girls and 32 boys with varying grades of reflux. The success rate increased to 79.4% at 3 months after treatment after subsequent reinjection. Reunanen [22] showed similar results, with a success rate of 82% in nonduplicated systems at 4 years of follow-up. Collagen, however, has been shown to lose volume over time, which has been correlated clinically with poor long-term results. Haferkamp and colleagues [23] showed that only 9% of 57 treated units remained reflux free at 37 months of follow-up. There have also been reports of development of serum antibodies to bovine collagen [24]. For

these reasons, collagen has not been approved by the FDA for the treatment of VUR.

Calcium hydroxyapatite (coaptite)

Calcium hydroxyapatite has been used as a biocompatible implant for orthopedic and dental procedures in humans for more than 25 years [25]. It was approved by the FDA for use in the treatment of SUI in women and girls in 2005. Mora Durban and colleagues [26] showed resolution of reflux in 75% of cases with a single injection of calcium hydroxyapatite, with 85% resolution after a second injection. A recent prospective multicenter trial demonstrated ureteral cure rates of 46% and 40% at 1 and 2 years, respectively. At the primary center, however, the 2-year cure rate was 66% of patients and 72% of ureters [27]. Merrot and colleagues [28] compared dextranomer and hyaluronic acid copolymer and calcium hydroxyapatite in the treatment of VUR and found no significant difference in terms of cure rate, regardless of grade, in a total of 44 refluxing units. To date, however, calcium hydroxyapatite has not received FDA approval for the treatment of VUR.

Dextranomer/hyaluronic acid copolymer

The need for a nonimmunogenic, biodegradable, injectable bulking agent for the treatment of reflux prompted Stenberg and Lackgren [29] to develop a system based on dextranomer microspheres suspended in a sodium hyaluronan solution in a 1:1 ratio. Dextranomer microspheres are made up of a network of cross-linked dextran polysaccharide molecules. After injection, the microspheres induce fibroblast and collagen deposition, leading to endogenous tissue augmentation. After 1 week, the microspheres disappear but the fibroblast and collagen ingrowth remains stable [30]. They are nonimmunogenic because of the lack of free circulating dextran molecules and nonmigratory because of their spherical shape and larger particle size (80–120 μm) [31]. After successful animal studies, these investigators injected 101 ureters in 75 consecutive patients and reported reduction or resolution of reflux in 81% of ureters at 3 months of follow-up. They followed 18 ureters for 1 year after treatment, and of these, 16 remained free of reflux [29]. Dextranomer and hyaluronic acid copolymer was approved by the FDA in 2001 for the treatment of VUR in children and is now approved for treatment of VUR grades 2 through 4 [32].

Technique of injection

O'Donnell and Puri popularized the classic suburetric transurethral injection (STING) technique in 1984. General anesthesia is administered, a urine culture is obtained, and prophylactic antibiotics are given. Cystoscopy is performed before opening any injection materials in case the procedure is cancelled because of bladder inflammation or infection. Their original description suggested entering the bladder mucosa 2 to 3 mm distal to the ureterovesical junction (UVJ) and advancing the needle in the submucosal plane for a distance of 4 to 5 mm [8]. To treat high-grade reflux and ureters without a submucosal tunnel, Chertin and colleagues [33] suggested inserting the needle directly into the affected ureteral orifice to increase the length of the intravesical ureter and create a slit-like orifice. This modified STING procedure was popularized by Kirsch and colleagues [34], for which they described ureteral success rates significantly greater for the modified STING (92%) versus the standard STING (79%). They describe inserting the needle approximately 4 mm in the submucosa of the mid- to distal ureteral tunnel at the 6 o'clock position, all under the aid of hydrodistention.

The hydrodistention-implantation technique (HIT) has evolved to now include two intraureteral submucosal injections proximal and distal HITs, or "double HIT," until total ureteral tunnel coaptation occurs [35]. The proximal HIT (site 1) should lead to coaptation of the proximal ureteral tunnel (Fig. 1A). The distal HIT (site 2) is performed by placing the needle to the same depth just within the ureteral orifice and injecting until the ureteral orifice is coapted and elevated to the height of the ureteral tunnel (see Fig. 1B). The end result should look like a mountain range appearance of the tunnel and orifice. If the ureteral orifice does not completely coapt with intraureteric injection, Kirsch [36] recommends that a classic suburetric implantation (STING; see Fig. 1C) be performed. In addition, he recommends that after each injection, an attempt at ureteral hydrodistention be done to ensure proper technique, because the ureter should remain coapted with irrigation.

Independent of the technique used, there exists a significant learning curve with endoscopic correction of VUR [37]. Kirsch [37] noted a lower success rate (60%) in his first 20 patients compared with an 80% success rate in his last 20 patients. Herz and colleagues [17] reported a success rate of 46% in 28 refluxing ureters during the first 6 months of their study. In the remaining 18 months, the correction rate was 93% in 84 refluxing ureters. Lorenzo and colleagues [38] reported that physician experience was predictive of VUR correction after endoscopic injection on multivariate analysis. This finding was confirmed by Routh and colleagues [39] in their study of 301 patients.

Clinical results

At the present time, dextranomer and hyaluronic acid copolymer is the only FDA-approved material for use in endoscopic correction of VUR. The authors, therefore, limit their review to series using dextranomer and hyaluronic acid copolymer. Lackgren and colleagues [40] published the first series using dextranomer and hyaluronic acid copolymer in 2001. A total of 221 patients (335 ureters, grades II–V) were followed 2 to 7.5 years. A voiding cystourethrogram (VCUG) was performed at 3 and 12 months after injections. They reported a 75% success rate (defined as grade I or less) at 1 year of follow-up. Puri and colleagues [41] reported on 113 children (166 ureters) and found that reflux was corrected in 86% of ureters after a single injection, which increased to 99% after a second injection. Follow-up VCUG was performed at 3 months. Of the 113 patients, only 11 completed 1 year, and none had evidence of reflux on VCUG. This was followed up by a larger series in 2006, in which Puri and colleagues [42] treated 692 children (1101 ureters) and reported success rates of 86.5% and 98% after first and second injections, respectively. In 2003, Kirsch and colleagues [37] reported a 72% success rate after a single treatment at 3 months of follow-up. In a large series, Capozza and colleagues [43] used dextranomer and hyaluronic acid copolymer to treat 788 patients (1050 ureters) endoscopically, and reported a success rate of 82% after a single injection. Kirsch and colleagues [34] reported improved success rates in 459 ureters using a modified STING approach, with ureteral success rates greater for the modified STING (92%) compared with the standard STING (79%). Of the 8% who failed using the modified STING technique, a second injection resolved reflux in 88% of ureters that had grade I to III reflux [44]. Please refer to Table 1 for a summary of results.

Complex cases

Endoscopic injection of dextranomer and hyaluronic acid copolymer after failed ureteroneocystotomy has been reported. Kitchens and colleagues [45] reported on 18 patients who had persistent

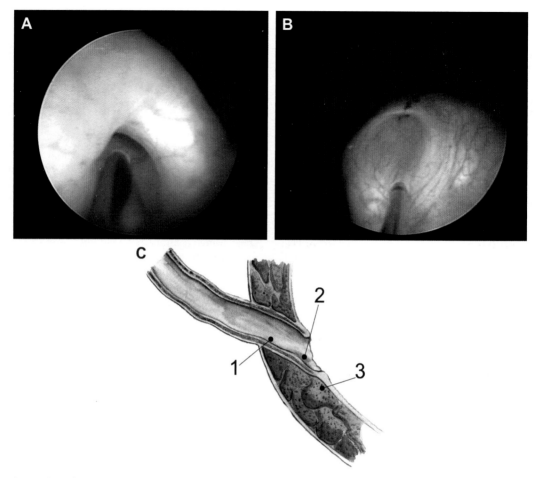

Fig. 1. Figure demonstrates the hydrodistention-implantation technique (HIT). (*A*) HIT in the proximal ureteral tunnel, leading to proximal coaptation. (*B*) Distal HIT site, performed by placing the needle just within the ureteral orifice. (*C*) Picture demonstrates proximal HIT (site 1), distal HIT (site 2), and classic subureteric implantation site (STING; site 3). (*From* Kirsch. AJ. Endoscopic management of vesicoureteral reflux. Hinman's atlas of urologic surgery. 3rd edition. Philadelphia: Elsevier. In press; with permission).

VUR or de novo ipsilateral VUR after attempted VUR correction and primary nonrefluxing mega-ureter or renal transplantation, respectively. Of the 20 renal units, 16 (80%) had complete resolution of VUR after a single injection. Similarly, Jung and colleagues [46] reported on dextranomer and hyaluronic acid copolymer injection for persistent VUR after ureteroneocystotomy, with a success rate of 70% and 90% after first and second injections, respectively. Chertin and colleagues [47] reported on endoscopic treatment of reflux in patients who had undergone ureterocele puncture. Of the patients with reflux into the lower moiety, 31 (70%) of 44 and 40 (91%) of 44 had resolution of reflux after one and two injections, respectively.

In a multi-institutional study, Perez-Brayfield and colleagues [48] reported on 72 patients (93 ureters) that they considered to be complex cases. Cases included persistent reflux after open surgery (n = 17), persistent reflux and neurogenic bladder (n = 11), ectopic ureters to bladder neck (n = 7), bilateral Hutch diverticulum (n = 6), stump reflux (n = 6), ureterocele after puncture or incision (n = 5), and ureteral duplication (n = 15). The overall success rate in their series was 68% after one endoscopic injection. Özok and colleagues [49] performed endoscopic injection of dextranomer and hyaluronic acid copolymer in 21 renal transplant candidates (29 ureters) with reflux grades I through IV and reported success rates of 79.3%

Table 1
Endoscopic outcomes

Published report	No. children/ No. ureters	VUR grade	Technique	Longest clinical follow-up (years)	Success rate (%)	Long-term follow-up (months)
Lackgren et al [40]	221/335	II–V	STING	7	75	72
Puri et al [41]	113/166	II–V	STING	1	86, 99[a]	N/A
Kirsch et al [37]	180/292	I–IV	STING	1	72	N/A
Capozza et al [43]	788/1050	II–V	STING	1	82	N/A
Kirsch et al [34]	70/119	I–IV	HIT	1	92	N/A
Puri et al [42]	692/1101	II–V	STING	3	86.5, 98[a]	N/A

Abbreviation: N/A.
[a] After first and second injections.

and 82.7% after one and two injections, respectively. They did not report any adverse effects.

Factors predicting success

It seems reasonable to state that dextranomer and hyaluronic acid copolymer injection is a safe and efficacious procedure, at least in the short term. What is less obvious, however, are what factors predispose patients to success or failure. Capozza and colleagues [50] noted that uncontrolled voiding dysfunction contributed to endoscopic failure with dextranomer and hyaluronic acid copolymer in their series of 320 children. In contrast, Lackgren and colleagues [51] reported that endoscopic treatment with dextranomer and hyaluronic acid copolymer was similarly effective in patients with and without bladder dysfunction (urge syndrome and dysfunctional voiding). The data demonstrating any affect of voiding dysfunction dextranomer and hyaluronic acid copolymer results, however, are weakened by the lack of standard assessment for voiding dysfunction. Lavelle and colleagues [52] examined 52 patients (80 ureters) and found that mound morphology was the only statistically significant factor predictive of a successful outcome, using Fisher's exact test. No difference was found in terms of volume injected or the presence or absence of voiding dysfunction. In a multivariate analysis on 168 patients (259 ureters), Yucel and colleagues [53] found that reflux grade, volume of dextranomer/hyaluronic acid injected, and mound appearance correlated with outcomes. Factors not correlated with outcomes included gender, age, unilateral versus bilateral, ureteral duplication, subureteral versus intraureteral, and presence of voiding dysfunction. Further prospective studies are required

to elucidate fully what determines outcomes in patients who undergo endoscopic correction of their VUR. Lackgren and colleagues [54] retrospectively reviewed 68 children with duplex ureters and 40 children with a small kidney (contributing 10%–35% of total renal function) and found similar results when compared with their main study population.

Complications of endoscopic injection

Recently, Elmore and colleagues [55] reported on new contralateral reflux after dextranomer and hyaluronic acid copolymer injection. Of 126 patients who underwent unilateral dextranomer and hyaluronic acid copolymer injection, 17 (13.5%) developed contralateral reflux on follow-up VCUG. They found that girls younger than 5 years of age had the highest incidence of new reflux. Similarly, in another series, de novo contralateral reflux was reported in 10 (8.3%) of 120 patients who had unilateral VUR [56]. Menezes and colleagues [57] reported that 10.1% of children developed new contralateral reflux after dextranomer and hyaluronic acid copolymer injection. They were unable to identify any risk factors and did not recommend prophylactic treatment of nonrefluxing contralateral ureters. As of yet, the natural history and clinical sequelae of new contralateral reflux have not been fully elucidated. In the future, high-risk groups may benefit from prophylactic injection of the contralateral side.

Ureteral obstruction after dextranomer and hyaluronic acid copolymer injection is a rare event. Snodgrass [58] reported persistent asymptomatic obstruction of a dysmorphic ureter after dextranomer and hyaluronic acid copolymer injection that required open reimplantation. A recent multi-institutional review reported on 745 patients (1155 ureters) and found postoperative obstruction in 7 ureters (0.6%) in 5 patients (0.7%). Four of the 5 patients were immediately symptomatic with nausea or vomiting in 2 patients and anuria within 24 hours in 2 patients. All patients had resolution of symptoms with stent placement, with no recurrence after stent removal [59].

Cost-effectiveness

Costs are assuming increasing importance in health care, and costs of new interventions must be considered. Benoit and colleagues [60] examined the cost-effectiveness of dextranomer/hyaluronic acid copolymer injection as a substitution to surgical management. They found that dextranomer and hyaluronic acid copolymer injection injection may be more cost-effective than ureteral reimplantation for children who meet standard criteria for surgical therapy, especially for lower grades of reflux. If an increased volume of dextranomer and hyaluronic acid copolymer injection is needed for higher grades of reflux, injection would then only be cost-effective for grades I and II unilateral and bilateral reflux, and possibly unilateral grade III reflux. Benoit and colleagues [61] also compared the cost-effectiveness of performing dextranomer and hyaluronic acid copolymer injection at the time of diagnosis with that of traditional management. Two models were used: injection at diagnosis proceeding to traditional management if injection failed (scenario 1) and injection at diagnosis proceeding to ureteral reimplantation if injection failed (scenario 2). They found that in both scenarios, dextranomer and hyaluronic acid copolymer injection can never achieve cost-effectiveness for grades I and II unilateral and bilateral reflux and that high success rates of dextranomer and hyaluronic acid copolymer injection are needed to achieve cost-effectiveness for higher grades of VUR.

Follow-up

The current follow-up paradigm for endoscopic injection of dextranomer and hyaluronic acid copolymer injection is variable. Most clinical studies recommend renal and bladder ultrasound 2 to 4 weeks after surgery [37,40] and VCUG at 3 months [37,40,41]. Yu and colleagues [62] believe that routine renal ultrasound scans are unnecessary after endoscopic injection of dextranomer and hyaluronic acid copolymer in uncomplicated cases of VUR. Because of the known risk for late recurrence, some advocate follow-up VCUG at 1 year, although few series document this type of long-term follow-up.

Laparoscopic and robotic ureteroneocystotomy

Ureteral reimplantation has proved to be the "gold standard" therapy for VUR. Traditional open ureterovesical reimplantation procedures have been extremely successful in children with success rates approaching 95% to 98% [63]. Recent efforts have been directed toward reducing the perioperative morbidity of open reimplantation, however, including hematuria, irritative bladder symptoms, and postoperative pain. Initially described in the mid-1990s [64,65], laparoscopic antireflux surgery has never achieved popular consensus because of the technical difficulty in dissection and suturing required. Proposed advantages of the laparoscopic approach include better cosmetic results, shorter hospitalization, decreased analgesic requirement, faster recovery, and improved visualization. These theoretic advantages are not always easy to demonstrate in the pediatric population, however, and early outcomes have not demonstrated the laparoscopic approach to be as efficacious as the open ureteral reimplant.

Percutaneous trigonoplasty

An alternative to open and endoscopic injection procedures, the percutaneous endoscopic trigonoplasty was introduced in the early 1990s. A combination of intravesical cystoscopy and laparoscopy, the bladder is filled with carbon dioxide through percutaneously placed ports to improve visibility and the reimplant is performed using a Gil-Vernet or Cohen technique. First described by Okamura and colleagues [66] in 6 children (mean age of 7 years) with grade II through V (bilateral reflux in 5 children), they reported a 100% reflux correction rate, a mean operative time of 149 minutes, and a mean postoperative catheterization time of 4.6 days. No major complications were observed at a median follow-up of 8.5 months. In a larger series of 22 children (mean age of 7 years) and 32 refluxing units (grades II–V), Cartwright and colleagues [67] reported a reflux correction rate of 62.5%, with follow-up ranging from 4 to 11 months. Operative time ranged between 60 and 240 minutes, and complications included a vesicovaginal fistula, hyponatremia, and perivesical fluid collection. In an extension of this series, Gatti and colleagues [68] reported outcomes in 29 children with 46 refluxing ureters using the Gil-Vernet and Cohen reimplantation techniques. Success rates improved from 63% to 83% with the Cohen technique, but the operative time nearly doubled as well. In a comparison of children and adults with reflux, Okamura and colleagues [69] reported a 59% success rate in 15 children and trigonal splitting in 13%, causing recurrence of reflux greater than grade II. To improve success rates, this technique was modified to elongate the intramural ureter with reliable muscular backing. The initial success rate in 8 female children with 14 refluxing ureters was 86%, with a mean operative time of 245 minutes [70]. Despite the proposed advantages of a reduction of postoperative urgency and a shorter recovery time, reduced success rates and increased operative times in these early series are clearly inferior to those of traditional open techniques and this procedure has largely been abandoned.

Pneumovesicoscopic cross-trigonal ureteroneocystotomy

In a more recent application of the pneumovesiscopic approach, the laparoscope is placed transabdominally instead of per urethra, which had previously limited mobility. First successfully described using a pig model [71,72], the increase in maneuverability facilitates a Cohen type cross-trigonal ureteral implantation using standard laparoscopic instruments (Table 2). In 2001, Gill and colleagues [73] described the use of this approach in 2 children and one adult demonstrating that this procedure was effective and technically feasible. Yeung and colleagues [74] reported their initial experience with this technique in 16 children (mean age of 4.1 years) with 23 refluxing ureters. They reported a mean operative time of 136 minutes (112 minutes unilateral, 178 minutes bilateral), and an overall success rate of 96% with one conversion to an open procedure after displacement of a port into the extravesical space [74]. In 32 children (mean age of 5 years), Kutikov and colleagues [75] reported 93% and 80% success rates in ureters treated for primary VUR with the Cohen cross-trigonal technique and primary megaureter obstruction treated with the Glenn-Anderson technique, respectively. Complications included urine leak in 12.5% of patients and ureteral stricture in 6.3% of patients, with most occurring in children 2 years of age or younger with a bladder capacity less than 130 mL. In the most recent series, Canon and colleagues [76] compared 52 children undergoing vesicoscopic ureteral reimplantation with 40 children undergoing open reimplantation. They reported a significantly decreased postoperative analgesic requirement in the vesicoscopic group and a similar hospital length of stay when compared with the open management group. The mean operative time was significantly elevated (199 versus 92 minutes; $P = .001$), however, with a higher complication rate (6% versus none), including 1 child with bilateral ureteral obstruction in the vesicoscopic group.

Challenges with this technique include gaining and maintaining bladder access [77]. Access sites must be well sealed to maintain optimal operative exposure and avoid carbon monoxide leakage into the retroperitoneum. Preplaced sutures are used to close these sites at the conclusion of the procedure to prevent urine leakage, which can be difficult in older children with more subcutaneous tissue. Other limitations include the significant learning curve inherent to working within the small working space of the bladder, need for extended postoperative catheterization, and need for intravesical laparoscopic freehand suturing. Although few studies have explored this technique's benefits compared with open surgery, it is unlikely that this more complex approach is going to replace an operation performed through a small bikini incision with high success and minimal complication rates unless some additional benefit is proved.

Laparoscopic extravesicular ureteroneocystotomy

Initially described in animal models [78–81], the most common laparoscopic approach used to date has been extravesicular reimplantation with ureteral advancement (detrusorrhaphy) by the Lich-Gregoir technique (Table 3). Assuming that the primary benefits of the laparoscopic approach are a shorter length of hospital stay, less morbidity, and better cosmesis, recent efforts have focused on minimal tissue dissection, achieving reliable detrusor closure, and downsizing ports and instruments. In a large series of 71 reimplants in 47 children (23 unilateral and 24 bilateral), Lakshmanan and colleagues [82] reported a 100% success rate with no persistent reflux or obstruction. They recommended careful selection of operative candidates, speculating that ureters requiring tapering are unsuitable and that the working space in the pelvis of children younger

Table 2
Pneumovesicoscopic ureteroneocystostomy outcomes

Report	No. children No. ureters	VUR grade	Technique	Mean OR time (minutes)	Success (%)	Complications (%)
Okamura et al [66]	6/11	II–V	G-V	149	100	Hematuria (16.7) Mechanical failure (16.7)
Cartwright et al [67]	22/32	II–V	G-V	60–240	62.5	Vesicovaginal fistula (4.5) Hyponatremia (4.5) Perivesical fluid collection (4.5)
Okamura et al [69]	15/27	II–V	G-V	201	59	Trigonal splitting (13.3)
Gatti et al [68]	29/42	I–V	G-V, C	60–240 (G-V) 197 (C)	47 (G-V), 83 (C)	Vesicovaginal fistula (3.4) Hyponatremia (3.4) Perivesical fluid collection (3.4) Hydronephrosis (6.8) Bilateral pneumothoraces (3.4)
Tsuji et al [70]	8/14	I–IV	G-V	245	86	Ureteral injury (14)
Yeung et al [74]	16/23	II–V	C	136	96	Scrotal and suprapubic emphysema (12.5) Port displacement (18.8)
Peters et al [77,87]	6/12	2.3	C[a]	210	91.7	Urine leak (16.7)
Kutikov et al [75]	27/54	II–V	C	168	92.6	Urine leak (7.4) Ureteral stricture (3.7)
Canon et al [76]	52/87	I–V	C	199	91	Urine leak (1.9) Bladder stones (1.9) Bilateral ureteral obstruction (1.9)

Abbreviations: C, Cohen cross-trigonal ureteral reimplantation; G-V, Gil-Vernet trigonoplasty.
[a] Robotic assisted.

than 4 years of age may be inadequate for laparoscopic techniques. In a series of 15 children with 19 refluxing ureters, Riquelme and colleagues [83] reported a 95% success rate with no major complications. Mean operative time was 110 minutes in cases of unilateral reflux and 180 minutes in cases of bilateral reflux, with 3 children requiring catheterization for 3 to 4 days for mucosal perforation. These results have been duplicated in a small cohort of postpubertal children with VUR. Shu and colleagues [84] reported a 100% reflux correction rate in 6 children (mean age of 18.7 years), with a mean of 11.4 months of follow-up. Mean operative times for unilateral and bilateral procedures were 1.75 and 3.75 hours, respectively, and mean hospital stay was 36 hours.

Although division of the lateral bladder pedicle is thought to contribute to transient postoperative urinary retention in some patients, proposed benefits of the extravesical repair include sparing a trigonal incision and anastomosis, resulting in fewer postoperative bladder irritative symptoms.

Using a combination of intra- and extravesical principles, Simforoosh and colleagues [85] have recently described a novel technique of extraperitoneal laparoscopic trigonoplasty. In their series of 27 children with 41 refluxing units, after gaining extraperitoneal access, the bladder was opened with laparoscopic scissors and the ureters were approximated in the midline after a trigonal incision. With a mean operative time of 147 minutes, a 93% success rate was reported with a mean of 8.2 months of follow-up. These investigators propose that their high success rate is a result of ease of intracorporeal free hand suturing afforded by the increased extraperitoneal space when compared with pneumovesiscopic procedures.

Robotic-assisted ureteroneocystostomy

The goal of robotic surgical assistance in pediatric urology is to gain the advantages of laparoscopy, including reduced pain and morbidity, while shortening the steep learning curve of

Table 3
Laparoscopic ureteroneocystostomy outcomes

Report	No. children/ No. ureters	VUR grade	Technique	Mean OR time (minutes)	Success	Complications(%)
Lakshmanan et al [82]	47/71	I–V	L-G	N/A	100	Ureteral injury (4.2)
Shu et al [84]	6/6	N/A	L-G	105	100	Hydronephrosis (16.7) Abdominal pain (16.7)
Peters et al [77]	17/17	2.9	L-G[a]	120	88.2	Urine leak (5.9)
Riquelme et al [83]	15/19	II-III	L-G	110 unilateral 180 bilateral	94.7	Mucosal perforation (15.8)
Simforoosh et al [85]	27/41	I–IV	G-V	147	93	Peritoneal tear (3.7)

Abbreviations: C, Cohen cross-trigonal ureteral reimplantation; G-V, Gil-Vernet trigonoplasty; L-G, Lich-Gregoir ureteral reimplantation.

[a] Robotic assisted.

traditional laparoscopy without sacrificing reconstructive precision. Potential advantages of robotic-assisted laparoscopy include an increased ability to perform precise suturing for reconstruction because of stereoscopic three-dimensional vision, increased instrument dexterity, and tremor-filtered instrument control with movement scaling. The chief deterrents include increased cost, lack of tactile feedback, and lack of pediatric-sized ports and instruments [86].

Initial efforts with robotic-assisted laparoscopy have focused on performing an extravesical transperitoneal Lich-Gregoir procedure in a similar manner to the described straight laparoscopic method in children with unilateral reflux. Because of concerns regarding increased risk for urinary retention with bilateral extravesical reimplantation [82] however, an intravesical robotically assisted bilateral ureteral reimplantation technique has been developed in a similar manner to the transtrigonal (Cohen) laparoscopic repair [87]. Ports are placed in the dome of the bladder, and after takedown of periureteral attachments to the bladder, submucosal transtrigonal tunnels are created with sharp dissection to the opposite side of the trigone. In a recent review of the applications of robotic technology to pediatric urology, Peters [77] described his unpublished outcomes in the robotically assisted treatment of VUR. Unilateral Lich-Gregoir procedures were performed in 17 children, intravesical cross-trigonal Cohen procedures were performed in 3 children with bilateral reflux, and contralateral nephrectomies were

performed in 4 children. Of these 24 children, correction of reflux was achieved in 89% of refluxing units, with two cases of bladder leak, one case of transient obstruction, and a mean operating room time ranging from 2 to 3.5 hours.

Summary

As management of VUR continues to evolve, laparoscopic and robotic-assisted reflux corrective procedures remain in their infancy. Overall, early results demonstrating feasibility with pneumovesiscopic-, laparoscopic-, and robotic-assisted techniques are encouraging and warrant further evaluation in the management of pediatric VUR. Nevertheless, limited patient numbers and lack of stratification by grade of reflux make interpreting these results difficult. Although theoretic benefits include reduction in postoperative bladder spasms, decreased incisional pain, more rapid catheter removal, and improved cosmesis, these have yet to be clearly demonstrated in available series, and significant improvement is needed to match the efficacy and cosmetic outcomes achieved with traditional open repairs.

Open ureteral reimplantation remains the gold standard in the surgical treatment of VUR. Endoscopic correction of VUR is a reasonable alternative to open surgical reimplantation, particularly in cases of low-grade VUR, although long-term results into adulthood remain unknown. Laparoscopic- and robotic-assisted techniques have shown encouraging early results and warrant further study in the surgical management of VUR.

References

[1] Smellie JM, Barratt TM, Chantler C, et al. Medical versus surgical treatment in children with severe bilateral vesicoureteric reflux and bilateral nephropathy: a randomised trial. Lancet 2001;357:1329–33.

[2] Weingarten J, Kauffman SL. Teflon embolization to pulmonary arteries. Ann Thorac Surg 1977;23: 371–3.

[3] Kasperbauer JL. Injectable Teflon for vocal cord paralysis. Otolaryngol Clin North Am 1995;28:317–23.

[4] Berg S. Polytef augmentation urethroplasty. Correction of surgically incurable urinary incontinence by injection technique. Arch Surg 1973;107:379–81.

[5] Politano VA, Small MP, Harper JM, et al. Periurethral Teflon injection for urinary incontinence. J Urol 1974;111:180–3.

[6] Politano VA. Transurethral polytef injection for post-prostatectomy urinary incontinence. Br J Urol 1992;69:26–8.

[7] Matouschek E. Treatment of vesicorenal reflux by transurethral Teflon-injection. Urologe A 1981;20: 263–4 [author's transl].

[8] O'Donnell B, Puri P. Treatment of vesicoureteric reflux by endoscopic injection of Teflon. Br Med J (Clin Res Ed) 1984;289:7–9.

[9] Puri P. Ten year experience with subureteric Teflon (polytetrafluoroethylene) injection (STING) in the treatment of vesico-ureteric reflux. Br J Urol 1995; 75:126–31.

[10] Puri P, Ninan GK, Surana R. Subureteric Teflon injection (STING). Results of a European survey. Eur Urol 1995;27:71–5.

[11] Malizia AA Jr, Reiman HM, Myers RP, et al. Migration and granulomatous reaction after periurethral injection of polytef (Teflon). JAMA 1984; 251:3277–81.

[12] Claes H, Stroobants D, Van Meerbeek J, et al. Pulmonary migration following periurethral polytetrafluoroethylene injection for urinary incontinence. J Urol 1989;142:821–2.

[13] Aaronson IA, Rames RA, Greene WB, et al. Endoscopic treatment of reflux: migration of Teflon to the lungs and brain. Eur Urol 1993;23:394–9.

[14] Radley SC, Chapple CR, Mitsogiannis IC, et al. Transurethral implantation of macroplastique for the treatment of female stress urinary incontinence secondary to urethral sphincter deficiency. Eur Urol 2001;39:383–9.

[15] Peeker R, Edlund C, Wennberg AL, et al. The treatment of sphincter incontinence with periurethral silicone implants (macroplastique). Scand J Urol Nephrol 2002;36:194–8.

[16] Dodat H, Valmalle AF, Weidmann JD, et al. Endoscopic treatment of vesicorenal reflux in children. Five-year assessment of the use of macroplastique). Prog Urol 1998;8:1001–6.

[17] Herz D, Hafez A, Bagli D, et al. Efficacy of endoscopic subureteral polydimethylsiloxane injection for treatment of vesicoureteral reflux in children: a North American clinical report. J Urol 2001;166: 1880–6.

[18] van Capelle JW, de Haan T, El Sayed W, et al. The long-term outcome of the endoscopic subureteric implantation of polydimethylsiloxane for treating vesico-ureteric reflux in children: a retrospective analysis of the first 195 consecutive patients in two European centres. BJU Int 2004;94:1348–51.

[19] Oswald J, Riccabona M, Lusuardi L, et al. Prospective comparison and 1-year follow-up of a single endoscopic subureteral polydimethylsiloxane versus dextranomer/hyaluronic acid copolymer injection for treatment of vesicoureteral reflux in children. Urology 2002;60:894–7 [discussion: 898].

[20] Henly DR, Barrett DM, Weiland TL, et al. Particulate silicone for use in periurethral injections: local tissue effects and search for migration. J Urol 1995; 153:2039–43.

[21] Frey P, Lutz N, Jenny P, et al. Endoscopic subureteral collagen injection for the treatment of vesicoureteral reflux in infants and children. J Urol 1995;154:804–7.

[22] Reunanen M. Correction of vesicoureteral reflux in children by endoscopic collagen injection: a prospective study. J Urol 1995;154:2156–8.

[23] Haferkamp A, Contractor H, Mohring K, et al. Failure of subureteral bovine collagen injection for the endoscopic treatment of primary vesicoureteral reflux in long-term follow-up. Urology 2000;55: 759–63.

[24] Leonard MP, Decter A, Hills K, et al. Endoscopic subureteral collagen injection: are immunological concerns justified? J Urol 1998;160:1012–6.

[25] Uchida A, Nade SM, McCartney ER, et al. The use of ceramics for bone replacement. A comparative study of three different porous ceramics. J Bone Joint Surg Br 1984;66:269–75.

[26] Mora Durban MJ, Navarro Sebastian FJ, Munoz Delgado MB, et al. [Endoscopic treatment of the vesicoureteral reflux in children: preliminary experience with the subureteral injection of Coaptite]. Arch Esp Urol 2006;59:493–9.

[27] Mevorach RA, Hulbert WC, Rabinowitz R, et al. Results of a 2-year multicenter trial of endoscopic treatment of vesicoureteral reflux with synthetic calcium hydroxyapatite. J Urol 2006;175:288–91.

[28] Merrot T, Ouedraogo I, Hery G, et al. [Preliminary results of endoscopic treatment of vesicoureteric reflux in children. Prospective comparative study of Deflux vs. Coaptite]. Prog Urol 2005;15:1114–9.

[29] Stenberg A, Lackgren G. A new bioimplant for the endoscopic treatment of vesicoureteral reflux: experimental and short-term clinical results. J Urol 1995; 154:800–3.

[30] Joyner BD, Atala A. Endoscopic substances for the treatment of vesicoureteral reflux. Urology 1997;50: 489–94.

[31] Stenberg AM, Sundin A, Larsson BS, et al. Lack of distant migration after injection of a 125iodine labeled dextranomer based implant into the rabbit bladder. J Urol 1997;158:1937–41.

[32] Dean GE, Doumanian LR. The extended use of Deflux (dextranomer/hyaluronic acid) in pediatric urology. Curr Urol Rep 2006;7:143–8.

[33] Chertin B, De Caluwe D, Puri P. Endoscopic treatment of primary grades IV and V vesicoureteral reflux in children with subureteral injection of polytetrafluoroethylene. J Urol 2003;169:1847–9 [discussion: 1849].

[34] Kirsch AJ, Perez-Brayfield M, Smith EA, et al. The modified sting procedure to correct vesicoureteral reflux: improved results with submucosal implantation within the intramural ureter. J Urol 2004;171:2413–6.

[35] McMann LP, Scherz HC, Kirsch AJ. Long-term preservation of dextranomer/hyaluronic acid copolymer implants after endoscopic treatment of vesicoureteral reflux in children: a sonographic volumetric analysis. J Urol 2007;177:316–20 [discussion: 320].

[36] Kirsch AJ. Endoscopic management of vesicoureteral reflux. In: Hinman F, editor. Hinman's atlas of urologic surgery. 3rd edition. St. Louis (MO): Elsevier Ltd.; 2007.

[37] Kirsch AJ, Perez-Brayfield MR, Scherz HC. Minimally invasive treatment of vesicoureteral reflux with endoscopic injection of dextranomer/hyaluronic acid copolymer: the Children's Hospitals of Atlanta experience. J Urol 2003;170:211–5.

[38] Lorenzo AJ, Pippi Salle JL, Barroso U, et al. What are the most powerful determinants of endoscopic vesicoureteral reflux correction? Multivariate analysis of a single institution experience during 6 years. J Urol 2006;176:1851–5.

[39] Routh JC, Reinberg Y, Ashley RA, et al. Multivariate comparison of the efficacy of intraureteral versus subtrigonal techniques of dextranomer/hyaluronic acid injection. J Urol 2007;178:1702–5 [discussion: 1705–6].

[40] Lackgren G, Wahlin N, Skoldenberg E, et al. Long-term follow up of children treated with dextranomer/hyaluronic acid copolymer for vesicoureteral reflux. J Urol 2001;166:1887–92.

[41] Puri P, Chertin B, Velayudham M, et al. Treatment of vesicoureteral reflux by endoscopic injection of dextranomer/hyaluronic acid copolymer: preliminary results. J Urol 2003;170:1541–4 [discussion: 1544].

[42] Puri P, Pirker M, Mohanan N, et al. Subureteral dextranomer/hyaluronic acid injection as first line treatment in the management of high grade vesicoureteral reflux. J Urol 2006;176:1856–9 [discussion: 1859–60].

[43] Capozza N, Lais A, Nappo S, et al. The role of endoscopic treatment of vesicoureteral reflux: a 17-year experience. J Urol 2004;172:1626–8 [discussion: 1629].

[44] Elmore JM, Scherz HC, Kirsch AJ. Dextranomer/hyaluronic acid for vesicoureteral reflux: success rates after initial treatment failure. J Urol 2006; 175:712–5.

[45] Kitchens D, Minevich E, DeFoor W, et al. Endoscopic injection of dextranomer/hyaluronic acid copolymer to correct vesicoureteral reflux following failed ureteroneocystostomy. J Urol 2006;176: 1861–3.

[46] Jung C, DeMarco RT, Lowrance WT, et al. Subureteral injection of dextranomer/hyaluronic acid copolymer for persistent vesicoureteral reflux following ureteroneocystostomy. J Urol 2007;177: 312–5.

[47] Chertin B, Mohanan N, Farkas A, et al. Endoscopic treatment of vesicoureteral reflux associated with ureterocele. J Urol 2007;178:1594–7.

[48] Perez-Brayfield M, Kirsch AJ, Hensle TW, et al. Endoscopic treatment with dextranomer/hyaluronic acid for complex cases of vesicoureteral reflux. J Urol 2004;172:1614–6.

[49] Ozok U, Eroglu M, Imamoglu A, et al. Subureteral dextranomer/hyaluronic acid copolymer injection for vesicoureteral reflux in transplant candidates. J Endourol 2005;19:1185–7.

[50] Capozza N, Lais A, Matarazzo E, et al. Influence of voiding dysfunction on the outcome of endoscopic treatment for vesicoureteral reflux. J Urol 2002; 168:1695–8.

[51] Lackgren G, Skoldenberg E, Stenberg A. Endoscopic treatment with stabilized nonanimal hyaluronic acid/dextranomer gel is effective in vesicoureteral reflux associated with bladder dysfunction. J Urol 2007;177:1124–8 [discussion: 1128–9].

[52] Lavelle MT, Conlin MJ, Skoog SJ. Subureteral injection of deflux for correction of reflux: analysis of factors predicting success. Urology 2005;65: 564–7.

[53] Yucel S, Gupta A, Snodgrass W. Multivariate analysis of factors predicting success with dextranomer/hyaluronic acid injection for vesicoureteral reflux. J Urol 2007;177:1505–9.

[54] Lackgren G, Wahlin N, Skoldenberg E, et al. Endoscopic treatment of vesicoureteral reflux with dextranomer/hyaluronic acid copolymer is effective in either double ureters or a small kidney. J Urol 2003;170:1551–5 [discussion: 1555].

[55] Elmore JM, Kirsch AJ, Lyles RH, et al. New contralateral vesicoureteral reflux following dextranomer/hyaluronic acid implantation: incidence and identification of a high risk group. J Urol 2006;175: 1097–100 [discussion: 1100–1].

[56] Routh JC, Vandersteen DR, Pfefferle H, et al. Single center experience with endoscopic management of vesicoureteral reflux in children. J Urol 2006;175: 1889–92 [discussion: 1892–3].

[57] Menezes M, Mohanan N, Haroun J, et al. New contralateral vesicoureteral reflux after endoscopic correction of unilateral reflux—is routine

contralateral injection indicated at initial treatment? J Urol 2007;178:1711–3.

[58] Snodgrass WT. Obstruction of a dysmorphic ureter following dextranomer/hyaluronic acid copolymer. J Urol 2004;171:395–6.

[59] Vandersteen DR, Routh JC, Kirsch AJ, et al. Postoperative ureteral obstruction after subureteral injection of dextranomer/hyaluronic acid copolymer. J Urol 2006;176:1593–5.

[60] Benoit RM, Peele PB, Docimo SG. The cost-effectiveness of dextranomer/hyaluronic acid copolymer for the management of vesicoureteral reflux. 1: substitution for surgical management. J Urol 2006;176:1588–92 [discussion: 1592].

[61] Benoit RM, Peele PB, Cannon GM Jr, et al. The cost-effectiveness of dextranomer/hyaluronic acid copolymer for the management of vesicoureteral reflux. 2. Reflux correction at the time of diagnosis as a substitute for traditional management. J Urol 2006;176:2649–53 [discussion: 2653].

[62] Yu RN, Jones EA, Roth DR. Renal ultrasound studies after endoscopic injection of dextranomer/hyaluronic acid copolymer for vesicoureteral reflux. Urology 2006;68:866–8 [discussion: 868–9].

[63] Jodal U, Smellie JM, Lax H, et al. Ten-year results of randomized treatment of children with severe vesicoureteral reflux. Final report of the International Reflux Study in children. Pediatr Nephrol 2006;21:785–92.

[64] Ehrlich RM, Gershman A, Fuchs G. Laparoscopic vesicoureteroplasty in children: initial case reports. Urology 1994;43:255–61.

[65] Janetschek G, Radmayr C, Bartsch G. Laparoscopic ureteral anti-reflux plasty reimplantation. First clinical experience. Ann Urol (Paris) 1995;29:101–5.

[66] Okamura K, Yamada Y, Tsuji Y, et al. Endoscopic trigonoplasty in pediatric patients with primary vesicoureteral reflux: preliminary report. J Urol 1996;156:198–200.

[67] Cartwright PC, Snow BW, Mansfield JC, et al. Percutaneous endoscopic trigonoplasty: a minimally invasive approach to correct vesicoureteral reflux. J Urol 1996;156:661–4.

[68] Gatti JM, Cartwright PC, Hamilton BD, et al. Percutaneous endoscopic trigonoplasty in children: long-term outcomes and modifications in technique. J Endourol 1999;13:581–4.

[69] Okamura K, Kato N, Tsuji Y, et al. A comparative study of endoscopic trigonoplasty for vesicoureteral reflux in children and in adults. Int J Urol 1999;6:562–6.

[70] Tsuji Y, Okamura K, Nishimura T, et al. A new endoscopic ureteral reimplantation for primary vesicoureteral reflux (endoscopic trigonoplasty II). J Urol 2003;169:1020–2.

[71] Lakshmanan Y, Mathews RI, Cadeddu JA, et al. Feasibility of total intravesical endoscopic surgery using mini-instruments in a porcine model. J Endourol 1999;13:41–5.

[72] Olsen LH, Deding D, Yeung CK, et al. Computer assisted laparoscopic pneumovesical ureter reimplantation a.m. Cohen: initial experience in a pig model. APMIS 2003;109(Suppl):23–5.

[73] Gill IS, Ponsky LE, Desai M, et al. Laparoscopic cross-trigonal Cohen ureteroneocystostomy: novel technique. J Urol 2001;166:1811–4.

[74] Yeung CK, Sihoe JD, Borzi PA. Endoscopic cross-trigonal ureteral reimplantation under carbon dioxide bladder insufflation: a novel technique. J Endourol 2005;19:295–9.

[75] Kutikov A, Guzzo TJ, Canter DJ, et al. Initial experience with laparoscopic transvesical ureteral reimplantation at the Children's Hospital of Philadelphia. J Urol 2006;176:2222–5 [discussion: 2225–6].

[76] Canon SJ, Jayanthi VR, Patel AS. Vesicoscopic cross-trigonal ureteral reimplantation: a minimally invasive option for repair of vesicoureteral reflux. J Urol 2007;178:269–73 [discussion: 273].

[77] Peters CA. Laparoscopy in pediatric urology. Curr Opin Urol 2004;14:67–73.

[78] Atala A, Kavoussi LR, Goldstein DS, et al. Laparoscopic correction of vesicoureteral reflux. J Urol 1993;150:748–51.

[79] Schimberg W, Wacksman J, Rudd R, et al. Laparoscopic correction of vesicoureteral reflux in the pig. J Urol 1994;151:1664–7.

[80] McDougall EM, Urban DA, Kerbl K, et al. Laparoscopic repair of vesicoureteral reflux utilizing the Lich-Gregoir technique in the pig model. J Urol 1995;153:497–500.

[81] Baldwin DD, Pope JC, Alberts GL, et al. Simplified technique for laparoscopic extravesical ureteral reimplantation in the porcine model. J Endourol 2005;19:502–7.

[82] Lakshmanan Y, Fung LC. Laparoscopic extravesicular ureteral reimplantation for vesicoureteral reflux: recent technical advances. J Endourol 2000;14:589–93 [discussion: 593–4].

[83] Riquelme M, Aranda A, Rodriguez C. Laparoscopic extravesical transperitoneal approach for vesicoureteral reflux. J Laparoendosc Adv Surg Tech A 2006;16:312–6.

[84] Shu T, Cisek LJ Jr, Moore RG. Laparoscopic extravesical reimplantation for postpubertal vesicoureteral reflux. J Endourol 2004;18:441–6.

[85] Simforoosh N, Nadjafi-Semnani M, Shahrokhi S. Extraperitoneal laparoscopic trigonoplasty for treatment of vesicoureteral reflux: novel technique duplicating its open counterpart. J Urol 2007;177:321–4.

[86] Smaldone MC, Sweeney DD, Ost MC, et al. Laparoscopy in paediatric urology: present status. BJU Int 2007;100:143–50.

[87] Peters CA, Woo R. Intravesical robotically assisted bilateral ureteral reimplantation. J Endourol 2005;19:618–21 [discussion: 621–2].

ELSEVIER
SAUNDERS

Urol Clin N Am 35 (2008) 489–504

UROLOGIC
CLINICS
of North America

Minimally Invasive Surgical Approaches and Management of Prostate Cancer

Mark L. Gonzalgo, MD, PhD[a], Nilesh Patil, MD[b],
Li-Ming Su, MD[a], Vipul R. Patel, MD[b],*

[a]Department of Urology, James Buchanan Brady Urological Institute, The Johns Hopkins Medical Institutions,
600 North Wolfe Street, Marburg 145, Baltimore, MD 21287, USA
[b]Global Robotics Institute, Florida Hospital, 601 East Rollins Street, Orlando, FL 32803, USA

Prostate cancer is the second most common cancer in men in the United States. It has been estimated that 218,890 men would be diagnosed with prostate cancer in 2007 and 27,050 would die from this disease [1]. Prostate-specific antigen (PSA) screening, which started in the 1980s, has brought about a significant increase in the detection of prostate cancers at an earlier stage. Urologists are now frequently treating younger men with less advanced disease who have excellent preoperative urinary and sexual function. Today, if a patient is diagnosed with prostate cancer, he is more likely to have clinically nonpalpable disease than his counterparts in the pre-PSA era.

For clinically localized prostate cancer, radical prostatectomy remains the "gold standard" treatment. New forms of minimally invasive therapies are sought out by patients, however, because of the potential morbidity associated with open surgery. With quality-of-life aspects influencing patient decision making, minimally invasive therapeutic modalities have generated great interest among patients. Laparoscopic radical prostatectomy (LRP), robotic-assisted laparoscopic prostatectomy (RALP), brachytherapy, cryotherapy, and high-intensity focused ultrasound (HIFU) are all considered to be minimally invasive treatment options for the management of clinically localized prostate cancer.

Laparoscopic radical prostatectomy

The first successful LRP in a man was performed in 1997 [2]. This initial experience was characterized by long operative times (8–11 hours) and an average hospitalization of 7.3 days. Based on a limited series of nine patients, it was initially believed that LRP provided no significant benefit compared with open radical prostatectomy for treatment of clinically localized prostate cancer. Widespread acceptance and application of LRP was made possible by the efforts of French urologists who published their experience and early results with this technique in 2000 [3,4]. These results demonstrated reduced operative times (4–5 hours per case), acceptable continence rates after surgery (72%–84%), and preservation of erections in approximately 45% of patients with a sufficient level of preoperative sexual function.

Patient selection

Indications for LRP are identical to those for open radical prostatectomy: patients who have clinically localized prostate cancer with no evidence of metastatic disease and are in sufficiently good health to undergo surgery. There are relatively few contraindications to LRP; however, the presence of uncorrectable bleeding diatheses or inability to tolerate general anesthesia or cardiopulmonary effects of laparoscopy may warrant pursuit of alternative treatment methods. LRP can be safely performed in patients who have a history of prior abdominal surgery, hormonal therapy, or morbid obesity [5]. The primary goals

* Corresponding author.
E-mail address: gonzalgo@jhmi.edu (V.R. Patel).

of LRP remain the same as those of open radical prostatectomy: (1) cancer control, (2) preservation of urinary continence, and (3) preservation of erectile function.

Transperitoneal technique

Anatomic principles and surgical dissection of the prostate are similar regardless of whether a pure laparoscopic or robotic-assisted approach is used. LRP is performed under general anesthesia with the patient in a supine position. The patient is secured to the table at the shoulder level to prevent movement when placed in a steep Trendelenburg position during a transperitoneal approach. LRP can also be performed in an extraperitoneal fashion; in that case, the patient can remain in a more neutral position. The legs are slightly spread apart to permit access to the perineum during the operation. A Foley catheter is inserted at the beginning of the procedure, and a nasogastric tube is used to decompress the stomach.

Pneumoperitoneum can be established with the use of a Veress needle and the abdominal cavity entered under direct vision through a periumbilical incision using a Visiport device. Additional trocars are placed inferiorly and laterally for passage of laparoscopic instrumentation (Fig. 1). Once all trocars have been inserted and the patient has been positioned in a steep Trendelenburg position to facilitate retraction of the small bowel out of the operative field, a transverse incision is made in the peritoneum below the base of the bladder in the region in which the vas deferens joins the seminal vesicles. The seminal vesicles are dissected free from surrounding tissues, and vascular pedicles are ligated with titanium or Hemolockclips (Movie 1: Dissection of seminal vesicles and vas deferentia*). Every attempt is made to avoid the use of electrocautery during lateral dissection of the seminal vesicles to prevent thermal injury to the nearby cavernous nerves responsible for erections.

Once the seminal vesicles have been mobilized, a transverse incision is made in Denonvilliers' fascia to dissect the plane between the prostate and rectum (Movie 2: Posterior prostatic dissection*) (Fig. 2). To maximize neurovascular bundle

preservation, a closer dissection to the prostate posteriorly can be performed that leaves Denonvilliers' fascia on top of the perirectal fat. Alternatively, a deeper plane of dissection between Denonvilliers' fascia and perirectal fat can be performed when more extensive or palpable cancer is present. Once the plane between the prostate and rectum has been developed, attention is then turned to the anterior prostatic dissection.

The space of Retzius is entered transperitoneally by dividing the urachus above the bladder and incising the peritoneum just medial to the medial umbilical ligaments (Movie 3: Developing the space of Retzius*) (Fig. 3). Mobilization of the bladder is performed, and the alveolar tissue anterior to the bladder within the extraperitoneal space is dissected to expose the prostate. The endopelvic fascia and puboprostatic ligaments are sharply divided to mobilize the prostate and expose the levator muscle fibers. The deep dorsal venous complex (DVC) can be suture ligated for hemostasis (Movie 4: Ligation of the deep dorsal venous complex*); however, the DVC is typically divided later during the operation before the apical dissection of the prostate and division of the urethra (Movie 5: Division of deep dorsal venous complex*).

At this point in the operation, a transverse incision is made in the anterior bladder neck (Movie 6: Bladder neck transection and prostatic pedicle ligation*). This plane of dissection is carried through the posterior bladder neck to expose the previously dissected seminal vesicles. The seminal vesicles can then be pulled through this working space to provide mobilization of the prostate for the remainder of the operation (Fig. 4). The vascular pedicles to the prostate can be ligated with titanium or Hemolock clips to avoid the use of electrocautery, which may damage the neurovascular bundles (Movie 7: Antegrade neurovascular bundle preservation*). Once the neurovascular bundles have been dissected away from the prostate, the DVC and urethra can be transected from the apex of the prostate (Movie 8: Prostatic apical dissection and division of urethra*). The vesicourethral anastomosis may be accomplished using an interrupted closure or a running continuous suture with a single knot (Movie 9: Interrupted vesicourethral anastomosis*) [6]. An anterior or posterior tennis racquet closure of the bladder neck may be required if there is a significantly sized discrepancy in the bladder neck urethral opening.

---

* Videos for this article can be accessed by visiting www.urologic.theclinics.com. In the online table of contents for this issue, click on "add-ons."

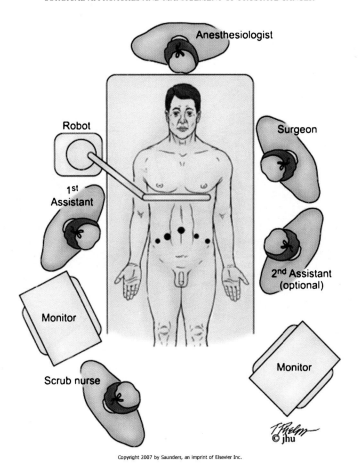

Copyright 2007 by Saunders, an imprint of Elsevier Inc.

Fig. 1. Operating room, port, and personnel configuration for laparoscopic radical prostatectomy. (*Courtesy of* Johns Hopkins University, Baltimore, MD; with permission. Copyright © 2005.)

Extraperitoneal technique

LRP can also be performed by means of an extraperitoneal approach. An infraumbilical incision is made, and the space of Retzius is entered under direct visualization with a Visiport device. The trocar and camera are removed, and the extraperitoneal space is developed using a trocar-mounted balloon dilator device (Movie 10: Extraperitoneal baloon access*) (Fig. 5). The balloon is inserted into the preperitoneal space and insufflated under direct vision. Additional trocars are inserted, and transection of the bladder neck occurs as one of the initial steps in this surgical approach. The remainder of

_____

* Videos for this article can be accessed by visiting www.urologic.theclinics.com. In the online table of contents for this issue, click on "add-ons."

the operation is similar to the transperitoneal approach.

Some studies have reported improved outcomes for extraperitoneal LRP compared with the transperitoneal approach. Extraperitoneal LRP has been associated with less operative time and has enabled faster recovery of continence compared with the transperitoneal approach [7]. Other groups have found no significant differences in clinicopathologic outcomes between the two techniques [8,9].

Pelvic lymphadenectomy

Laparoscopic pelvic lymphadenectomy may be performed in patients when indicated (ie, Gleason score ≥ 7, palpable disease, preoperative PSA ≥ 10). Laparoscopic PLND can be performed by the transperitoneal or extraperitoneal approach and using a pure laparoscopic technique or with

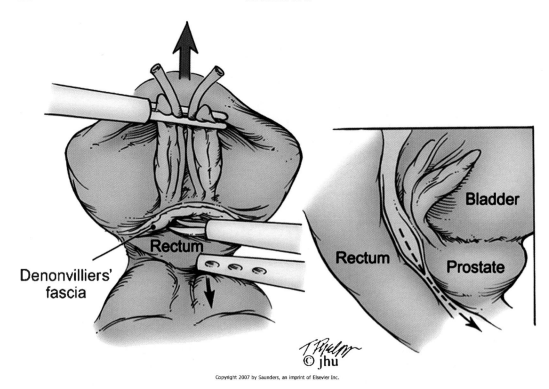

Copyright 2007 by Saunders, an imprint of Elsevier Inc.

Fig. 2. Posterior dissection of the prostate. The bedside assistant retracts the seminal vesicles and prostate in an upward direction. A transverse incision is made in Denonvilliers' fascia, and the plane between the prostate and rectum is developed. The plane of dissection toward the prostate is indicated by the dashed arrow. (*Courtesy of* Johns Hopkins University, Baltimore, MD; with permission. Copyright © 2005.)

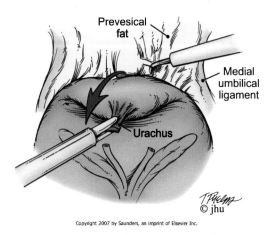

Copyright 2007 by Saunders, an imprint of Elsevier Inc.

Fig. 3. Division of urachus and entry into the space of Retzius. The urachus is retracted in a cephalad direction to assist with identification of the alveolar tissue anterior to the bladder. The medial umbilical ligaments demarcate the lateral extent of the bladder dissection. (*Courtesy of* Johns Hopkins University, Baltimore, MD; with permission. Copyright © 2005.)

robot assistance (Movie 11: Laparoscopic pelvic lymph node dissection*). The same limits of lymphadenectomy are respected as with open surgery, including the external iliac vein, pubis, obturator nerve, and bifurcation of the iliac vessels. Thermal energy and sharp dissection should be minimized to avoid vascular and neural injury. Clips should be applied to lymphatic channels to prevent postoperative lymphocele.

Pathologic outcomes after laparoscopic radical prostatectomy

The primary goal of radical prostatectomy is complete removal of the entire prostate. The most common site of a positive margin during LRP is at the prostatic apex [10]. Positive margin rates for pT2 and pT3 disease have been reported to range

---

* Videos for this article can be accessed by visiting www.urologic.theclinics.com. In the online table of contents for this issue, click on "add-ons."

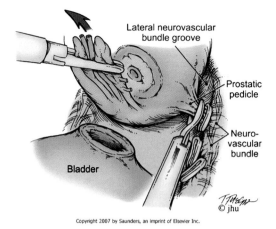

Fig. 4. Ligation of the prostatic pedicles and antegrade dissection of the neurovascular bundle. Anterior traction can be applied to the seminal vesicles and vasa to identify the prostatic pedicles. Titanium or Hemolock clips can be used for hemostasis to avoid the use of electrocautery. The direction and course of antegrade neurovascular bundle dissection can be guided by initially defining the lateral neurovascular bundle groove. (*Courtesy of* Johns Hopkins University, Baltimore, MD; with permission. Copyright © 2005.)

from 4.7% to 18.4% and from 26.2% to 45.7%, respectively [11–14]. Increasing experience has been shown to be associated with a decrease in the rate of positive surgical margins, suggesting that inexperience with the laparoscopic surgical approach may contribute to a higher rate of positive surgical margins.

A recent prospective analysis of clinical and pathologic outcomes of 508 men who underwent LRP at Johns Hopkins Medical Institutions

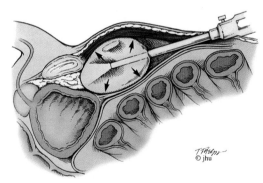

Fig. 5. Extraperitoneal approach for LRP by creation of working space with a trocar-mounted balloon dilator device. (*Courtesy of* Johns Hopkins University, Baltimore, MD; with permission. Copyright © 2005.)

demonstrated positive margin rates of 8.2% for pT2 disease and 39.3% for pT3 disease [15]. Three-year actuarial biochemical recurrence-free survival was 98.2% for pT2N0/Nx disease, 78.7% for pT3N0/Nx/N1 disease, and 94.5% overall.

Potency after laparoscopic radical prostatectomy

Avoidance of energy sources, such as monopolar or bipolar electrocautery and harmonic scalpel, during dissection of the neurovascular bundles has been associated with improved return of potency after surgery [16,17]. Potency rates after LRP have been reported to range from 46% to 88% (Table 1). Hemolock clips can be used to ligate vessels during dissection of the neurovascular bundles to minimize or eliminate the use of thermal energy.

A combined antegrade and retrograde laparoscopic approach for neurovascular bundle dissection with minimization of thermal energy can be accomplished with minimal blood loss and with excellent anatomic nerve preservation. The authors' experience with this technique has demonstrated that approximately 76% of patients engaging in sexual intercourse before surgery who underwent bilateral nerve preservation reported the ability to engage in sexual intercourse 1 year after LRP [11]. Improved potency outcomes have also been reported with a technique that incorporates temporary control of the lateral prostatic pedicle with bulldog clamps and real-time intraoperative transrectal ultrasound to visualize pulsations of the cavernous vessels within the neurovascular bundle [18,19]. Among patients with excellent preoperative potency (SHIM ≥ 22), the 1-year intercourse rate when using this technique was 88%. Faster recovery of erectile function using this technique was also observed and was found to be correlated with preserved pulsatile blood vessels within the neurovascular bundle on power Doppler transrectal ultrasonography [19].

Continence after laparoscopic radical prostatectomy

Urinary incontinence after LRP is typically manifested by stress incontinence attributable primarily to intrinsic sphincter deficiency. Differences in surgical technique may account for variability in the levels of continence after LRP; however, the exact physiologic mechanisms that contribute to urinary control after surgery are not entirely understood. Continence rates after LRP

Table 1
Potency rates after laparoscopic radical prostatectomy

Reference	Total patients	Evaluable patients	Definition used	Method of assessment	Assessment time	Potency rate
Hoznek et al [80]	200	82	Intercourse	Questionnaire	1 month	46%
Turk et al [81]	125	44	Intercourse	Physician	12 months	59%
Salomon et al [82]	235	43	Intercourse	Questionnaire	12 months	58.8%
Eden et al [83]	100	100	Erections	Physician	12 months	62%
Guillonneau et al [84]	550	47	Intercourse	Physician	1.5 months	66%
Anastasiadis et al [85]	230	230	Intercourse	Questionnaire	12 months	53%
Roumeguere et al [14]	85	85	Intercourse	Questionnaire	12 months	65.3%
Stolzenburg et al [86]	700	185	Intercourse	Questionnaire	6 months	47%
Rassweiler et al [12]	5824	NA	Intercourse	Questionnaire	12 months	52.5%
Su et al [11]	177	177	Intercourse	Questionnaire	12 months	76%
Goeman et al [87]	550	NA	Intercourse	Questionnaire	12 months	56%
Gill and Ukimura [19]	76	54	Intercourse	Questionnaire	12 months	88%

Data from Su LM, Smith JA. Laparoscopic and robotic-assisted laparoscopic radical prostatectomy and pelvic lymphadenectomy. In: Wein AJ, editor. Campbell-Walsh Urology, 9th ed. Philadelphia: Elsevier, 2007.

have been reported to range from 71% to 92% at various follow-up times (Table 2). It has been demonstrated that reconstruction of the posterior rhabdomyosphincter may lead to more rapid recovery of continence after radical prostatectomy [20]. At the time of catheter removal, 74.2% of patients were continent using this reconstructive technique after LRP [21].

Evolution of robotic surgery

In 1495, Leonardo da Vinci designed a "mechanized" mannequin in the form of an armed knight. During the Renaissance, this became a model from which numerous other mannequins were constructed for entertainment [22]. The term *robot* was first coined by Karel Capek in the 1923 book, *Rossum's Universal Robots* and relates to the Czech word for slave labor, *robota* [23]. The word robot and its practical applications increased only in the twentieth and twenty-first centuries, however.

The earliest uses of robots were for military purposes. The first surgical application was in 1985 in a neurosurgical procedure [24]. It was used to orient a needle for a brain biopsy under CT guidance. In 1992, International Business Machines (IBM) and associates developed a prototype for orthopedic surgery. The "ROBODOC" was used to assist surgeons in milling out a hole in the femur for total hip replacements [25]. A new era was beginning, and the concept of telepresence technology, which would allow the surgeon to operate at a distance from the operating room,

was being intensively researched simultaneously at the Stanford Research Institute, Department of Defense, and National Aeronautics and Space Administration (NASA). Intuitive Surgical acquired the prototype and commercialized the system. Soon thereafter, Computer Motion unveiled the first laparoscopic camera holder. Computer Motion later created a surgical system, which is an integrated robotic system [26]. In March 2003, the fusion of both companies was announced under the name of Intuitive Surgical, Inc.

The Intuitive Surgical system's main components are a control console that is operated by the surgeon and the surgical cart, which consists of four arms. The arms are operated by manipulation of two master controls on the surgeon console. The Intuitive Surgical system has tremor filtration, movement scaling, increased range of motion, three-dimensional vision, and ergonomic advantages. All these features make it ideal for complex laparoscopic movements in an anatomically confined space.

Binder and Kramer [27] from Germany reported on the first RALP in 2001. In 2002, a team from Henry Ford Hospital in Detroit reported on their initial experience with the use of the Intuitive Surgical robot [28]. Since then, a tremendous growth has been seen all around the world in adoption of this technique. In the year 2007, it was estimated that more than 40,000 radical prostatectomies would be performed robotically (personal communication, Intuitive Surgical).

Table 2
Continence rates after laparoscopic radical prostatectomy

Reference	Total patients	Definition used	Method of assessment	Follow-up (months)	Continence rate
Hoznek et al [80]	200	No pad	Questionnaire	12	86%
Turk et al [81]	125	0–1 pad	Physician	9	92%
Olsson et al [88]	228	No pad	Questionnaire	12	78.4%
Salomon et al [82]	235	No pad	Questionnaire	12	90%
Eden [83]	100	No pad	Physician	12	90%
Guillonneau et al [84]	550	No pad	Physician	12	82.3%
Anastasiadis et al [85]	230	No pad	Questionnaire	12	71.6%
Roumeguere et al [14]	85	No pad	Questionnaire	12	80.7%
Stolzenburg et al [86]	700	No pad	Questionnaire	12	92%
Rassweiler et al [12]	5824	No pad	Questionnaire	12	84.9%
Goeman et al [87]	550	No pad	Questionnaire	12	82.9%

Data from Su LM, Smith JA. Laparoscopic and robotic-assisted laparoscopic radical prostatectomy and pelvic lymphadenectomy. In: Wein AJ, editor. Campbell-Walsh Urology, 9th ed. Philadelphia: Elsevier, 2007.

Robotic-assisted laparoscopic prostatectomy

Similar to LRP, RALP can be performed transperitoneally or extraperitoneally. Pneumoperitoneum is generated using a Veress needle or Hasson technique. The abdomen is insufflated using carbon dioxide at 15 mm Hg, and trocars are placed under direct vision. The patient is placed in a lithotomy position and in a steep Trendelenburg position. The robot is docked to the trocars, and the procedure is begun using a 0° binocular lens, monopolar scissors in the right arm, PK dissecting forceps in the left arm, and the Prograsp in the fourth arm.

The anterior peritoneum is incised (bladder takedown) to enter the retropubic space of Retzius. The endopelvic fascia is then incised, and the levator ani fibers are separated from the prostate. The DVC is ligated, and a suspension stitch is placed with a 1-0 Monocryl suture on a CT-1 needle.

To proceed with the bladder neck dissection, a scope with a 30° down angle is used. Dissection proceeds in a downward direction until the urethra and catheter are visualized. The posterior wall of the bladder neck is dissected, and the vas deferens and the seminal vesicles are exposed. The seminal vesicle is dissected by approaching its medial wall initially in an atraumatic and athermal fashion.

Denonvilliers' fascia is then incised, and the posterior rectal plane is developed distally toward the urethra. The pedicles are ligated with hemostatic clips, and an athermal early retrograde release of the neurovascular bundle is performed.

Apical dissection is then performed using cold scissors to divide the DVC and urethra. The vesicourethral anastomosis is performed using a modified technique by Van Velthoven and colleagues [6]. A single continuous running suture is used by tying two separate 20-cm length 3-0 Monocryl sutures together with 10 knots. The posterior anastomosis is performed with one arm of the suture beginning at the 5 o'clock position running clockwise to the 10 o'clock position. The anterior anastomosis is completed with the second arm of the suture starting in the 5 o'clock position and proceeding in a counterclockwise fashion. Both sutures are tied in the 10 o'clock position on the urethral stump. A Foley catheter is left in place for 4 to 7 days. As with LRP, pelvic lymphadenectomy may be performed using robotic assistance when indicated.

Operative outcomes

Operative time

Comparing operative times is difficult in large series because they include setup time and pelvic lymph node dissection (Table 3). Operative times may also vary according to the learning curve. The operative time decreases as surgeon experience grows. In a previously reported series by Patel and colleagues [29], mean operative time was 130 minutes in their first 500 cases. With the authors' experience now having passed 1500 cases, the operative time has been reduced to 90 minutes [30]. This decrease in time has been noted despite adding a few new surgical variations to the authors' previously described technique (ie, DVC

Table 3
Operative time, blood loss, and transfusion data for robotic-assisted laparoscopic prostatectomy

Authors	No. cases	Operative time (minutes)	Blood loss (mL)	Transfusion rate (%)	In-hospital stay (days)	Catheter removal (days)
Patel et al [29]	500	130	50	0%	1	6.9
Joseph et al [89]	325	130	196	1%	1	—
Bhandari et al [90]	300	177	109	0%	1.2	6.9
Ahlering et al [38]	60	231	103	0%	1	7
Farnham et al [37]	176	—	191	0.5%	—	—
Cathelineau et al [91]	105	180	500	6%	5.5	7
Menon et al [31]	200	160	153	0%	1.2	7

and urethral suspension, posterior rhabdosphincter reconstruction). The mean operative time reported by Menon and colleagues [28] in 2002 was 274 minutes in their first 40 patients. In recently published data by the same investigators, the mean operative time reported was 154 minutes [31].

Blood loss

Decreased blood loss is one of the key advantages of minimally invasive surgery (see Table 3). Because most blood loss arises from the venous sinuses, the tamponade effect of pneumoperitoneum helps to diminish blood loss. Improved three-dimensional vision and precise ligation of vessels are contributing factors to the decreased amount of blood loss in RALP.

The overall transfusion rate reported in series beyond the learning curve varies from 0% to 12% [32–34]. Decreased blood loss has been a distinguishing feature of LRP and RALP. In many series, the rate of transfusion has been 0% [35,36]. Patel and colleagues [29] reported a blood transfusion rate of 0.4% in their initial RALP series. Farnham and colleagues [37] have reported in a prospective comparative study between RALP and radical retropubic prostatectomy (RRP) that the median serum discharge hematocrit was higher with RALP (38%) than after open radical prostatectomy (33%).

Hospital stay

Health care policies practiced in different centers around the world influence the duration of hospitalization (see Table 3). It is considered an important feature of patient recovery, however, and a measure of cost expenditure on the part of the hospital and patient likewise. The advantage of LRP and RALP is with respect to less postoperative pain and blood loss. The mean length of stay in larger series has been shown to be 1.08 to 1.5 days. Ahlering and colleagues [38] reported

a shorter length of stay in patients after RALP compared with RRP (25.9 versus 52.8 hours). It is becoming increasingly evident that a large number of patients undergoing RALP can be discharged within 24 hours of the surgery. In a prospective evaluation of short-term impact and recovery of health-related quality of life in men undergoing RALP versus open radical prostatectomy, Miller and colleagues [39] showed that there was decreased morbidity associated with RALP. Physical Component Score scores returned to baseline sooner in the RALP group compared with the open surgical group. Smith and colleagues [40] showed that discharge on the first postoperative day can also be achieved in most patients who undergo open radical prostatectomy, however.

Continence

RALP has the potential to allow for an earlier return of continence in patients (Table 4). Earlier return of continence is thought to be possible because of improved preservation of urethral sphincter and urethral length. The hypothesis is that better visualization of the apex allows the surgeon to sweep away urethral sphincter muscular tissue from the anterior prostate gently and improved hemostasis prevents blood from obscuring the apex, leading to inadvertent injury to the sphincter [38].

Urinary continence recovery, defined as use of no protection system or use of a single liner for security reasons, has been reported to vary from 72% to 95% [34,41,42]. A comparative study between RRP and RALP by Tewari and colleagues [43] showed that robotic surgery allowed earlier continence recovery compared with the traditional retropubic approach. Walsh and colleagues [44] reported their continence results in open RRP to be 54% at 3 months, 80% at 6 months, 93% at 12 months, and 93% at 18 months. Patel and

Table 4
Continence data for robotic-assisted laparoscopic prostatectomy

Authors	No. cases	Continence definition	Method of data collection	Continence rates (%)		
				3 months	6 months	12 months
Patel et al [29]	500	No pad	Questionnaire	89%	95%	—
Joseph et al [89]	325	No pad	Questionnaire	93%	96%	—
Ahlering et al [51]	90	No pad	Questionnaire	81%	—	—
Bentas et al [52]	41	0–1 pad ("safety pad")	Questionnaire	—	—	84%

colleagues [29] reported their continence data in 500 patients to be 89%, 95%, and 97% at 3, 6, and 12 months, respectively. Continence in this study was defined as no pad use. Body mass index (BMI) has been shown to be closely related to recovery of continence. Patients who had a BMI greater than 30 had a 6-month continence rate of 47% compared with 91% observed in patients who had a BMI less than 30 [45].

Posterior reconstruction of the rhabdosphincter or pelvic floor has been described in open prostatectomy and LRP, in which it was found to improve early postoperative urinary continence rates [20,21]. The authors use a modification of this technique for RALP with an aim to improve early continence after surgery. At 1 week, of 50 patients, 29 (58%) were completely continent, 7 (14%) had mild incontinence, 8 (16%) had moderate incontinence, and 6 (12%) had severe incontinence (unpublished data).

Potency

Factors like age, preoperative potency, nerve sparing, and individual surgical technique all seem to affect postoperative recovery of erectile function (Table 5). The anatomic basis for nerve sparing during RRP was initially described by Walsh and Donker [46]. After their description, a large number of modifications and different techniques have been described. Series with follow-up of data for more than 12 months have reported potency percentages ranging from 20% to 78% [29,33]. This is the percentage of patients who are able to have intercourse after nerve-sparing RALP. Patel and colleagues [47] described the Ohio State technique of early retrograde release of NVB while using an antegrade approach for nerve sparing. The early retrograde release helps in identifying the prostatic pedicle and prevents undue traction on the NVB. This allows a more efficient nerve-sparing procedure to be performed.

Ahlering and colleagues [48] have reported on a prospective, nonrandomized, comparative study adopting a cautery-free technique for neurovascular bundle preservation that allows for a higher potency rate at 3 months of follow-up compared with standard techniques. Chien and colleagues [49] have demonstrated that avoiding the use of clips or monopolar cautery during robotic LRP may result in early return of sexual function. Potency was defined as return to baseline function, and they reported 3-, 6-, and 12-month potency rates of 54%, 66%, and 59%, respectively.

The team at Henry Ford Hospital has described a "veil of Aphrodite" technique for nerve preservation. A plane of dissection between the prostatic fascia and the prostate capsule is established to enhance nerve preservation. Among patients with no preoperative erectile dysfunction (SHIM >21) who underwent bilateral veil nerve-sparing surgery, intercourse was successful in 70% and 97% of the patients at 12 and 48 months of follow-up, respectively. Approximately half of these patients attained a normal SHIM score without medication [50].

Table 5
Potency data for robotic-assisted laparoscopic prostatectomy

Authors	No. cases	Potency definition	Data collection	Potency rates (%)		
				3 months	6 months	12 months
Chien et al [49]	56	Return to baseline	UCLA-PCI	54%	66%	69%
Menon et al [31]	200	Sexual intercourse	IIEF-5	25%	64%	—
Ahlering et al [42]	23	Sexual intercourse	IIEF-5	47%	—	—

Oncologic data

Surgical technique and expertise are considered to be important factors in the progressive reduction in the rates of positive surgical margins (Table 6). Positive margin rates vary in reported series from 2% to 36% [50,51]. After data are stratified by pathologic staging, positive margin rates are between 4.7% and 27% for pT2 and 26% and 67% for pT3 disease [33,52]. It has been shown that as surgeon experience increases, the rate of positive margins decreases. Patel and colleagues [33] have reported a reduction in overall positive margin rates from 13% in the first 100 patients to 8% in the next 100 patients. Positive margin was defined as presence of cancer cells at the inked margin.

One of the criticisms of RALP has been that there is no tactile feedback from the robotic arms to the surgeon. The fear was that this would lead to poorer oncologic results compared with open surgery. In two prospective, nonrandomized, comparative studies, Ahlering and colleagues [38] and Tewari and colleagues [43] have shown that the positive surgical margin rates were higher in patients who underwent RRP compared with RALP [38,43]. The 5-year actuarial biochemical free survival rate among 2766 patients who underwent RALP at a single institution was reported to be 84% [53].

Conclusions about laparoscopic radical prostatectomy and robotic-assisted laparoscopic prostatectomy

Minimally invasive surgery has considerably changed the surgical treatment of prostate cancer. Critical analysis of the data available for LRP and RALP suggests that results are similar to open retropubic prostatectomy. Reduced blood loss, decreased postoperative pain and convalescence, and possibly early return to continence are their main advantages. Midterm results of LRP and RALP are encouraging. These excellent outcomes have to await long-term oncologic and functional data, however, to define the precise role of LRP and RALP as alternative surgical treatments to open radical prostatectomy.

Radiation therapy and brachytherapy

External beam radiation therapy (EBRT) typically requires multiple administration doses referred to as fractions. Simulation is performed as part of pretreatment planning to generate a model of the patient that is used for radiation therapy. Intensity-modulated radiation therapy (IMRT) uses three-dimensional conformal reconstruction to optimize angles and shapes for radiation delivery. This technique provides more accurate delivery of radiation to prostate tissue and is currently the most widely used form of external beam radiation for definitive management of prostate cancer [54].

Prostate brachytherapy is typically performed under spinal or general anesthesia as an outpatient procedure. The most commonly used isotopes for brachytherapy seeds are iodine-125 (^{125}I) or palladium-103 (^{103}Pd). Pretreatment imaging may include transrectal ultrasound and CT-based volumetric studies to assist with planning three-dimensional seed distribution. Brachytherapy seeds are placed under direct transrectal ultrasound guidance during the procedure. Low-energy radiation is emitted from implanted seeds for a period of weeks to months to destroy prostate cancer cells. Relative contraindications for prostate brachytherapy include large prostate size (>50–60 cm^3), prior history of transurethral resection of the prostate (TURP), and irritative or obstructive voiding symptoms. A trial of androgen deprivation may be used for men with larger prostates to reduce the size of the gland to an acceptable range for brachytherapy.

Table 6
Positive margin data for robotic-assisted laparoscopic prostatectomy

Authors	No. cases	Pathologic stage			Overall PSM rate (%)
		pT2	pT3a	pT3b	
Patel et al [29]	500	78%	15%	5%	9.4%
Bentas et al [52]	41	63%	22%	15%	30%
Costello et al [92]	122	80%	16%	4%	16%
Ahlering et al [51]	50	62%	36%		36%
Chien et al [49]	56	82%	18%		11%

High-intensity focused ultrasound

HIFU is a technology that causes thermal tissue destruction with precision and minimum damage to the surrounding structures. It was discovered in the early 1940s and has been used to destroy tumors. Its use to treat localized prostate cancer has been increasing in Europe. A probe is inserted transrectally, and a high-energy ultrasound beam is focused into the prostate. Acoustic energy absorbed by the prostate tissue is converted into thermal energy, with intraprostatic temperatures reaching upward of 98.6 °C. The result is a focal area of coagulative necrosis. Tissue outside the focal zone, including rectal mucosa and serosa, has no significant temperature increase, and therefore no tissue damage.

The mechanism of action of HIFU is based on mechanical and thermal effects to achieve destruction of prostate tissue. Thermal energy is associated with absorption of ultrasound energy by the prostate and generation of heat. Ultrasound waves are delivered by a transducer. As they travel through tissues, ultrasound waves deposit energy into tissues. HIFU uses a high intensity of the waves and focuses them on a single point to deposit large amounts of energy into a focal area, thus resulting in tissue destruction [55]. Tissue damage occurs by two different mechanisms: thermal effect and cavitation [56]. Absorption of ultrasound energy into the tissue gets converted into heat, causing the thermal effect. An increase in temperature of up to 70 °C to 100 °C can be achieved in a few seconds with each pulse. The interaction of ultrasound and microbubbles in the sonicated tissue is responsible for the cavitation mechanism. Both of these mechanisms cause the destruction of the cells by coagulative necrosis.

HIFU is generally indicated for patients who have localized prostate cancer and are not candidates for surgery because of age, medical comorbidities, or preference. HIFU has largely been used and is typically recommended for patients who have localized prostate cancer with clinical stage T1 to T2 NxM0 to N0M0 prostate cancer who are not suitable candidates for radical prostatectomy (eg, age >70 years, life expectancy ≤10 years, major comorbidities precluding surgery) or who refuse to undergo surgery [57,58]. HIFU can also be used for local recurrence of prostate cancer after radiation or brachytherapy failure.

Unlike other nonsurgical treatments for clinically localized prostate cancer, HIFU treatment can be repeated for local recurrence and can also be used as salvage therapy. Prostate gland size greater than 40 cm^3 is a relative contraindication for the use of this technique because of the focal length of HIFU [59]. Larger glands can be treated with certain HIFU devices after downsizing by means of TURP or hormonal therapy. Because treatment is administered by means of a transrectal probe, any rectal pathologic finding is a relative contraindication. Finally, major prostatic calcifications can lead to ultrasonic wave transmission impairment and should be considered a contraindication unless TURP can remove them.

High-intensity focused ultrasound devices

Two commercially available devices for HIFU are currently in use: the Sonablate and Ablatherm. Both devices use transrectal ultrasound-guided imaging for treatment with a probe that is encased within a degassed fluid-filled coupling balloon to cool the rectum. Several differences between the two devices exist with respect to patient positioning, treatment, planning, ultrasound frequency, intraprostatic treatment mode, and rectal wall control.

The Ablatherm has imaging (7.5 MHz) and therapeutic (3 MHz) transducers included in a unique endorectal probe focused at 40 mm. It requires a specific bed with a patient in the lateral position. It includes three treatment protocols with specifically designed treatment parameters depending on the clinical use (standard, HIFU retreatment, and radiation failure).

The Sonablate uses a single transducer (4 MHz) for imaging and treatment. Several probes are available with many focal lengths (25–45 mm). The procedure is conducted in a dorsal position with the patient lying on a regular operating table. It uses a single treatment protocol in which the power is manually modified by the operator. This visually directed HIFU treatment is based on gray-scale ultrasonographic changes observed during treatment, which allows the operator to change the power level for each HIFU pulse [60].

Both devices offer real-time ultrasonic monitoring of the treatment. Because the rectal wall is sensitive to temperature changes, precise rectal monitoring is required. Hence, both devices provide active cooling of the rectal wall during treatment, continuous temperature monitoring of the rectal wall, and constant distance measuring between the rectal wall and the prostate.

Early data regarding the use of HIFU for treatment of prostate cancer is primarily from Europe (Table 7). There are no randomized controlled studies available to compare the outcomes of HIFU with those of other therapies. Various studies have reported a disease-free survival rate ranging from 66% to 84% [61,62]. The first long-term study of 140 patients who had clinically localized prostate cancer treated with the Ablatherm demonstrated actuarial biochemical failure-free survival rates at 5 and 7 years of 77% and 69%, respectively. The actuarial disease-free survival rates at 5 and 7 years were 66% and 59%, respectively [63]. In summary, HIFU is still evolving as a treatment modality for clinically localized prostate cancer. The main advantages of HIFU seem to be its low morbidity and the possibility of repeated treatments.

Cryotherapy

Cryotherapy involves the freezing and thawing of tissue with the use of probes inserted into prostate tissue. Isotherms are created around each probe that radially extend into surrounding tissues until a normothermic temperature is attained. Temperatures can reach as low as -190 °C at the cryoprobe and warm to 0 °C at the periphery of the ice ball [64]. The freeze margin can be visualized under direct ultrasound guidance by the hyperechoic appearance of the cold zone. Tissues transition to normothermic temperatures beyond this margin. Cellular tissue near the probe is cooled more rapidly and to a lower temperature than tissue further away from the probe. Cellular injury and death are attributable to mechanical destruction from ice formation and cellular biochemical injury resulting from ischemic effects, endovascular cell death, and apoptosis.

There are two mechanisms responsible for direct cellular injury during cryotherapy. The first results from rapid cooling of cells closest to the cryoprobe, with formation of intracellular ice crystals that cause mechanical disruption of cell membranes [65]. The critical temperature for cellular destruction has been reported to be -40 °C [66,67]. The second mechanism for cellular injury and cell death involves slow cooling and a dehydration effect resulting from ice formation in the extracellular space further away from the cryoprobe [65]. This process is cumulative, time-dependent, and most damaging during the thaw phase. Biochemical effects from this process lead to cell membrane injury and an increase in cellular ion permeability; they also weaken the cytoskeleton, leading to increased sensitivity to mechanical injury. Damaged endothelial cells can also become more permeable and increase the likelihood of platelet aggregation and microthrombus formation [68].

Cryoablation has been used for primary treatment of clinically localized prostate cancer and also as salvage therapy. Robinson and colleagues [69] have shown excellent quality-of-life outcomes using validated questionnaires after cryoablation. A total of 69 men were studied and found to have a high level of return to baseline quality of life in all domains by 12 months, except for sexual functioning. At 3 years after cryoablation, quality of life was found to be stable with no new complications [70]. Approximately 13% of men returned to baseline levels of sexual function, with an additional 34% of patients able to resume sexual activity with treatment [70]. Another retrospective study of 223 patients managed with primary cryoablation found a 4.3% incidence of incontinence, an 85% incidence of erectile dysfunction, and 10% of men who required a subsequent procedure to manage urethral sloughing. Despite these reported complications, 96% of the men in this study reported a high degree of satisfaction with their choice of cryotherapy as treatment [71].

One of the earliest studies examining the efficacy of salvage prostate cryoablation demonstrated an 86% negative biopsy rate at 3 months after treatment but was associated with a high complication rate because of the early use of liquid nitrogen–based cooling systems [72]. Other

Table 7
High-intensity focused ultrasound data

Authors	No. patients	Clinical stage	Mean pre-HIFU PSA	Mean follow-up	Mean follow-up	Disease-free survival rate (%)
Poissonnier [61]	227	T1–2N0M0	6.99	27	27	66%
Blana et al [62]	146	T1–2N0M0	11.3	22.5	22.5	84%
Chaussy and Thuroff [59]	271	T1–2N0M0	8.3	14.8	14.8	82.1%

studies demonstrated negative biopsy rates for salvage cryoablation as high as 93% [73]. The introduction of gas-based cryoablation equipment has been shown to achieve similar oncologic efficacy as earlier systems with a significant reduction in the incidence of complications, such as rectourethral fistula formation and urinary incontinence [74]. The incidence of rectourethral fistula has been reduced to 0% to 3%, and urinary incontinence has been reported to range from to 0% to 13% after treatment [75,76]. The negative prostate biopsy rate for salvage cryoablation has been shown to range from 86% to 95% and is associated with a 5- to 7-year biochemical disease-free survival rate of 40% to 68% for a PSA cutoff less than 0.5 ng/mL [77–79].

References

[1] Jemal A, Siegel R, Ward E, et al. Cancer statistics, 2007. CA Cancer J Clin 2007;57(1):43–66.

[2] Schuessler WW, Schulam PG, Clayman RV, et al. Laparoscopic radical prostatectomy: initial short-term experience. Urology 1997;50(6):854–7.

[3] Guillonneau B, Vallancien G. Laparoscopic radical prostatectomy: the Montsouris technique. J Urol 2000;163(6):1643–9.

[4] Abbou CC, Salomon L, Hoznek A, et al. Laparoscopic radical prostatectomy: preliminary results. Urology 2000;55(5):630–4.

[5] Eden CG, Chang CM, Gianduzzo T, et al. The impact of obesity on laparoscopic radical prostatectomy. BJU Int 2006;98(6):1279–82.

[6] Van Velthoven RF, Ahlering TE, Peltier A, et al. Technique for laparoscopic running urethrovesical anastomosis: the single knot method. Urology 2003;61(4):699–702.

[7] Porpiglia F, Terrone C, Tarabuzzi R, et al. Transperitoneal versus extraperitoneal laparoscopic radical prostatectomy: experience of a single center. Urology 2006;68(2):376–80.

[8] Erdogru T, Teber D, Frede T, et al. Comparison of transperitoneal and extraperitoneal laparoscopic radical prostatectomy using match-pair analysis. Eur Urol 2004;46(3):312–9 [discussion: 320].

[9] Rozet F, Galiano M, Cathelineau X, et al. Extraperitoneal laparoscopic radical prostatectomy: a prospective evaluation of 600 cases. J Urol 2005; 174(3):908–11.

[10] Touijer K, Kuroiwa K, Saranchuk JW, et al. Quality improvement in laparoscopic radical prostatectomy for pT2 prostate cancer: impact of video documentation review on positive surgical margin. J Urol 2005; 173(3):765–8.

[11] Su LM, Link RE, Bhayani SB, et al. Nerve-sparing laparoscopic radical prostatectomy: replicating the open surgical technique. Urology 2004;64(1):123–7.

[12] Rassweiler J, Stolzenburg J, Sulser T, et al. Laparoscopic radical prostatectomy—the experience of the German Laparoscopic Working Group. Eur Urol 2006;49(1):113–9.

[13] Guillonneau B, el-Fettouh H, Baumert H, et al. Laparoscopic radical prostatectomy: oncological evaluation after 1,000 cases at Montsouris Institute. J Urol 2003;169(4):1261–6.

[14] Roumeguere T, Bollens R, Vanden Bossche M, et al. Radical prostatectomy: a prospective comparison of oncological and functional results between open and laparoscopic approaches. World J Urol 2003;20(6): 360–6.

[15] Pavlovich CP, Trock BJ, Sulman A, et al. 3-Year actuarial biochemical recurrence-free survival following laparoscopic radical prostatectomy: experience from a tertiary referral center in the United States. J Urol, in press.

[16] Ahlering TE, Eichel L, Chou D, et al. Feasibility study for robotic radical prostatectomy cautery-free neurovascular bundle preservation. Urology 2005;65(5):994–7.

[17] Ahlering TE, Skarecky D, Borin J. Impact of cautery versus cautery-free preservation of neurovascular bundles on early return of potency. J Endourol 2006;20(8):586–9.

[18] Gill IS, Ukimura O, Rubinstein M, et al. Lateral pedicle control during laparoscopic radical prostatectomy: refined technique. Urology 2005;65(1):23–7.

[19] Gill IS, Ukimura O. Thermal energy-free laparoscopic nerve-sparing radical prostatectomy: one-year potency outcomes. Urology 2007;70(2):309–14.

[20] Rocco F, Carmignani L, Acquati P, et al. Restoration of posterior aspect of rhabdosphincter shortens continence time after radical retropubic prostatectomy. J Urol 2006;175(6):2201–6.

[21] Rocco B, Gregori A, Stener S, et al. Posterior reconstruction of the rhabdosphincter allows a rapid recovery of continence after transperitoneal videolaparoscopic radical prostatectomy. Eur Urol 2007; 51(4):996–1003.

[22] Hegarty N, Gill IS. Robotic urologic surgery: an introduction and vision for the future. In: Pater VR, editor. Robotic urologic surgery. Springer; 2007. p. 1–14.

[23] Capek K. Rossum's universal robots. New York: Doubleday; 1923.

[24] Kwoh YS, Hou J, Jonckheere EA, et al. A robot with improved absolute positioning accuracy for CT guided stereotactic brain surgery. IEEE Trans Biomed Eng 1988;35:153–60.

[25] Bann S, Khan M, Hernandez J, et al. Robotics in surgery. J Am Coll Surg 2003;196(5):784–95.

[26] Satava RM. Robotic surgery: from past to future—a personal journey. Surg Clin North Am 2003;83(6): 1491–500, xii.

[27] Binder J, Kramer W. Robotically-assisted laparoscopic radical prostatectomy. BJU Int 2001;87(4): 408–10.

[28] Menon M, Shrivastava A, Tewari A, et al. Laparo-scopic and robot assisted radical prostatectomy: establishment of a structured program and prelimi-nary analysis of outcomes. J Urol 2002;168(3):945–9.

[29] Patel VR, Thaly R, Shah K. Robotic radical prosta-tectomy: outcomes of 500 cases. BJU Int 2007;99(5): 1109–12.

[30] Palmer KJ, Shah K, Thaly R, et al. Robotic assisted laparoscopic radical prostatectomy: perioperative outcomes of 1500 consecutive cases. Urology 2007; (Suppl 3a):136.

[31] Menon M, Shrivastava A, Kaul S, et al. Vattikuti In-stitute prostatectomy: contemporary technique and analysis of results. Eur Urol 2007;51(3):648–57 [dis-cussion: 657–8].

[32] Menon M, Tewari A. Robotic radical prostatectomy and the Vattikuti Urology Institute technique: an interim analysis of results and technical points. Urol-ogy 2003;61(4 Suppl 1):15–20.

[33] Patel VR, Tully AS, Holmes R, et al. Robotic radical prostatectomy in the community setting—the learn-ing curve and beyond: initial 200 cases. J Urol 2005; 174(1):269–72.

[34] Wolfram M, Brautigam R, Engl T, et al. Robotic-assisted laparoscopic radical prostatectomy: the Frankfurt technique. World J Urol 2003;21(3): 128–32.

[35] Menon M, AS A, Kaul S, et al. Vattikuti Institute prostatectomy: contemporary technique and analy-sis of results. Eur Urol 2007;51:648–58.

[36] Joseph JV, Vicente I, Madeb R, et al. Robot-assisted vs pure laparoscopic radical prostatectomy: are there any differences? BJU Int 2005;96(1):39–42.

[37] Farnham SB, Webster TM, Herrell SD, et al. Intra-operative blood loss and transfusion requirements for robotic-assisted radical prostatectomy versus radical retropubic prostatectomy. Urology 2006; 67(2):360–3.

[38] Ahlering TE, Woo D, Eichel L, et al. Robot-assisted versus open radical prostatectomy: a comparison of one surgeon's outcomes. Urology 2004;63(5):819–22.

[39] Miller J, Smith A, Kouba E, et al. Prospective evaluation of short-term impact and recovery of health related quality of life in men undergoing robotic assisted laparoscopic radical prostatectomy versus open radical prostatectomy. J Urol 2007; 178(3 Pt 1):854–8 [discussion: 859].

[40] Nelson B, Kaufman M, Broughton G, et al. Com-parison of length of hospital stay between radical retropubic prostatectomy and robotic assisted lapa-roscopic prostatectomy. J Urol 2007;177(3):929–31.

[41] Menon M, Shrivastava A, Sarle R, et al. Vattikuti Institute prostatectomy: a single-team experience of 100 cases. J Endourol 2003;17(9):785–90.

[42] Ahlering TE, Skarecky D, Lee D, et al. Successful transfer of open surgical skills to a laparoscopic environment using a robotic interface: initial experi-ence with laparoscopic radical prostatectomy. J Urol 2003;170(5):1738–41.

[43] Tewari A, Srivasatava A, Menon M. A prospective comparison of radical retropubic and robot-assisted prostatectomy: experience in one institution. BJU Int 2003;92(3):205–10.

[44] Walsh PC, Marschke P, Ricker D, et al. Patient-reported urinary continence and sexual function af-ter anatomic radical prostatectomy. Urology 2000; 55(1):58–61.

[45] Ahlering TE, Eichel L, Edwards R, et al. Impact of obesity on clinical outcomes in robotic prostatec-tomy. Urology 2005;65(4):740–4.

[46] Walsh PC, Donker PJ. Impotence following radical prostatectomy: insight into etiology and prevention. J Urol 1982;128(3):492–7.

[47] Obek C, Kural AR. Alternative approaches to nerve sparing: techniques and outcomes. In: Patel VR, ed-itor. Robotic urologic surgery. London: Springer-Verlag; 2007;124–30.

[48] Ahlering TE, Eichel L, Skarecky D. Rapid commu-nication: early potency outcomes with cautery-free neurovascular bundle preservation with robotic lap-aroscopic radical prostatectomy. J Endourol 2005; 19(6):715–8.

[49] Chien GW, Mikhail AA, Orvieto MA, et al. Modi-fied clipless antegrade nerve preservation in robotic-assisted laparoscopic radical prostatectomy with validated sexual function evaluation. Urology 2005;66(2):419–23.

[50] Menon M, Kaul S, Bhandari A, et al. Potency follow-ing robotic radical prostatectomy: a questionnaire based analysis of outcomes after conventional nerve sparing and prostatic fascia sparing techniques. J Urol 2005;174(6):2291–6 [discussion: 2296].

[51] Ahlering TE, Eichel L, Edwards RA, et al. Robotic radical prostatectomy: a technique to reduce pT2 positive margins. Urology 2004;64(6):1224–8.

[52] Bentas W, Wolfram M, Jones J, et al. Robotic technology and the translation of open radical prostatectomy to laparoscopy: the early Frank-furt experience with robotic radical prostatec-tomy and one year follow-up. Eur Urol 2003; 44(2):175–81.

[53] Badani KK, Kaul S, Menon M. Evolution of robotic radical prostatectomy: assessment after 2766 proce-dures. Cancer 2007;110(9):1951–8.

[54] Leibel SA, Fuks Z, Zelefsky MJ, et al. Technological advances in external-beam radiation therapy for the treatment of localized prostate cancer. Semin Oncol 2003;30(5):596–615.

[55] Madersbacher S, Pedevilla M, Vingers L, et al. Effect of high-intensity focused ultrasound on human pros-tate cancer in vivo. Cancer Res 1995;55(15):3346–51.

[56] Chapelon JY, Margonari J, Vernier F, et al. In vivo effects of high-intensity ultrasound on prostatic ade-nocarcinoma Dunning R3327. Cancer Res 1992; 52(22):6353–7.

[57] Uchida T, Ohkusa H, Nagata Y, et al. Treatment of localized prostate cancer using high-intensity focused ultrasound. BJU Int 2006;97(1):56–61.

[58] Blana A, Walter B, Rogenhofer S, et al. High-intensity focused ultrasound for the treatment of localized prostate cancer: 5-year experience. Urology 2004; 63(2):297–300.

[59] Chaussy C, Thuroff S. The status of high-intensity focused ultrasound in the treatment of localized prostate cancer and the impact of a combined resection. Curr Urol Rep 2003;4(3):248–52.

[60] Murat FJ, Poissonnier L, Pasticier G, et al. High-intensity focused ultrasound (HIFU) for prostate cancer. Cancer Control 2007;14(3):244–9.

[61] Poissonnier L, Chapelon JY, Rouviere O, et al. Control of prostate cancer by transrectal HIFU in 227 patients. Eur Urol 2007;51(2):381–7.

[62] Blana A, Rogenhofer S, Ganzer R, et al. Morbidity associated with repeated transrectal high-intensity focused ultrasound treatment of localized prostate cancer. World J Urol 2006;24(5):585–90.

[63] Blana A, Murat FJ, Walter B, et al. First analysis of the long-term results with transrectal HIFU in patients with localised prostate cancer. Eur Urol Nov 5 2007.

[64] Baust J, Gage AA, Ma H, et al. Minimally invasive cryosurgery—technological advances. Cryobiology 1997;34(4):373–84.

[65] Mazur P. Cryobiology: the freezing of biological systems. Science 1970;168:939.

[66] Tatsutani K, Rubinsky B, Onik G, et al. Effect of thermal variables on frozen human primary prostatic adenocarcinoma cells. Urology 1996;48(3): 441–7.

[67] Bischof JC, Smith D, Pazhayannur PV, et al. Cryosurgery of dunning AT-1 rat prostate tumor: thermal, biophysical, and viability response at the cellular and tissue level. Cryobiology 1997;34(1): 42–69.

[68] Hoffmann NE, Bischof JC. The cryobiology of cryosurgical injury. Urology 2002;60(2 Suppl 1):40–9.

[69] Robinson JW, Saliken JC, Donnelly BJ, et al. Quality-of-life outcomes for men treated with cryosurgery for localized prostate carcinoma. Cancer 1999; 86(9):1793–801.

[70] Robinson JW, Donnelly BJ, Saliken JC, et al. Quality of life and sexuality of men with prostate cancer 3 years after cryosurgery. Urology 2002;60(2 Suppl 1):12–8.

[71] Badalament RA, Bahn DK, Kim H, et al. Patient-reported complications after cryoablation therapy for prostate cancer. Arch Ital Urol Androl 2000; 72(4):305–12.

[72] Bales GT, Williams MJ, Sinner M, et al. Short-term outcomes after cryosurgical ablation of the prostate in men with recurrent prostate carcinoma following radiation therapy. Urology 1995;46(5): 676–80.

[73] Pisters LL, von Eschenbach AC, Scott SM, et al. The efficacy and complications of salvage cryotherapy of the prostate. J Urol 1997;157(3):921–5.

[74] de la Taille A, Hayek O, Benson MC, et al. Salvage cryotherapy for recurrent prostate cancer after radiation therapy: the Columbia experience. Urology 2000;55(1):79–84.

[75] Anastasiadis AG, Sachdev R, Salomon L, et al. Comparison of health-related quality of life and prostate-associated symptoms after primary and salvage cryotherapy for prostate cancer. J Cancer Res Clin Oncol 2003;129(12):676–82.

[76] Ismail M, Ahmed S, Kastner C, et al. Salvage cryotherapy for recurrent prostate cancer after radiation failure: a prospective case series of the first 100 patients. BJU Int 2007;100(4):760–4.

[77] Chin JL, Pautler SE, Mouraviev V, et al. Results of salvage cryoablation of the prostate after radiation: identifying predictors of treatment failure and complications. J Urol 2001;165(6 Pt 1):1937–41 [discussion: 1941–2].

[78] Bahn DK, Lee F, Silverman P, et al. Salvage cryosurgery for recurrent prostate cancer after radiation therapy: a seven-year follow-up. Clin Prostate Cancer 2003;2(2):111–4.

[79] Ng CK, Moussa M, Downey DB, et al. Salvage cryoablation of the prostate: followup and analysis of predictive factors for outcome. J Urol 2007; 178(4 Pt 1):1253–7 [discussion: 1257].

[80] Hoznek A, Salomon L, Olsson LE, et al. Laparoscopic radical prostatectomy. The Creteil experience. Eur Urol 2001;40(1):38–45.

[81] Turk I, Deger S, Winkelmann B, et al. Laparoscopic radical prostatectomy. Technical aspects and experience with 125 cases. Eur Urol 2001;40(1):46–52 [discussion: 53].

[82] Salomon L, Anastasiadis AG, Katz R, et al. Urinary continence and erectile function: a prospective evaluation of functional results after radical laparoscopic prostatectomy. Eur Urol 2002;42(4):338–43.

[83] Eden CG, Cahill D, Vass JA, et al. Laparoscopic radical prostatectomy: the initial UK series. BJU Int 2002;90(9):876–82.

[84] Guillonneau B, Rozet F, Cathelineau X, et al. Perioperative complications of laparoscopic radical prostatectomy: the Montsouris 3-year experience. J Urol 2002;167(1):51–6.

[85] Anastasiadis AG, Salomon L, Katz R, et al. Radical retropubic versus laparoscopic prostatectomy: a prospective comparison of functional outcome. Urology 2003;62(2):292–7.

[86] Stolzenburg JU, Rabenalt R, Do M, et al. Endoscopic extraperitoneal radical prostatectomy: oncological and functional results after 700 procedures. J Urol 2005;174(4 Pt 1):1271–5 [discussion: 1275].

[87] Goeman L, Salomon L, La De Taille A, et al. Long-term functional and oncological results after retroperitoneal laparoscopic prostatectomy according to a prospective evaluation of 550 patients. World J Urol 2006;24(3):281–8.

[88] Olsson LE, Salomon L, Nadu A, et al. Prospective patient-reported continence after laparoscopic radical prostatectomy. Urology 2001;58(4):570–2.

[89] Joseph JV, Rosenbaum R, Madeb R, et al. Robotic extraperitoneal radical prostatectomy: an alternative approach. J Urol 2006;175(3 Pt 1):945–50 [discussion: 951].

[90] Bhandari A, McIntire L, Kaul SA, et al. Perioperative complications of robotic radical prostatectomy after the learning curve. J Urol 2005; 174(3):915–8.

[91] Cathelineau X, Cahill D, Widmer H, et al. Transperitoneal or extraperitoneal approach for laparoscopic radical prostatectomy: a false debate over a real challenge. J Urol 2004;171(2 Pt 1):714–6.

[92] Costello AJ, Haxhimolla H, Crowe H, et al. Installation of telerobotic surgery and initial experience with telerobotic radical prostatectomy. BJU Int 2005; 96(1):34–8.

ELSEVIER
SAUNDERS

Urol Clin N Am 35 (2008) 505–518

UROLOGIC
CLINICS
of North America

Minimally Invasive Treatment of Male Lower Urinary Tract Symptoms

Jean J.M.C.H. de la Rosette, MD, PhD[a],*,
Stavros Gravas, MD, PhD[b],
John M. Fitzpatrick, MCh, FRCSI, FC Urol (SA), FRCSGlas, FRCS[c]

[a]Department of Urology, Academic Medical Center, University of Amsterdam,
Meibergdreef 9, 1105 AZ Amsterdam, The Netherlands
[b]Department of Urology, University Hospital of Larissa, Mezourlo 411 10, Larissa, Greece
[c]Department of Surgery, Mater Misericordiae Hospital, University College, 47 Eccles Street, Dublin, Ireland

Scientific and technological advances during the last years have challenged the established surgical treatment patterns regarding lower urinary tract symptoms (LUTS) caused by benign prostatic obstruction (BPO) such as transurethral resection of the prostate (TURP) and open prostatectomy (OP). The driving forces behind the development of minimally invasive methods were:

The rather unchanged morbidity of transurethral resection of prostate in terms of early (bleeding, TURsyndrome)
Late complications (particularly relating to sexual dysfunction)
The need for anesthesia and hospitalization

Various minimally invasive treatments (MITs) have been developed using new techniques including thermal-based therapies, laser therapy, and other treatment modalities such as prostatic ethanol injection.

Most of MITs use thermal energy to coagulate and not really ablate prostate tissue. Nonablative thermal therapies include hot water-induced thermotherapy (WIT), transurethral microwave thermotherapy (TUMT), transurethral needle ablation (TUNA), and high-intensity focused ultrasound (HIFU). Injectables (including anhydrous ethanol

and Botox) into the prostate result in improvement of lower urinary tract obstruction with a different mechanism. On the other hand, ablative surgical treatments alternative to TURP include laser prostatectomy with the most dominants being the holmium enucleation and the emerging photoselective vaporization of the prostrate (PVP), bipolar TURP, and laparoscopic prostatectomy. It is obvious that the minimally invasive nature of these treatments significantly varies from true ambulatory ones to surgical procedures that require anesthesia, but they are less invasive than TURP.

Transurethral microwave thermotherapy

During the last decade, numerous studies have been published presenting the clinical results from the application of TUMT. These studies have used different devices with different treatment protocols and have had different follow-up periods.

Recently, a systematic review of all available randomized comparative trials (RCTs) on TUMT attempted to quantify the therapeutic efficacy [1]. TUMT was somewhat less effective than TURP in reducing LUTS. The weighted mean difference (WMD) for the symptom score at the 12-month follow-up was −1.83, favoring TURP. TURP achieved a greater improvement in Qmax than TUMT (WMD of 5.37 mL/s in favor of resection) [1]. Data on TUMT efficacy from this study are presented in Table 1. Gravas and colleagues [2]

---

* Corresponding author.
E-mail address: j.j.delarosette@amc.uva.nl
(J.J.M.C.H. de la Rosette).

Table 1
Efficacy of minimally invasive treatments 12 months after therapy

Treatment	Patients	Symptom score			Maximum flow rate (mL/s)			Type of study	Level of evidence
		Preop	Postop	Change	Preop	Postop	Change		
TURP [100]	1480	NA	NA	70.6%	NA	NA	125%	Systematic review	1a
HoLEP [29]	100	22.1	1.7	20.4[a] (92%)	4.9	27.9	23.0 (469%)	RCT	1b
TUMT [1]	322	19.4	6.7	12.7 (65%)	7.9	13.5	5.6 (70%)	Systematic review	1a
TUNA [12]	182	NA	NA	12.1 (55%)	NA	NA	6.5 (76%)	Meta-analysis	1a
Bipolar [78]	120	23.0	4.0	19.0 (83%)	7.2	19.5	12.3 (171%)	RCT	1b
PVP [45]	60	27.2	12.2	15.0 (54%)	8.5	20.6	12.1 (167%)	RCT	1b
WIT [19]	125	24.0	12.0	12.0 (50%)	8.7	15.7	7.0 (80%)	Noncomparative	3
Ethanol [64]	93	20.6	10.3	10.3 (50%)	9.9	13.4	3.5 (35%)	Noncomparative	3
BONT-A [70]	17	23.2	8.9	14.3[a] (62%)	8.1	15.0	6.9 (85%)	RCT[c]	1b
HIFU [22]	20	14.7	4.3	10.4 (71%)	9.2	13.1	3.9 (42%)	nRCT	2a
LapProst [57]	20	20.9	2.5[b]	18.4 (88%)	8.8	34.5[b]	25.7 (292%)	nRCT	2a

Abbreviations: BONT-A, botulinum toxin type A; HIFU, high-intensity focused ultrasound; HoLEP, holmium laser enucleation of the prostrate; LapProst, laparoscopic prostatectomy; NA, not available; nRCT, nonrandomized clinical trial; postop, postoperative; preop, preoperative; RCT, randomized clinical trial; TUMT, transurethral microwave thermopathy; TUNA, transurethral needle ablation; TURP, transurethral resection of the prostrate; WIT, water-induced thermotherapy.

[a] American Urological Association (AUA) Symptom Index.
[b] Patents who reached follow-up.
[c] Placebo controlled.

performed a pooled analysis of three studies (two RCTs and one open-label study) of ProstaLund Feedback TUMT with 12-month follow-up. The responder rate was 85.3% and 85.9% in the ProstaLund Feedback Treatment (PLFT) and TURP groups, respectively.

High-quality data regarding morbidity come from the pooled analysis of published randomized studies comparing TUMT with TURP [1,3,4]. For patients treated with TURP, the mean length of hospitalization and catheterization time was 4.0 days and 3.6 days, respectively, while in the TUMT group, the corresponding mean values were 0 days and 13.7 days, respectively. More patients treated with TUMT developed dysuria/urgency and urinary retention compared with the TURP subjects. The incidence of hematuria, clot retention, transfusions, TUR syndrome, is reported to be significantly less for TUMT than for TURP. The impact of TUMT on sexual function in terms of erectile dysfunction and retrograde ejaculation also has been studied in comparison with pooled data to be in favor of TUMT [3].

Retreatment of TUMT is related to treatment failure, whereas retreatment of TURP is related to complications of resection. Reported retreatment rates after TUMT range from 19.8% to 29.3%, but with different mean follow-up durations (from 30 to 60 months) [5–8]. Hoffman and colleagues found that TUMT patients (7.54 events/100 person–years) were more likely than TURP patients (1.05 events/100 person–years) to require additional treatment for benign prostatic hyperplasia

(BPH) symptoms, while in contrast, the retreatment rate for strictures (meatal, urethral, or bladder neck) was found to be 5.85/100 person–years and 0.63/100 person–years for the TURP and TUMT groups, respectively [1].

It is very difficult to identify predictive baseline parameters for TUMT, because different devices have been used, and studies suggest that a predictive factor for a particular device cannot be applied to the other devices necessarily [9]. Advanced age of the patient, small prostate volume, mild-to-moderate bladder outlet obstruction, and low amount of energy delivered during treatment, however, are considered to be independent baseline parameters predicting unfavorable outcome [10].

The reported low morbidity and the absence of any anesthesia (spinal or general) needs make TUMT a true outpatient procedure representing an excellent option for patients in high operative risk (American Society of Anesthiologists classifications 3 and 4) who are unsuitable for an invasive treatment [11]. Recommendations from the most popular BPH guidelines on the use of TUMT are given in Table 2.

Transurethral needle ablation

A significant number of clinical studies on TUNA have been published with different number of patients in each study and different follow-up period. A recent meta-analysis provides high level of evidence on the efficacy and safety of TUNA [12]. Results on Qmax and International Prostate

Table 2
Recommendations for minimally invasive therapies from clinical practice guidelines

Minimally invasive therapy	Sixth International Consultation on Prostate Cancer and Prostate Diseases 2006 [98]	European Association of Urology 2004 [26]	American Urological Association 2003 [99]
HoLEP	R	R	R
TUMT	R	R	R
TUNA	R	R	R
Bipolar TURP	IS	ND	E
PVP	IS	ND	ND
WIT	I	ND	E
Ethanol injections	I	ND	I
HIFU	ND	NR-I	I
BONT-A	ND	ND	ND
LapProst	ND	ND	ND

Abbreviations: BONT-A, botulinum toxin type A; E, emerging; HoLEP, holmium laser enucleation of the prostrate; I, investigational; IS, inadequately studied; LapProst, laparoscopic prostatectomy; NR, not recommended; ND, not discussed; PVP, photoselective vaporization of the prostate; R, recommended; TUMT, transurethral microwave thermopathy; TUNA, transurethral needle ablation; WIT, water-induced thermotherapy.

Symptom Score (IPSS) are listed in Table 1. Comparisons with TURP showed that in the short term, TUNA achieves a similar level of efficacy, but at 12 months the degree of improvement in both subjective and objective variables was significantly lower than of TURP [12]. An older meta-analysis reached to similar conclusions [13].

TUNA can be performed as an outpatient procedure under local anesthesia and sedation in most patients. The excellent adverse effect and safety profile of TUNA has been documented in several short- and long-term studies. Analysis of pooled data showed that TUNA resulted in a significantly lower number of complications than TURP [12]. The estimated odds ratio of experiencing an adverse event (AE) following TUNA is 0.14 (95% CI 0.05 to 0.41) compared with TURP. This indicates that TUNA has an absolute risk reduction of complications of 19.4% [12].

The only post-treatment complications having a higher incidence in patients undergoing TUNA include transient urinary retention (from 13.3% to 41.6%) and dysuria [12]. All the other AEs, including mild hematuria, urinary infections, strictures, and sexual dysfunction (erectile dysfunction and ejaculation disorders), are more common in patients undergoing TURP than in those undergoing TUNA.

The combined results of the available studies demonstrated that TUNA had a retreatment rate significantly higher than that of TURP, given that 10% (21/206) of patients undergoing TUNA versus only 1% (3/282) of patients undergoing TURP required new treatments [12].

Few selection criteria have been identified. TUNA is not suitable for patients who have prostate volumes exceeding 75 mL or isolated bladder neck obstruction [14]. Other studies, however, found that prostate size and shape were not related to treatment response [15,16]. TUNA is not recommended in patients who have metallic pelvic prosthesis and pacemaker [17].

Available data suggest that TUNA is an effective and safe MIT for men with even severe symptoms who do not wish to undergo long-term medical therapy, or who are poor candidates for surgery or who are concerned about the adverse effects of TURP [13].

Water-induced thermotherapy

WIT is another thermal-based therapy for BPO that aims to produce heat-induced coagulative necrosis using heated water as a source. The treatment is performed as a 45-minute outpatient procedure without requiring systemic analgesia, because topical lidocaine jelly provides sufficient analgesia [18].

Limited data on WIT efficacy and morbidity are available [18]. Evidence comes mainly from a single international, uncontrolled, multicenter trial demonstrating symptom reduction and safety (see Table 1) [19]. Overall, short-term results seem to be inferior to TURP. No significant ablation is achieved, because the procedure has been associated with a median post-treatment prostate shrinkage of 3.2 cc at 12 months compared with baseline [19].

Published studies have not reported significant morbidity [18]. Main AEs included prolonged or excessive dysuria (11.2%), prolonged and excessive hematuria (22.4%), bacteriuria or urinary tract infection (32.8%), and urinary retention subsequent to the post-treatment catheterization period (12.0%). No patient suffered from newly occurring permanent erectile dysfunction or retrograde ejaculation, while interest in sex and sexual activity were not affected or were slightly improved by WIT [20].

Data regarding durability are lacking. On an intention-to-treat basis, the retreatment rates were higher: 10.4% after 12 months, 23.2% after 24 months, and 36% after 36 months [21]. No predicting parameters have been identified using logistic regression models to evaluate baseline parameters for successful outcome [19]. Protrusion of a median prostate lobe is a relative contraindication for this therapy [18].

It is obvious that randomized studies against one of the standard treatments are required, thus WIT is not recommended by clinical guidelines and is considered to remain investigational (see Table 2).

Transrectal high-intensity focused ultrasound

Randomized controlled studies comparing HIFU to the standard therapy have not been published. A non-RCT comparing TURP with four MITs including transurethral electrovaporization (TUVP), visual laser ablation of the prostate (VLAP), TUNA, and HIFU has performed [22]. The clinical results of HIFU are presented in Table 1. Increase in Qmax after HIFU was smaller than the improvement achieved after TURP. Data analysis from a study with the longer follow-up showed that 43.8% (35/80) of the patients required TURP within 4 years [23]. In the group of responders, IPSS improved from 19.6 to 8.5 after 12 months and remained practically unchanged during the 4-year follow-up, while Qmax increased from 9.1 mL/s to 11.8 mL/s at 12 months and subsequently deteriorated to 10.2mL/s at 4 years.

In general, the treatment is tolerated well but requires general or regional anesthesia. The most prominent AE is prolonged urinary retention, thus a suprapubic catheter is offered to the patients postoperatively [24]. Complication rates are low because of absence of any urethral manipulation. Effects on erectile and antegrade ejaculation are uncommon. Hematospermia can be noticed up to 4 to 6 weeks in up to 80% of sexually active men [25].

Predictors of unfavorable outcome include large prostates (greater than 75 mL), presence of a pronounced middle lobe, presence of prostatic calculi (caused by attenuation of ultrasound), and higher grades of bladder outlet obstruction [26].

To date, the interest for treating BPH patients with HIFU has declined while there is a shift toward the use of HIFU for the treatment of prostate cancer. Because of the lack of high-quality data, HIFU is considered as an investigational treatment modality by most of the guidelines (see Table 2).

Holmium laser enucleation of the prostate

Several clinical studies have shown the efficacy and safety of holium laser enucleation of the prostate (HoLEP) [27–30]. A recent meta-analysis of the available RCTs comparing HoLEP with TURP showed that there was no statistically significant difference between HoLEP and TURP in terms of Qmax (WMD was 0.59) at 12 months after treatment [31]. Unfortunately, this meta-analysis does not provide the pooled values of Qmax and IPSS at baseline and during follow-up; therefore it has not included in Table 1. Thus the results from the largest RCT comparing HoLEP with TURP are presented there [29]. On the other hand, this meta-analysis offers significant information regarding perioperative variables and AEs [31]. No statistically significant differences between pooled estimates were noted between HoLEP and TURP for urethral stricture (2.6 versus 4.4%), blood transfusion (0 versus 2.2%), and reintervention (4.3 versus 8.8%). The overall complication rate, however, was 19 of 232 (8.1%) in the HoLEP group and 37 of 228 (16.2%) in the TURP group, with a statistically significant difference in the pooled estimates. Pooled data suggest that HoLEP is superior to

TURP in terms of catheterization time, hospital stay, and blood loss. In contrast, pooled estimates showed a benefit of TURP over HoLEP for duration of operation [31]. Montorsi and colleagues [32] reported that there was no TUR syndrome in the HoLEP group, versus 2.2% of patients in the TURP group.

The impact on erectile dysfunction and retrograde ejaculation is very similar between the two groups. The erectile function did not show a decrease from baseline in either group. In addition, Kuntz and colleagues [29] reported that 74% of sexually active patients in the HoLEP group and 70.3% in the TURP group had retrograde ejaculation.

Gilling and colleagues [33] performed a meta-analysis of four RCTs comparing HoLEP and TURP. They found that urodynamic relief of obstruction (PdetQmax and Schaffer grade) was superior with HoLEP compared with TURP, but only when prostate volumes were greater than 50 g. Studies evaluating durability of HoLEP are now available. Recently, Gilling and colleagues [34] reported the results from a series of patients with a mean follow-up of 6.1 years. HoLEP achieved durable results in terms of Qmax, quality of life (QOL), and IPSS, while the reoperation rate was 1.4%. Similarly, Elzayat and Elhilali [35] found that the objective and subjective improvements after HoLEP remained sustained at 6 years, with a reoperation rate of 4.2% for recurrent BPH obstruction.

HoLEP has no size limitation and has been shown to be effective for large prostates that traditionally have been treated by open prostatectomy [36–38]. The main evident advantages are reduced blood loss and shorter catheterization and hospitalization time. Recent, long-term (5 years) data from a RCT comparing HoLEP with OP demonstrated similar durable subjective and objective improvement for both groups and a reoperation rate of 5% in the HoLEP group and 6.7% in the OP group [39].

HoLEP is recommended by the guidelines (see Table 2); however, the main criticism of HoLEP includes a significant learning curve (requiring 30 to 50 cases), purchase cost, and the difficulty in tissue removal.

Photoselective vaporization of the prostate

PVP using the high-power (80 W) potassium-titanyl-phosphate (KTP) laser represents the latest evolutionary development in laser and is attracting the interest of urologists.

Initial studies on the 80 W setting have shown promising outcomes [40–44]. Mean increase in Qmax ranged from 106% to 253%, and mean IPSS improvement varied from 59% to 84%. Reduction in prostate volume ranged from 37% [40] to 53% [44]. There is only one randomized study; however, that compares PVP with TURP, and results are displayed in Table 1 [45].

Catheterization time is generally less than 24 hours, while in one study, 44 patients (32%) were left without a catheter at the end of the procedure [40]. The perioperative morbidity is low, with the most frequent complications being the need for recatheterization (range from 1% to 15.4%), dysuria (from 6.2% to 30%), and minor hematuria (up to 18%). One of the main advantages of PVP is the virtually bloodless tissue ablation, resulting in absence of significant bleeding and need for blood transfusion. No TUR syndrome rate was reported in any study. Between 36% and 55% of sexually active men experienced retrograde ejaculation after treatment [40–44]. In the only RCT, PVP was superior to TURP in terms of blood loss, catheter time, and duration of hospital stay [45].

Long-term results of this technique are still missing. A study with the longest follow-up (5 years) showed that a significant improvement in American Urological Association (AUA) symptom index and Qmax after PVP that remained durable during follow-up [46]. This study, however, suffered from a very high attrition rate (68% and 85% at 3 and 5 years, respectively).

Published studies also demonstrated that the 80 W KTP laser seems to be a safe and effective means for treating men who have large prostates (mean volume greater than 100 mL) [47–49]. The mean lasing time ranged from 79 to 123 minutes. Qmax, IPSS, and QOL scores showed significant improvements without the presence of TUR syndrome or the need for blood transfusions. The new 120 W high-performance system (HPS) recently was introduced, aiming at a faster tissue removal in less lasing time and the ability to treat large glands in an acceptable time. A consideration, however, is that the high-power settings may result in higher complication rates including capsule perforation, bladder perforation, or injury of the orifices and decreased haemostatic capability [50].

KTP laser vaporization has a relatively short learning curve, but caution is required when the prostate gland or the median lobe is very large. Another consideration is that the recently introduced 120 W HPS with the high-power settings may require a longer leaning curve.

The lack of randomized studies and long-term data does not allow definitive recommendations about the position of PVP for managing LUTS (see Table 2).

Laparoscopic simple prostatectomy

The laparoscopic prostatectomy for large benign prostatic adenomas causing bladder outlet obstruction recently was introduced [51]. Several studies have shown the feasibility of the technique (either the Millin's or transvesical procedure) [52–59] with functional outcome comparable with those of open prostatectomy (see Table 1).

The main advantage of laparoscopic simple prostatectomy over the conventional open approach is the significantly lower blood loss [57,58]. In a study presenting the 6-year experience with laparoscopic prostatectomy, the most frequent long-term complication was retrograde ejaculation, which occurred in all patients after 6 months of follow-up [59]. The erectile function was preserved in all those patients who were potent before surgery, while none of the patients experienced urinary incontinence.

Laparoscopic prostatectomy, however, requires a long learning curve and significant laparoscopic expertise; therefore it is performed in centers with considerable experience in laparoscopic urology. In addition, the reported results regarding operative time, hospitalization time, and length of hospital stay were controversial [57,58] and have questioned the position of laparoscopic prostatectomy as a true minimally invasive alternative to open prostatectomy.

Therefore, further randomized studies with long follow-up are required to evaluate laparoscopic prostatectomy for managing patients who have very large adenomas, in comparison with OP and endoscopic methods including HoLEP. Guidelines do not discuss laparoscopic prostatectomy yet.

Transurethral ethanol ablation of the prostate

Transurethral ethanol ablation of the prostate (TEAP) aims at effectively treating patients who have symptomatic BPO by injecting anhydrous ethanol into the prostate under continuous urethroscopic irrigation. The exact mechanism is not known, but it seems that there is coagulative tissue necrosis with associated protein denaturation, and cell membrane lysis and a neurolytic role likely exist also.

Although there are no randomized studies, available data show that there is a significant improvement in terms of IPSS and Qmax after TEAP that remains durable at 12 months [60–64]. Table 1 presents the clinical results from a multicenter, noncomparative study [64].

It recently has been shown that TEAP can be performed in an outpatient setting using local anesthesia and oral-only sedation [65]. Patients require a catheter after TEAP, but more than 90% of them are able to void after 96 hours. The most commonly reported AE (of mild or moderate severity) included hematuria (42.9%), irritative voiding symptoms (40.3%), pain/discomfort (25.6%), and urinary retention (22.1%). Erectile dysfunction occurred in less than 5% of the patients. The most serious complication was ethanol-induced bladder necrosis, which occurred in three cases [66].

Long-term studies are limited. Goya and colleagues [64] followed 17 patients and found that IPSS and Qmax improved after TEAP and were stable at 3-year follow-up without any major complications associated with the procedure. Durable improvement, however, was reported in only 59% of patients. The reported reintervention rate after TEAP ranged from 7% by 1 year to 26% by 3 years [63,64].

Again, the main limitation of this MIT is the lack of randomized studies comparing this procedure with other minimally invasive procedures or with TURP. TEAP seems to be effective up to 12 months, but long-term data are required to define its potential role for managing lower urinary tract obstruction.

Injection of botulinum toxin type A

The use of intraprostatic injection of botulinum toxin type A (BONT-A), an exotoxin produced by *Clostridium botulinum*, very recently has been introduced for treating BPH [67–71]. The exact mechanism of action remains unknown, but possible mechanisms include neurotoxin-induced denervation atrophy, induction of apoptosis, and decreased proliferation and down-regulation of α1A-adrenergic receptors [72].

BONT-A has been injected into the prostate using transperineal, transurethral, or transrectal approaches [71,73–75]. The transurethral application requires cystoscopy under anesthesia, when transperineal (most commonly reported) or

transrectal approaches can be used without even local anesthesia. In these studies, different therapeutic doses have been reported (range from 100 to 300 U Botox) in different volumes (from 4 to20 mL) [71,73–75]. To date, the number of available published studies is limited, and they suffer from the small patient numbers, short follow-up, and differences in study design. The preliminary results, however, seem to be encouraging, because injection of BONT-A achieves significant improvement with persistent effects for 6 to 12 months after treatment. The clinical outcomes from the double-blinded placebo-controlled study by Maria and colleagues [70] with the larger follow-up (19.8 months) are listed in Table 1. The procedure also has proven safe without report of any serious AE. Intraprostatic BONT-A, however, has not been approved formally by the US Food and Drug Administration (FDA) for treating BPH [72].

Controversial results have been reported regarding the impact of BONT-A in prostate volume. Chuang and colleagues [68] also found no change in prostate volume in 12 of 41 patients, while seven had improved IPSS, QOL, and Qmax indices, suggesting that BONT-A may affect not only the static but also the dynamic component of BPH.

It is obvious that intraprostatic injection of BONT-A has to run a long distance before one can define its position into the armamentarium of urologists for managing LUTS obstruction. Understanding of the mechanism of action, standardization of both technique and doses, large randomized comparative studies against established MIT, and longer follow-up of the patients are required.

Bipolar resection of the prostate

To date, five types of bipolar resection devices, with technical differences in delivering bipolar current flow to achieve the plasma effect, have been used:

Plasma kinetic (PK) system (Gyrus International, Ltd., Berkshire, United Kingdom)
Vista Coblation/CTR (controlled tissue resection) system (ACMI, Maple Grove, Minnesota)
Transurethral resection in saline (TURIS) system (Olympus, Center Valley, Pennsylvania)
Karl Storz (Karl Storz GmbH & Company KG, Tuttlingen, Germany)

Wolf [76] (Richard Wolf GmbH, Knittlingen, Germany)

The efficacy and safety of those bipolar devices have been demonstrated by RCTs and case series [76–80]. All studies found that the clinical efficacy, in terms of Qmax and IPSS, was similar in both bipolar and monopolar TURP. The results of the largest RCT comparing bipolar (PK system) with monopolar TURP are listed in Table 1 [78].

Main advantages of bipolar resection include the reduced blood loss and the decreased incidence of postoperative clot retention and blood transfusion requirement [78,79]. TUR syndrome had not been observed with bipolar TURP because of the use of saline irrigation and the reduced fluid absorption during bipolar TURP. Both the postoperative catheterization and hospitalization time were significantly less (40% on average) in the bipolar arm of RCTs compared with monopolar TURP [76,79,80] and were attributed to the reduced bleeding associated with improved coagulation. Postoperative irritative LUTS, particularly dysuria, was observed less commonly with bipolar TURP. Urethral stricture is observed more commonly with bipolar TURP (range from 4.0 %to 6.1%). Larger resectoscope size (27 F), the type of return electrode, and the higher current densities may contribute to this risk [76,79].

In a RCT comparing bipolar TURP with plasma kinetic energy and monopolar TURP with a mean follow-up of 18.3 months, the reoperation rate was 4.1% and 2.1% for the PK system and TURP groups, respectively [81].

Available data suggest that bipolar resection devices seem to achieve results comparable to conventional TURP, with decreased bleeding and shorter catheterization and hospital stay and without the occurrence of TUR syndrome.

Longer-term outcomes on the durability and incidence of urethral strictures are required to strengthen the position of bipolar resection as a less-invasive alternative to TURP.

Specific conditions

Retention

Historically, patients in retention are considered to be associated with a higher complication rate and sometimes a poorer outcome in terms of voiding parameters. In the first studies on the efficacy of most MITs, urinary retention was one of the exclusion criteria. Urologists, however, have become more confident and offered MIT to this specific group of patients. Table 3 presents the success rate of MITs on patients in retention, defined as the percentage of patients who regained the ability to void spontaneously [12,82–87]. All these studies reported the short-term results and it should be underlined that long-term results for this group of patients are limited. Gravas and colleagues [88] followed 213 patients with or without retention treated with the TUMT 3.5 protocol for up to 5 years. It was found that 28.6% of patients without urinary retention required additional treatment, while treatment failure was 37.8% in the retention group. Additionally, the cumulative risk at 5 years was 42.3% and 58.8%, respectively. Therefore, long-term studies are required to evaluate the durability of MITs on patients who have retention.

Anticoagulated men with medical comorbidities

With the growing life expectancy, urologists face with an increasing number of patients requiring prostatectomy, who suffer from serious comorbidities. Nonablative MITs require minimal

Table 3
Success rate of minimally invasive therapy in patients with retention

Minimally invasive therapy	Success rate	Follow-up (FU)	Type of study
HoLEP [84]	164/164 (100%)	24 mo	Noncomparative
TUMT [82]	48/61 (79%)	6 mo	RCT
TUNA [12]	78/112 (70%)	NA	Systematic review
PVP [85]	68/70 (97%)	12 mo[b]	Noncomparative
WIT [83]	12/13 (92%)	12 mo	Noncomparative
Ethanol injections [86]	17/21(81%)	16 mo[a]	Noncomparative
BONT-A [87]	17/21 (81%)	3 mo	Noncomparative

Abbreviations: BONT-A, botulinum toxin type A; HoLEP, holium laser enucleation of the prostrate; PVP, photoselective vaporization of the prostrate; RCT, randomized clinical trial; TUMT, transurethral microwave thermotherapy; TUNA, transurethral needle ablation; WIT, water-induced thermotherapy.
[a] mean FU.
[b] median FU.

anesthesia/analgesia and offer low morbidity, low incidence of adverse events, and low potential mortality for those at high surgical risk.

Recently, studies on the 80 W KTP laser have indicated that the procedure seems to be safe and beneficial for patients who have coagulopathies, platelet disorders, and those considered to be of high cardiopulmonary surgical risks who could not discontinue oral anticoagulant therapy [89–91]. Similarly, HoLEP has been performed successfully in patients who normally are considered unfit for a TURP, including those with significant comorbidities, such as coagulopathy, anticoagulant dependency, and significant anemia [92].

Cost

The introduction of new technology in health care sometimes is charged as one of the major causes of escalating costs because of the purchase of the capital equipment and failure in terms of efficacy, morbidity, and durability. High costs frequently are cited as a major drawback of the new laser techniques. Different economic models evaluating the cost-effectiveness of MITs for BPO have been introduced [93,94]. Performance of treatment on an outpatient basis represents a critical factor that reduces the direct cost and renders MITs economically advantageous compared with surgical treatments. This benefit, however, may be balanced by the higher retreatment rate of most ambulatory MITs.

Data from the Urologic Diseases in America BPH project showed that BPH therapy trends are moving away from the gold standard operation of TURP and toward less- invasive pharmacologic options and MIT in an outpatient setting [95]. Reimbursement policy encourages the outpatient performance of MITs. TUMT and TUNA have an extremely high in-office reimbursement, with Medicare rates of $4272 and $4098, respectively, compared with $552 and $585 for the respective hospital procedures [96].

Disantostefano and colleagues [97] showed that the best treatment for BPO varies depending on the value that individuals and society place on costs and consequences, including disease progression, clinical outcomes, hospitalization, and catheterization time.

In addition, the cost-effectiveness of all techniques depends on the existence of long- term data, costs of complications, and the different reimbursement systems in different countries.

Therefore, it is difficult to draw solid conclusions that are applicable to every country.

Overview

The range of therapeutic options for the management of BPO continues to widen as technology continues to evolve and improve. Increased choice creates the increased need for clarity in selection and application of various treatment options based on the clinical outcomes, morbidity, and technical improvement of these technologies. Clinical practice guidelines (CPGs) have been developed to help practitioners and patients decide about appropriate health care for specific clinical circumstances. Table 2 presents the current recommendations of the most popular CPGs [26,98,99]. Recently introduced MITs, however, have not been included, or data were insufficient when CPGs were released, underlying the need for regular updating of guidelines.

TURP remains the gold standard for surgical treatment, and indeed new MITs have not demonstrated better outcomes than TURP in terms of efficacy and retreatment rate. Table 1 presents the clinical results at 12 months after treatment based on the highest quality study for each of the treatment options. The available type of study also indicates how extensively these MITs have been studied. TUNA and TUMT are the best-studied MITs; thus data come from meta-analyses of RCTs. An ablative therapy like TURP or ablative laser therapy therefore should be advocated as first-line treatment for patients with an absolute surgical indication. In terms of minimal morbidity however, MITs are considered to be superior. In general, an increased ablative power results in increased relief of BPO at the expense of higher morbidity.

The algorithm for the instrumental treatment of lower urinary tract obstruction outlines the authors' approach to this controversial issue (Fig. 1). Patients are classified on the basis of operative risk of patients, because TURP morbidity was the main reason for the search of alternative treatment modalities. Grades (1, 2, 3, 4) have been allocated to the procedures based on clinical efficacy, morbidity, durability, and strength of evidence. When two procedures were considered to be equally useful, were been graded with the same number. The first alternative has the number 1. WIT, HIFU, BONT-A, and laparoscopic prostatectomy were not included in this algorithm because of limited data or decline in their use in

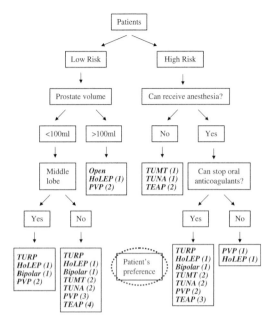

Fig. 1. Algorithm for instrumental treatment of lower urinary tract obstruction.

the clinical practice. In the future, modifications of this algorithm may prove necessary as more RCTs and studies on the long-term outcome of MIT will come into light.

The present algorithm is indicative, but patients also should be involved in treatment selection. It also should be underlined that best data and clinical expertise should be combined with patients' preferences (including interest in sexual function and perioperative morbidity). In addition, management is influenced by other factors, including availability of MIT and urologists' beliefs.

Summary

In line with many other urological diseases, the treatment of prostate-related pathologies has undergone numerous improvements during the last decades, with a major impact on the incidence of intra- and postoperative complications. On one hand, these improvements are because of the introduction of new minimally invasive technologies, whereas on the other hand, the established technologies have evolved. At present, TUNA and TUMT have been established as valuable ambulatory treatments, and clinical outcomes are in between medical management and surgical treatments. HoLEP and Greenlight laser

treatment, however, have challenged the so-called gold standard, and at present, the balance between clinical outcomes versus morbidity seems to swing in their favor. The different minimally invasive treatment modalities currently available, however, have paved the way for further improvements of TURP. For 80 years, TURP has been the cornerstone of minimally invasive surgical management of BPO. With the introduction of bipolar technology, TURP has reinforced its position.

References

[1] Hoffman RM, Monga M, Elliot S, et al. Microwave thermotherapy for benign prostatic hyperplasia. Cochrane Database Syst Rev 2007;17(4):CD004135.

[2] Gravas S, Laguna P, Ehrnebo M, et al. Seeking for evidence that cell kill-guided thermotherapy gives results not inferior to transurethral resection of prostate: results of a pooled analysis of 3 studies on feedback transurethral microwave thermotherapy. J Urol 2005;174(3):1002–6.

[3] Walmsley K, Kaplan S. Transurethral microwave thermotherapy for benign prostatic hyperplasia: separating truth from marketing hype. J Urol 2004;172:1249–55.

[4] de la Rosette JJ, Laguna MP, Gravas S, et al. Transurethral microwave thermotherapy: the gold standard for minimally invasive therapies for patients with benign prostatic hyperplasia? J Endourol 2003;17:245–51.

[5] Floratos DL, Kiemeney LA, Rossi C, et al. Long-term follow-up of randomized transurethral microwave thermotherapy versus transurethral prostatic resection study. J Urol 2001;165:1533–8.

[6] d'Ancona FC, Francisca EA, Witjes WP, et al. Transurethral resection of the prostate vs high-energy thermotherapy of the prostate in patients with benign prostatic hyperplasia: long-term results. Br J Urol 1998;81:259–64.

[7] Thalmann GN, Mattei A, Treuthardt C, et al. Transurethral microwave therapy in 200 patients with a minimum follow-up of 2 years: urodynamic and clinical results. J Urol 2002;167:2496–501.

[8] Miller PD, Kastner C, Ramsey EW, et al. Cooled thermotherapy for the treatment of benign prostatic hyperplasia: durability of results obtained with the Targis system. Urology 2003;61:1160–4.

[9] Tubaro A, d'Ancona FCH. Case selection for high-energy transurethral microwave thermotherapy. World J Urol 1998;16:124–30.

[10] d'Ancona FCH, Francisca EAE, Debruyne FMJ, et al. High-energy transurethral microwave thermotherapy in men with lower urinary tract symptoms. J Endourol 1997;11:285–9.

[11] d'Ancona FCH, van der Bij AK, Francisca EAE, et al. The results of high-energy transurethral

microwave thermotherapy in patients categorized according to the American Society of Anaesthiologists operative risk classification (ASA). Urology 1999;54:18–22.

[12] Bouza C, López T, Magro A, et al. Systematic review and meta-analysis of transurethral needle ablation in symptomatic benign prostatic hyperplasia. BMC Urol 2007;6:14, p. 1–17.

[13] Boyle P, Robertson C, Vaughan ED, et al. A meta-analysis of trials of trnasurethral needle ablation for treating symptomatic benign prostatic obstruction. BJU Int 2004;94(1):83–8.

[14] Schulman CC, Zlotta AR. Transurethral needle ablation of the prostate for the treatment of benign prostatic hyperplasia: early clinical experience. Urology 1995;45:28–33.

[15] Steele GS, Sleep DJ. Transurethral needle ablation of the prostate: a urodynamic-based study with 2-year follow-up. J Urol 1997;158:1834–8.

[16] Kahn S, Alphonse P, Tewari A, et al. An open study on the efficacy and safety of transurethral needle ablation of the prostate in treating symptomatic benign prostatic hyperplasia: the University of Florida experience. J Urol 1998;160: 1695–700.

[17] Barmoshe S, Zlotta AZ. How do I treat and follow my TUNA patients. World J Urol 2006;24: 397–404.

[18] Muschter R. Conductive heat: hot water-induced thermotherapy for ablation of prostatic tissue. J Endourol 2003;17(8):609–16.

[19] Muschter R, Schorsch I, Danielli L, et al. Transurethral water-induced thermotherapy for the treatment of benign prostatic hyperplasia: a prospective multicenter clinical trial. J Urol 2000;164: 1565–9.

[20] Muschter R, Schorsch I, Matalon G, et al. Two-year follow-up of a multicenter clinical study using water-induced thermotherapy (WIT) for benign prostatic hyperplasia (BPH) [abstract]. J Endourol 2000;14(Suppl):A74.

[21] Muschter R, Schorsch I, Matalon G, et al. Water-induced thermotherapy (WIT): a prospective multicenter study with three-year follow-up results. J Urol 2001;165(Suppl):A296.

[22] Schatzl G, Madersbacher S, Djavan B, et al. Two-year results of transurethral resection of the prostate versus four less invasive treatment options. Eur Urol 2000;37(6):695–701.

[23] Madersbacher S, Schatzl G, Djavan B, et al. Long-term outcome of transrectal high-intensity focused ultrasound therapy for benign prostatic hyperplasia. Eur Urol 2000;37(6):687–94.

[24] Bihrle R, Foster RS, Sanghvi NT, et al. High-intensity focused ultrasound for the treatment of benign prostatic hyperplasia: early United States clinical experience. J Urol 1994;151(5):1271–5.

[25] Schatzl G, Madersbacher S, Lang T, et al. The early postoperative morbidity of transurethral resection of the prostate and four minimally invasive treatment alternatives. J Urol 1997;158:105–11.

[26] de la Rosette J, Alivizatos G, Madersbacher S, et al. EAU guidelines on benign prostatic hyperplasia (BPH). Available at: www.uroweb.org. Accessed June 29, 2008.

[27] Gilling PJ, Kennett K, Das AK, et al. Holmium laser enucleation of the prostate (HoLEP) combined with transurethral tissue morcellation: an update on the early clinical experience. J Endourol 1998;12:457–9.

[28] Hurle R, Vavassori I, Piccinelli A, et al. Holmium laser enucleation of the prostate combined with mechanical morcellation in 155 patients with benign prostatic hyperplasia. Urology 2002;60:449–53.

[29] Kuntz RM, Ahyai S, Lehrich K, et al. Transurethral holmium laser enucleation of the prostate vs transurethral electrocautery resection of the prostate: a randomized prospective trial in 200 patients. J Urol 2004;172:1012–6.

[30] Vavassori I, Hurle R, Vismara A, et al. Holmium laser enucleation of the prostate combined with mechanical morcellation: two years of experience with 196 patients. J Endourol 2004;18(1):109–12.

[31] Tan A, Liao C, Mo Z, et al. Meta-analysis of holmium laser enucleation versus transurethral resection of the prostate for symptomatic prostatic obstruction. Br J Surg 2007;94:1201–8.

[32] Montorsi F, Naspro R, Salonia A, et al. Holmium laser enucleation versus transurethral resection of the prostate: results from a 2-center, prospective, randomized trial in patients with obstructive benign prostatic obstruction. J Urol 2004;172: 1926–9.

[33] Gilling PJ, Kennett K, Westenberg AM, et al. Relief of symptoms and obstruction following HoLEP and TURP-size matters: a meta-analysis. J Endourol 2005;19(Suppl 1) MP24-14, A119.

[34] Gilling PJ, Aho TF, Frampton CM, et al. Holmium laser enucleation of the prostate: results at 6 years. Eur Urol 2008;53(4):744–9.

[35] Elzayat EA, Elhilali MM. Holmium laser enucleation of the prostate (HoLEP): long-term results, reoperation rate, and possible impact of the learning curve. Eur Urol 2007;52(5):1465–72.

[36] Kuntz RM, Lehrich K, et al. Transurethral holmium laser enucleation of the prostate compared with transvesical open prostatectomy: 18-month follow-up of a randomized trial. J Endourol 2004; 18:189–91.

[37] Elzayat EA, Elhali MM. Holmium laser enucleation of the prostate (HoLEP): the endourologic alternative to open prostatectomy. Eur Urol 2006;49: 87–91.

[38] Matlaga BR, Kim SC, Kuo RL, et al. Holmium laser enucleation of the prostate for prostates of > 125 mL. BJU Int 2006;97:81–4.

[39] Kuntz RM, Lehrich K, Ahyai SA. Holmium laser enucleation of the prostate versus open

prostatectomy for prostates greater than 100
grams: 5-year follow-up results of a randomised
clinical trial. Eur Urol 2008;53(1):160–6.

[40] Te AE, Malloy TR, Stein BS, et al. Photoselective
vaporization of the prostate for the treatment of benign prostatic hyperplasia: 12-month results from
the first United States multicenter prospective trial.
J Urol 2004;172:1404–8.

[41] Sulser T, Reich O, Wyler SF, et al. Photoselective
KTP laser vaporization of the prostate: first experiences with 65 procedures. J Endourol 2004;18:
976–81.

[42] Volkan T, Tasci AI, Ordekci Y, et al. Short-term
outcomes of high-power (80 W) potassium-titanyl-phosphate laser vaporization of the prostate.
Eur Urol 2005;48:608–61.

[43] Bachmann A, Schurch L, Ruszat R, et al. Photoselective vaporization (PVP) versus transurethral
resection of the prostate (TURP): a prospective
bi-centre study of perioperative morbidity and
early functional outcome. Eur Urol 2005;48:
965–71.

[44] Sarica K, Alkan E, Luleci H, et al. Photoselective
vaporization of the enlarged prostate with KTP
laser: long-term results in 240 patients. J Endourol
2005;19:1199–202.

[45] Bouchier-Hayes DM, Anderson P, van Appledorn
S, et al. KTP Laser versus transurethral resection:
early results of a randomized trial. J Endourol
2006;20:580–5.

[46] Malek R, Kuntzman R, Barrett D. Photoselective potassium-titanyl-phosphate laser vaporization of the benign obstructive prostate:
observations on long-term outcomes. J Urol
2005;174:1344–8.

[47] Sandhu JS, Ng C, Vanderbrink BA, et al. High-
power potassium-titanyl-phosphate photoselective
laser vaporization of prostate for treatment of
benign prostatic hyperplasia in men with large
prostates. Urology 2004;64:1155–9.

[48] Ruszat R, Wyler S, Seifert HH, et al. Photoselective
vaporization of the prostate: experience with
prostate adenomas >80 cm^3. Urologe A 2006;45:
858–64.

[49] Rajbabu K, Chandrasekara SK, Barber NJ, et al.
Photoselective vaporization of the prostate with
the potassium-titanyl-phosphate laser in men with
prostates >100 mL. BJU Int 2007;100:593–8.

[50] Te AE. The next generation in laser treatments and
the role of the greenlight high-performance system
laser. Rev Urol 2006;8(Suppl 3):S24–30.

[51] Mariano MB, Graziottin TM, Tefilli MB. Laparoscopic prostatectomy with vascular control for
benign prostatic hyperplasia. J Urol 2002;167:
2528–9.

[52] Van Velthoven RFP, Peltier A, Laguna MP, et al.
Laparoscopic extraperitoneal adenomectomy
(Millin): pilot study on feasibility. Eur Urol 2004;
45:103–9.

[53] Nadler RB, Blunt LW Jr, User HM, et al. Preperitoneal laparoscopic simple prostatectomy. Urology
2004;63:778–9.

[54] Rehman J, Khan SA, Sukkarieh T, et al. Extraperitoneal laparoscopic prostatectomy (adenomectomy) for obstructing benign prostatic hyperplasia:
transvesical and transcapsular (Millin) techniques.
J Endourol 2005;19:491–8.

[55] Sotelo R, Spalivieiro M, Garcia-Segui A, et al. Laparoscopic retro-pubic simple prostatectomy. J Urol
2005;173:757–60.

[56] Rey D, Ducarme G, Hoepffner JL, et al. Laparoscopic adenectomy: a novel technique for managing
benign prostatic hyperplasia. BJU Int 2005;95:
676–8.

[57] Porpiglia F, Terrone C, Renard J, et al. Transcapsular adenomectomy (Millin): a comparative study,
extraperitoneal laparoscopy versus open surgery.
Eur Urol 2006;49:120–6.

[58] Baumert H, Ballaro A, Dugardin F, et al. Laparoscopic versus open simple prostatectomy: a comparative study. J Urol 2006;175:1691–4.

[59] Mariano MB, Tefilli MV, Graziottin TM, et al.
Laparoscopic prostatectomy for benign prostatic
hyperplasia—a six-year experience. Eur Urol
2006;49:127–32.

[60] Plante KM, Bunnel ML, Trotter SJ, et al.
Transurethral prostatic tissue ablation via a single-
needle delivery system: initial experience with
radio-frequency energy and ethanol. Prostate
Cancer and Prostatic Dis 2002;5:183–8.

[61] DiTrolio JV, Patel P, Watson RA, et al. Chemo-
ablation of the prostate with dehydrated alcohol
for the treatment of prostatic obstruction. J Urol
2002;67:2100–4.

[62] Gutierrez-Aceves J, Gilling P, Schettini M, et al.
Transurethral ethanol ablation of the prostate
(TEAP), initial long-term report of two prospective
multicenter studies. J Urol 2003;169(Suppl):466.

[63] Grise P, Plante M, Palmer J, et al. Evaluation of the
transurethral ethanol ablation of the prostate
(TEAP) for symptomatic benign prostatic obstruction: a european multi-center evaluation. Eur Urol
2004;46:496–502.

[64] Goya N, Ishikawa N, Ito F, et al. Transurethral
ethanol injection therapy for prostatic obstruction:
3-year results. J Urol 2004;172:1017–20.

[65] Plante MK, Marks LS, Anderson R, et al. Phase I/
II examination of transurethral ethanol ablation of
the prostate for the treatment of symptomatic
benign prostatic hyperplasia. J Urol 2007;177:
1030–5.

[66] Plante MK, Palmer J, Martinez-Sagarra J, et al.
Complications associated with transurethral
ethanol ablation of the prostate for the treatment
of benign prostatic obstruction: a worldwide
experience. J Urol 2003;169(Suppl):392, A1466.

[67] Chuang YC, Chiang PH, Huang CC, et al. Botulinum toxin type A improves benign prostatic

hyperplasia symptoms in patients with small prostates. Urology 2005;66:775–9.

[68] Chuang YC, Chiang PH, Yoshimura N, et al. Sustained beneficial effects of intraprostatic botulinum toxin type A on lower urinary tract symptoms and quality of life in men with benign prostatic hyperplasia. BJU Int 2006;98:1033–7.

[69] Geurcini F, Giannantoni A, Bard R. Intraprostatic botulin toxin injection in patients with severe benign prostatic hyperplasia: a multicenter feasibility study [abstract]. J Urol 2005; 173(Suppl):376.

[70] Maria G, Brisinda G, Civello IM, et al. Relief by botulinum toxin of voiding dysfunction due to benign prostatic hyperplasia: results of a randomized, placebo-controlled study. Urology 2003;62:259–64 [discussion: 264–5].

[71] Park DS, Cho TW, Lee YK, et al. Evaluation of short-term clinical effects and presumptive mechanism of botulinum toxin type A as a treatment modality of benign prostatic hyperplasia. Yonsei Med J 2006;47:706–14.

[72] Saemi AM, Plante MK. Injectables in the prostate. Curr Opin Urol 2008;18(1):28–33.

[73] Chuang YC, Huang CC, Kang HY, et al. Novel action of botulinum toxin on the stromal and epithelial components of the prostate gland. J Urol 2006;175:1158–63.

[74] Kuo HC. Prostate botulinum A toxin injection—an alternative treatment for benign prostatic obstruction in poor surgical candidates. Urology 2005;65: 670–4.

[75] Chuang YC, Giannantoni A, Chancellor MB. The potential and promise of using botulinum toxin in the prostate gland. BJU Int 2006;98:28–32.

[76] Rassweiller J, Schulze M, Stock C, et al. Bipolar transurethral resection of the prostate—technical modifications and early clinical experience. Minim Invasive Ther Allied Technol 2007;16(1)):11–21.

[77] Ho HS, Yip SK, Lim KB, et al. A prospective randomized study comparing monopolar and bipolar transurethral resection of prostate using transurethral resection in saline (TURIS) system. Eur Urol. 2007;52(2):517–24.

[78] Erturhan S, Erbagci A, Seckiner I, et al. Plasmakinetic resection of the prostate versus standard transurethral resection of the prostate: a prospective randomized trial with a 1-year follow-up. Prostate Cancer Prostate Dis 2007;10(1):97–100.

[79] Ho H, Cheng CWS. Bipolar TURP: a new reference standard? Curr Opin Urol 2008;18(1):50–5.

[80] de Sio M, Autorino R, Quarto G, et al. Gyrus bipolar versus standard monopolar transurethral resection of the prostate: a randomized prospective trial. Urology 2006;76:69–72.

[81] Tefekli A, Muslumanoglu AY, Baykal M, et al. A hybrid technique using bipolar energy in transurethral prostate surgery: a prospective, randomized comparison. J Urol 2005;174(4):1339–43.

[82] Schelin S, Geertsen U, Walter S, et al. Feedback microwave thermotherapy versus TURP/prostate enucleation surgery in patients with benign prostatic hyperplasia and persistent urinary retention: a prospective, randomized, controlled, multicenter study. Urology 2006;68(4):795–9.

[83] Brausi M, Breda G, Isgro A. Transurethral water-induced thermotherapy: is it a therapeutic option for patients in urinary retention? [abstract]. J Urol 2000;165(Suppl):294.

[84] Peterson MD, Matlaga BR, Kim SC, et al. Holmium laser enucleation of the prostate for men with urinary retention. J Urol 2005;174(3): 998–1001.

[85] Ruszat R, Wyler S, Seifert HH, et al. Photoselective vaporization of the prostate: subgroup analysis of men with refractory urinary retention. Eur Urol 2006;50(5):1040–9.

[86] Mutaguchi K, Matsubara A, Kajiwara M, et al. Transurethral ethanol injection for prostatic obstruction: an excellent treatment strategy for persistent urinary retention. Urology 2006;68: 307–11.

[87] Silva J, Silva C, Saraiva L, et al. Intraprostatic botulinum toxin type A injection in patients unfit for surgery presenting with refractory urinary retention and benign prostatic enlargement. Effect on prostate volume and micturition resumption. Eur Urol 2008;53(1):153–9.

[88] Gravas S, Laguna P, Kiemeney LA, et al. Durability of 30 minutes high-energy transurethral microwave therapy for the treatment of BPH: a study of 213 patients with and without urinary retention. Urology 2007;69(5):854–8.

[89] Reich O, Bachmann A, Siebels M, et al. High-power (80 W) potassium-titanyl-phosphate laser vaporization of the prostate in 66 high-risk patients. J Urol 2005;173:158–60.

[90] Sandhu JS, Ng CK, Gonzalez RR, et al. Photoselective laser vaporization prostatectomy in men receiving anticoagulants. J Endourol 2005;19: 1196–8.

[91] Ruszat R, Wyler S, Forster T, et al. Safety and effectiveness of photoselective vaporization of the prostate (PVP) in patients on ongoing oral anticoagulation. Eur Urol 2007;51:1031–41.

[92] Pedraza R, Samadi A, Eshghi M. Holmium laser enucleation of the prostate in critically ill patients with technique modification. J Endourol 2004;18: 795–8.

[93] Manyak MJ, Ackerman SJ, Blute ML, et al. Cost-effectiveness of treatment for benign prostatic hyperplasia: an economic model for comparison of medical, minimally invasive, and surgical therapy. J Endourol 2002;16:51–6.

[94] Stovsky MD, Griffiths RI, Duff SB. A clinical outcomes and cost analysis comparing photoselective vaporization of the prostate to alternative minimally invasive therapies and transurethral prostate

resection for the treatment of benign prostatic hyperplasia. J Urol 2006;176:1500–6.

[95] Wei JT, Calhoun E, Jacobsen SJ. Urologic diseases in America. Project: benign prostatic hyperplasia. J Urol 2005;173:1256–61.

[96] Lotan Y, Cadeddu JA, RoehrbornCG, et al. The value of your time: evaluation of effects of changes in Medicare reimbursement rates on the practice of urology. J Urol 2004;172:1958–62.

[97] Disantostefano RL, Biddle AK, Lavelle JP. An evaluation of the economic costs and patient-related consequences of treatments for benign prostatic hyperplasia. BJU Int 2006;97:1007–16.

[98] Baba S, Badlani G, Elhilali M, et al. New minimally invasive and surgical developments in the management of BPO. In: Mc Connell J, Abrams P, Akaza H, Roerborn C, editors. 6th International consultation on prostate cancer and prostate diseases. HEALTH Publications, Paris, France; 2006.

[99] AUA Practice Guideline Committee. AUA guidelines on management of benign prostatic hyperplasia. Chapter 1: diagnosis and treatment recommendations. J Urol 2003;170:530–47.

[100] Madersbacher S, Marberger M. Is transurethral resection of the prostate still justified? BJU Int 1999;83(3):227–37.

ELSEVIER
SAUNDERS

Urol Clin N Am 35 (2008) 519–531

UROLOGIC
CLINICS
of North America

Simulation and Computer-Animated Devices: The New Minimally Invasive Skills Training Paradigm

Robert M. Sweet, MD[a,b], Elspeth M. McDougall, MD, FRCSC[c,d],*

[a]Simulation PeriOperative Resource for Training and Learning, University of Minnesota,
D509 Mayo Memorial Building, 420 Delaware Street SE, Minneapolis, MN 55455, USA
[b]Department of Urologic Surgery, University of Minnesota, D509 Mayo Memorial Building,
420 Delaware Street SE, Minneapolis, MN 55455, USA
[c]Surgical Education Center, University of California, Irvine, USA
[d]Department of Urology, University of California, Irvine Medical Center, Building 55,
Route 81, Room 302, 101 The City Drive South, Orange, CA 92868-3201, USA

The rapid development of complex surgical technologies, particularly in minimally invasive therapy, has resulted in challenging learning curves for surgeons. In addition, limited case experience as a result of restricted resident work hours and limited case volumes in surgical practice add additional challenges to surgical education in the 21st century. Meanwhile, surgeons are finding it increasingly important to not just maintain skills, but to develop new skills, especially those new technically challenging skills related to minimally invasive surgical therapies. In addition, minimally invasive therapies are highly dependent on uniquely specialized teams of health care workers. For all of these reasons, simulation is gaining increasing attention as an additional component to the surgical education armamentarium for the development and refinement of minimally invasive surgical skills and technique [1].

Technical skills education in urology, as in many of the technically oriented fields has its primary roots in the operating room, augmented by cadaver and live animal models and, in select cases, inanimate artificial tissues. In fact "simulators" were used by Susrutha in ancient India in the form of inanimate artificial tissues and physical models [2]. With the advent of digital imaging techniques (CT and MRI), visual-spatial anatomic understanding and "preoperative" planning rose to a whole new level both from a clinical and an education standpoint. With the advent of fiber optics and the video monitor, the trainee and trainer were able to comfortably view the same endoscopic image simultaneously, allowing for more rapid training. Renewed interest in urologic simulation and a paradigm shift in surgical education came about with a series of closely related events. The "To Err is Human" report and the increased public awareness of surgical errors have brought medical care in general under greater scrutiny [3]. Restrictions on residency work hours, the surge of minimally invasive training procedures in urology, and the acute rise in health care costs have all led administrators to seek alternative learning environments to the operating room for training. Technologies offering virtual reality, a term coined in 1987 by Jaron Lanier, opened up new possibilities in medicine for creating a practice environment with intelligent data-collection and mentoring. Unfortunately, this concept was overpromised and underdelivered for many reasons: limitations of computer processing, lack of organized structure and understanding around curriculum design, lack of defined "standards" and metrics, the high cost of development, the multidisciplinary nature of such projects, and

* Corresponding author. University of California, Irvine Medical Center, Department of Urology, 101 The City Drive, Building 55, Room 302, Route 81, Orange, CA 92868-3201, USA.

E-mail address: elspethm@uci.edu (E.M. McDougall).

a lack of fundamental modeling and validation data during the development process. One of the largest technical challenges is the application of this technology. As much as we like to make the analogy with flight simulation, the human body is not an airplane. The human body is a very complex "model," with many unknown components, and so is difficult to accurately and consistently simulate. Such complexity becomes magnified when one considers the relatively unknown dynamic impact that the brain has on the body at the microcellular, macrocellular, tissue, physiologic, and behavioral levels.

Simulation is the technique of imitating the behavior of some situation or process by means of a suitable analogous situation or apparatus especially for the purpose of study or training [4]. This has been used extensively in economics, the military, and the aeronautics and space industry and is now becoming an important part of medical education. Learning devices that produce simulation are training simulators. The terms *low*- and *high-fidelity* refer to how closely the simulator itself and the environment in which the training occurs represent reality. To be most effective, high-fidelity simulation must lead learners to suspend their disbelief. To do this, the interactive sights, sounds, smells, and feel of the simulated experience must mimic reality and subsequently elicit the emotions and generate the behaviors that would be observed in a real situation. The difference between a low-fidelity simulation and a high-fidelity simulation can be significant. A low-fidelity trainer, for example, may be a simple abstract box-model for use in a nonclinical environment, such as a living room, to practice a procedure. By contrast, the highest-fidelity simulation currently for the same procedure would involve an operation on a live animal in a real operating room under supervision. Anatomic models made in virtual reality represent an attempt to recreate the environment of real tissue. However, unlike either the abstract box model or the live-animal situation, they have the exciting capability of generating data on everything the user does in the environment and of incorporating a virtual instructor. These simulation formats can be used for skills training, task training, and procedure training. They can also provide high reliability team training for such environments as the operating room, the intensive care unit, and the emergency department. Many surgical courses now rely on simple abstract material-based trainers to teach novice surgeons basic skills and techniques.

These are excellent tools as long as proper techniques are conveyed. Courses use higher-fidelity tissue or virtual reality trainers to make assessments and provide training for tasks requiring higher-level skills and to provide a means to practice acquired skills. Virtual reality trainers that are software-based and can incorporate curricula, assess formative metrics, recognize errors, and contain management features are gaining more interest as a means of learner-centered, independent, and deliberative practice with feedback.

One of the newest additions to continuing medical education is high reliability team training [5,6]. Much can be learned by experiencing errors as they occur and studying how these errors can be successfully managed by the team vis-à-vis a debrief exercise. As such, simulation has a profound ability to provide significant advantages as a platform for repetitive practice by both the team and the individual in a no-risk environment away from patients. Simulation technologies can build in every potential error and thereby provide acute-scenario training so that the trainees can learn to recognize, avert, and resolve these events in a no-risk environment. This better prepares them for a similar clinical situation. In addition, virtual reality and other dry-laboratory simulation exercises are helping to reduce the reliance on animal and cadaver laboratories, and have shown the capability to reduce operative times and errors in the operating room [7].

In clinical teaching, it is essential that the teacher be focused on the patient first and the trainee second. Dedicated facilities with a curriculum embedded with simulation enable teachers to focus all of their attention on learners. The curriculum involves creating a comprehensive knowledge base so that the trainee understands what is to be learned, why it should be learned, and how it can be learned. Of equal importance is teaching the trainee how to recognize an error, why it is an error, and what to do to avoid and recover from the error. It is the combination of basic knowledge and manipulative skills, along with the development of judgment during clinical experiences, that creates the master surgeon. Simulation provides both an opportunity to study and commit to memory how master surgeons attain and perform their skills and an environment by which learners can refine and perfect their skills to achieve such mastery.

The adult learner is a unique student in the environment of health care education. These learners tend to have a problem-centered orientation to their learning and a readiness to learn, as well as increased self-directedness [8]. Residents and fellows as a group of learners comprise a unique group of students who are in Erickson's seventh stage of development [9]. These middle adult learners have a significant need to develop knowledge and skills, and to be able to apply them effectively to their clinical practice as part of their quest for generativity rather than stagnation. However, as learners, they also have weaknesses and therefore strategies must be devised to overcome these. Research has shown that physicians are pretty awful at self-assessment. It is part of the human condition to suppress our inadequacies to both others and ourselves. As such, these learners like the reward that comes from success and, left to their own devices, gravitate to studying things they enjoy and are already good at. While self-directed learning may be appropriate for an evening pottery class, it is less appropriate for the learning and application of medicine and surgical skills. People increasingly expect doctors to have a reasonable amount of cognitive and technical skill before embarking on the practice of medicine and surgery.

An effective curriculum must clearly identify the goals of the educational program. This is based on a defined desired outcome and a needs assessment that directs the development of the educational program. This assessment generates the specific learning objectives of the curriculum as they relate to the cognitive and skills performance that is to be learned in the training program. The objectives clearly outline not only the material to be covered but also the format that will be used to assess the student for each of the curricular objectives. The curriculum will include a clear delineation of all teaching methods and strategies as they relate to the curricular objectives. Appropriate formative student assessment must be incorporated into the curriculum to provide ongoing feedback to help guide and shape learning. The curriculum must also include summative assessment opportunities to determine if the student has achieved the required level of proficiency before advancing to the next stage of training. Finally, the curriculum must be subject to ongoing evaluation by both the students and the instructors to direct curriculum growth and improvement.

Several researchers have shown that didactic lectures by themselves do not play a significant role in immediately changing physician performance or improving patient care [10]. Education programs that use interactive techniques are generally more effective in changing physician performance or improving patient care outcomes. In addition, educational sessions delivered in a longitudinal or sequenced manner also appear to have a more beneficial impact on physician learning [11]. The provision of enabling methods to facilitate implementation of the new knowledge or skill in the practice setting appears to have a positive effect on the success of medical education programs.

Gallagher and colleagues [12] have clearly shown the importance of the knowledge and psychomotor curriculum in surgical education. Humans have a limited capacity for attention. This limitation becomes extremely important in planning the education of novice surgeons or in learning a new surgical technique. These surgeons are trying to gain additional knowledge while comprehending instruction from their mentor in the operating room. At the same time, they are dealing with the challenges of depth and spatial judgment as this affects their psychomotor performance, especially during minimally invasive therapy. Add to this the demand for operative judgment and decision-making and they may well exceed their attention capacity, which results in their inability to cope with an error or complication. In contrast, the master surgeon has the fundamental knowledge, requires less attention for already well-developed spatial judgment and surgical skills, and therefore can devote more attention to a situation in which an error may be about to occur. Simulation can provide an opportunity for trainees to gain the knowledge and develop better psychomotor and spatial judgment skills so that they too can apply more attention to other skills and learn more about operative judgment and decision–making in the clinical setting. As surgeons, we have long understood our lifelong commitment to education and this concept must be further instilled in our trainees as they become self-directed learners. "Practice makes perfect" is a concept that is well understood by pilots learning to fly, dancers rehearsing complex dance routines, and golfers perfecting their swings. The concept is just as valid in the field of surgery.

Surgical practice is a concept that has been highlighted in a recent report by Kahol and colleagues [13] in their study on the effect of short-term, pretrial practice on surgical proficiency in simulated environments. In this study, subjects performed standardized exercises as a preoperative warm-up, after which the standardized exercises were repeated in a random order. The experimental group was allowed to warm up with the standardized exercises, after which a different task (electrocautery stimulation) was performed. The study participants included experienced laparoscopic surgeons, fellows, and residents. The results of this study provide substantial evidence that short-term practice (warm-up) with exercises designed to target both the psychomotor and cognitive skills involved in surgical procedures can greatly enhance surgical proficiencies during a follow-up procedure. Similar practice techniques enhanced gesture proficiency and made general movements and movements involving tools smoother. Interestingly, the participants of varying experience levels all benefited from the warm-up exercises. Perhaps most importantly, error rates fell significantly following the warm-up exercises. The time required to complete a task, which is one important indicator of efficiency, was also reduced significantly in this study population.

Simulation is also being proposed as an assessment and credentialing tool similar to that in the aviation industry [14]. This proposal comes from a need to measure more than just knowledge, to model real-life situations, and to standardize the assessment of surgeons. Simulation has the potential to provide the "vehicle" to measure skills. However, for simulation assessment to be of value, it must have a scoring system that aligns with expert agreement on what and how a task should be performed and that is subject to strict research to confirm construct and predictive validity. As an appropriate device for surgical evaluation, the curriculum must be able to distinguish the novice from the expert laparoscopic surgeon, or have construct validity. In addition, the simulation-embedded curriculum must be able, on the basis of the performance of the trainee, to predict the surgeon's performance in the corresponding clinical setting and predict the student's likelihood of eventual success if being used for screening applicants.

The demonstration of consistent performance at validated criterion levels within the curriculum is a clear indicator that the trainee is ready to advance to the operating room to perform the procedure. The establishment of such criterion levels is often done by having experts go through the curriculum and adjust these based on their performance and consensus [15]. The curriculum will judge proficiency based on such factors as economy of motion, target acquisition, and procedural judgment, rather than just operative time and subjective performance assessment. Hence a surgeon's advancement up the training ladder would be more precisely determined, thereby providing clarity to trainees and their teachers as to trainees' skill levels and learning needs, and ensuring that patients are cared for by doctors with documented expertise in the procedures they are planning to perform. Confirmation of predictive validity then allows a simulator device to be used in the certifying and recertifying processes for the subspecialty to determine surgeon competency. Validation studies are essential to determine whether a simulation-embedded curriculum can teach what it is supposed to teach, to demonstrate whether the data generated can distinguish between the novice and the experienced surgeon, and, most importantly, to predict the current and future performance of the surgeon in the clinical operating room.

The development of a comprehensive and effective teaching program depends on the collaborative efforts of many educators across multiple institutions to ensure a robust curriculum that addresses all the needs of the learner, teacher, and end user or patient. Multiple, interactive educational encounters that are longitudinally sequenced will provide more productive learning for the health profession student. Such encounters, combined with immediate, task-specific feedback as to performance and errors, will allow these learners to better learn new skills and effectively integrate them into their clinical practice. However, simultaneous curriculum evaluation is essential to the creation of durable and relevant education programs. It is through evaluation combined with discussion and deliberative inquiry that curriculum development will be achieved. Continuous curriculum revision and renewal can be expected to meet the educational demands of a rapidly advancing, technology-oriented, surgical subspecialty [16]. Curriculum development should be considered a long-term, dynamic, and continuous process that anticipates many revisions and changes to the initial curriculum template. Sustaining the effort of curricular reform will only happen from a combined bottom-up and top-down approach. Commitment at the departmental level by academicians who recognize the advantages of a standardized curriculum and the importance of collaborative communication will lead to the development of robust surgical curricula. The incorporation of appropriate curricular evaluation will allow constructive, proactive response to the expectations of society and the policies of the boards mandating such standardization. The American College of Surgeons' recent Accreditation of Education Institutes program is an example of this association's commitment to the incorporation of simulation for surgical residency training programs and the development of dedicated skills training curricula [17,18].

The creation of a simulator for training begins with agreement on what is the desired outcome and the development of learning goals and objectives. Learning objectives are specific and contain action verbs describing what learners should be able to do once they have completed the exercise. The simulation tool is designed specifically to meet these objectives [19]. The process of task deconstruction into the learning domains described in Fig. 1 allows for the development and application of the appropriate simulated experience.

The cognitive domain is underappreciated in surgical education and simulation. It has been estimated that performing an operation properly is 75% decision-making and 25% dexterity [20]. Bloom's taxonomy [21] describes the transition from the baseline memorization of material (knowledge) to synthesis (comprehension). The ability to appropriately apply this knowledge represents the next level in ascent toward the higher-cognitive functions of analysis, synthesis, and evaluation associated with self-reflection and teaching. Cognitive "simulation" in surgery has existed in a "passive form" for over a century in the form of surgical atlases, for decades in the form of videos, and more recently in the form of the Fundamentals of Laparoscopic Surgery, with its well-validated curriculum and strong cognitive component [22]. It is widely used across the United States in skills centers. With interactive video technology, SimPraxis (Red Llama, Seattle Washington; www.redllamainc.com) has designed a novel platform that integrates an entire cognitive curriculum for procedures into an interactive multimedia trainer that provides virtual mentorship, error tracking, and scoring [23].

The technical domain has been a focus of computer-based simulation devices. With a stepwise curricular approach that is not procedure-specific, such basic skills as camera navigation precedes more complex manipulative skills, such as transfer and cutting exercises [24]. Box trainers and abstract virtual reality models have been found to be useful for training these skills. Subsequently, such simple tasks as dissection, clipping, and dividing a vessel can be performed on slightly more complex virtual reality models, inanimate or animate tissue, or human cadaver models. It is only when combined with the cognitive and judgment components of a curriculum that a full procedural trainer can be created. Outside of the standard training on actual anesthetized patients, live animal models remain the gold standard. The role of virtual reality for training advanced surgical procedures continues to evolve. The traditional method of evaluating surgical competence has been the In-Training Evaluation Report, which is filled out at the end of rotations by faculty. Unfortunately, these reports do not provide formative feedback to the trainee. Many programs are shifting toward the Objective Structured Assessment of Technical Skills evaluation whereby the learner is evaluated on multiple domains, such as tissue handling and flow of the operation. This type of assessment is being done in both the operating room and in skills-training laboratories [25]. While operating room competency evaluation in urology residency training programs is encouraged but not required by the Accreditation Council for Graduate Medical Education [26], programs struggle with whether or not to use the Objective Structured Assessment of Technical Skills (OSATS) evaluation, which is

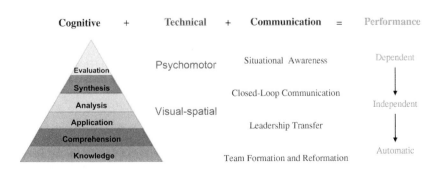

Fig. 1. Learning domains in surgical training. (*Courtesy of* RM Sweet and C Schmitz.)

an effective, reliable tool for formative feedback provided immediately in the form of a debrief. OSATS is more effective for guiding the surgical trainee than the less labor-intensive method of summative end-of-the-rotation feedback. Criterion levels and standards are yet to be established by the governing bodies and societies for urology as to competence for specific procedures and, therefore, these are currently established at the individual or institutional level.

If one were to mention the word *simulation* to an anesthesiologist or an emergency medicine physician, a much different image would come to mind than would come to the mind of the surgeon. Dozens of truly "high-fidelity" simulation scenarios have been designed for mass-casualty and emergent crisis situations. The most common domain studied and practiced in these scenarios pertains to communication. The standardized Objective Structured Clinical Examination allows this domain to be assessed and is commonly used in medical school curricula [27]. Its use during urology residency/credentialing for this domain has been described and is encouraged by the Accreditation Council for Graduate Medical Education [28]. Gettman and colleagues [29] recently published a study using a high-fidelity simulation environment to assess the "communication" domain for delivering the news of an unexpected death to a urology patient's family. These scenarios can either be done in a simulation center, which has the advantage of a more "standardized" and controlled environment like that of Gettman's study, or they can be done in situ, as described in work by Riley and colleagues [30], whereby situational awareness, closed-loop communication, leadership transfer, and team formation and reformation are studied and practiced with artificial scenarios at the actual location where real events normally occur. This approach increases the fidelity and has value for discovering latent conditions.

All of these domains ultimately contribute to performance where the trainee makes the transition from dependence toward independence and finally can perform skills automatically. This process of learning establishes the ability of the trainee to shift more of his or her attention toward more advanced decision-making or "judgment." While all skill sets have a cognitive component, some clearly rely on the judgmental aspect more than others.

"Skill sets" specific to urology that have been successfully simulated include such cognitive skill sets as pelvic lymph node dissection skills and laparoscopic skills. The fundamentals of laparoscopic surgery contain cognitive training modules to accompany their skills modules that have been well validated by the American College of Surgeons. More recently Red Llama has built and validated an interactive video-based trainer for training pelvic lymph node dissection [31] (Movie 1: SimPraxis® open pelvic lymph node trainer*). Technical skills trainers focusing on the Seldinger technique; endoscopic procedures, such as cystoscopy, transurethral resection, and ureteroscopy; and basic laparoscopic and robotic skills have been designed and are being integrated into curricula primarily focused at the junior urology resident level. Basic open and laparoscopic surgery skills simulation exercises in the form of Objective Structured Assessment of Technical Skills examinations are being administered at select institutions and typically use inanimate tissue models with proctors.

Until recently, there has been a general lack of training tools and curriculum development for even the most basic of skill sets in urology. Simulation has primarily consisted of manikin-based catheterization simulators for the female and male urethra as well simulators for digital rectal examinations (Simulution, Prior Lake, Minnesota; www.simulution.com). However, validation studies are lacking.

The skills necessary to perform flexible ureteroscopy, not unlike skills for other endoscopic procedures, are quite amenable to simulation. Current systems reported in the curriculum of training programs and courses include low-fidelity bench models, such as the one described by Matsumoto [32], which consists of a urethra represented by a Penrose drain, a bladder represented by an inverted polystyrene plastic cup, and ureters modeled with latex-embedded straws. Commercially available bench models include the Uro-Scopic Trainer (Limbs & Things, Bristol, United Kingdom; www.limbsandthings.com) and the Scope Trainer (Medi Skills, Edinburgh, United Kingdom; www.mediskills.com) [33]. McDougall and colleagues have developed a bench-top ureteroscopic model that is being validated (Movie 2: University of California Irvine (UCI) ureteroscopy trainer*). Uro Mentor (Simbionix, Lod, Israel; www.simbionix.com) is the only currently available virtual reality simulator for ureteroscopy

---

* Videos for this article can be accessed by visiting www.urologic.theclinics.com. In the online table of contents for this issue, click on "add-ons."

(Movie 3: Uromentor® ureteteroscopy trainer*). It allows the user to navigate the ureter and perform various upper urinary tract procedures, such as lithotripsy, laser incision of a stricture, and tumor ablation with tools, including baskets, graspers, intracorporeal lithotripters, guide wires, catheters, stents, biopsy devices, and dilation devices. Several studies have examined its validity and have established that it has educational value at the novice end of the learning curve, but less on the more experienced end [34,35]. Matsumoto [36] compared performance on Uro Mentor with a high-fidelity bench model and showed a similar level of skill improvement using either training device. Chou and colleagues [37] demonstrated a similar finding in comparing the bench model Uro-Scopic trainer with the Uro Mentor in a group of 16 medical students for teaching basic ureteroscopy skills.

Only 11% of urologists obtain their own renal access [38], even though it has been shown that stone-free rates are higher when a fellowship-trained urologist obtains access compared with rates when a radiologist obtains access [39]. Three training methods have been presented as options for training to acquire the skills needed for using two-dimensional fluoroscopic images to understand three-dimensional space. Such skills are essential for performing percutaneous access to the kidney. Hammond and colleagues [40] describe an innovative model using porcine kidneys with preimplanted artificial stone material in an intact chicken carcass. Using real-time C-arm fluoroscopy, the residents gain needle access, perform dilation, and do fragmentation/extraction of the stone material. Hacker and colleagues [41] took this model one step further by cannulating the ureter, renal artery, and renal vein for continuous perfusion. They surround the "perfused" kidney with ultrasound gel before putting it in the chicken carcass. Acceptability studies of Hammond's model were encouraging. However, again validation studies are lacking. Strohmaier and Giese [42] also use a porcine renal unit, but describe embedding it in silicone for teaching percutaneous renal access. Medi Skills offers a manikin-based percutaneous-access model. The PercMentor (Simbionix) is a hybrid manikin–virtual reality simulator focused on training the percutaneous renal access portion of the procedure. The force-feedback interface consists of a manikin silicone flank with ribs underneath. The learner controls a virtual C-arm with corresponding virtual fluoroscopic images and a needle is tracked in virtual space with respect to the model. This training model also collects data on cognitive decision-making with regards to choice of instrumentation and choice of calyceal access. Once the needle access is obtained, guidewires, catheters, and tubes are also employed to gain access to the collecting system. These are registered in the virtual space. Knudsen and colleagues [43] prospectively randomized 63 trainees into training versus no training using the PercMentor simulator as the pre- and posttest assessment tool. Performance was assessed using a subjective global rating scale and key metrics generated by the simulator. Subjects who underwent 60 minutes of training on the PercMentor outperformed their peers on PercMentor for both the subjective and objective parameters.

Transurethral resection of the prostate and bladder remain the mainstay skill sets for urologists. Virtual reality cystoscopy models are present as modules in both the Uro Mentor (Simbionix) validated by Gettman and colleagues [44], the Uro-Trainer (Karl Storz, Tuttlingen, Germany; www.karlstorz.com), and the SurgicalSIM transurethral resection of the prostate (TURP) simulator (Medical Education Technologies, Inc. [METI], Sarasota, Florida; www.meti.com). A physical model by Limbs & Things, proposes to train TURP cutting skills on a disposable model and is primarily used for booth demonstrations by endoscopic vendors. Validation of this simulator in educational programs has not been reported. A full TURP skills curriculum is available on the METI's SurgicalSIM TURP, the commercially available version of the University of Washington TURP trainer designed and validated at the American Urological Association by Sweet and colleagues [14,45–49]. This simulator logs important metrics, such as grams resected, blood loss, irrigation used, and critical errors. (Movie 4: Virtual reality transurethral resection of the prostate skills trainer*). The Uro-Trainer simulator includes simulation capabilities for TURP and transurethral resection of bladder tumor, but lacks a standardized curriculum. Like the University of Washington TURP trainer, however, the Uro-Trainer has force-feedback and simulates bleeding. Preliminary validity studies have been conducted [50]. Simulation offers a third virtual reality system, PelvicVision for training TURP. Validation studies for this trainer are currently lacking.

The development and validation of trainers for laparoscopic psychomotor skills have primarily stemmed from the general surgery literature, driven by the establishment of laparoscopic cholecystectomy as the standard-of-care procedure for removing gallbladders. The Fundamentals of Laparoscopic Surgery program provides a well-validated, standardized curriculum comprised of cognitive and psychomotor tasks. It has been incorporated into the curricula of many of the American College of Surgeons–accredited simulation centers of excellence. Video-box trainers are also popular and useful for basic tasks, such as navigation, transferring, suturing, and knot tying. These skills can then be transferred to the cadaver models [51] and the human patient [52,53]. Unfortunately, these low-fidelity models require a trained observer to be in attendance to provide assessment and formative feedback for the trainee. ProMis (Haptica, Dublin, Ireland; www.haptica.com) also offers a hybrid video box–virtual reality trainer that has undergone rigorous validation studies and has been found to be more acceptable than many of the pure virtual reality trainers [54–57] (Movie 5: ProMis® laparoscopic skills trainer*). METI's SurgicalSIM LTS offers a video-box trainer with a self-contained computer assessment component [58,59] (Movie 6: Surgical Sim LTS® laparoscopic skills trainer*). The exercises include peg manipulation, ring manipulation, ductal cannulation, lasso-loop formation and cinching, knot tying, knot integrity, and circle cutting. Virtual reality–based simulation trainers have the distinct advantage of both formative and summative assessment capability. The Minimally Invasive Surgical Trainer–Virtual Reality (MIST-VR; Mentice, Göteborg, Sweden; www.mentice.com) consists of six abstract tasks focused on training navigation, grasping, translocation, and diathermy. Seymour and colleagues [7] showed for the first time that training on a virtual reality laparoscopic trainer (MIST-VR's diathermy task) translated to improved performance in diathermy tasks in the operating room. Their randomized blinded-design

using videotapes and blinded evaluators was a model study-design for simulation validation studies to follow. While procedure-specific virtual reality models are now only available for general surgery and gynecologic applications, most of the laparoscopic virtual reality platforms provide skills exercises that translate to basic skill sets in urology. Examples of such virtual reality platforms include the SurgiSIM platform (METI) (Movie 7: Surgical Sim VR laparascopic skills trainer*). Surgical Science AB's LapSim (Surgical Science, Göteborg, Sweden; www.surgical-science.com), the LaparoscopyVR System (Immersion Medical, Gaithersburg, Maryland; www.immersion.com), and LapMentor (Simbionix) (Table 1).

The American Urological Association is collaborating with METI to build a dedicated laparoscopic transperitoneal nephrectomy simulator. The team assembled to deliver the final learning module represents a professional society, led by members of the American Urological Association's Laparoscopy Committee and Surgical Simulation Group, which created the curriculum and assessment methods; the University of Minnesota, which serves as the academic partner responsible for building the models; and METI as the industry partner and integrator. The American Urological Association has established the learning objectives, is developing the corresponding metrics, is creating the didactic content, and has committed to performing the validation studies on the final module. The University of Minnesota is using novel advanced modeling techniques to deliver models that look and behave like real tissue using real tissue properties, and METI is responsible for developing the architecture, providing all simulated scenarios, integrating all aspects of the curriculum into the learning module, and bringing the product to market.

The "intuitive" wrist interface and stereoscopic vision of the da Vinci robot (Intuitive Surgical, Sunnyvale, California; www.intuitivesurgical.com) has enabled the wide dissemination of the laparoscopic approach to radical prostatectomy and to other reconstructive urologic procedures. Dry laboratory exercises, including those for passing rings, suturing pads, and tying knots, have been developed for use with the surgical robot for training. The advantage of three-dimensional over

---

* Videos for this article can be accessed by visiting www.urologic.theclinics.com. In the online table of contents for this issue, click on "add-ons."

Table 1
Commercially available laparoscopic technical-skills trainers

Trainer	Manufacturer	Type	Built-in assessment	Cognitive components	Force-feedback	Urology procedural application
SurgicalSim [59]	METI (www.meti.com)	Virtual reality	Yes	Yes	No	In pipeline
LapSim [60–64]	Surgical Science (www.surgical-science.com/)	Virtual reality	Yes	No	No	No
LapVR [65,66]	Immersion Med (www.immersion.com/medical/)	Virtual reality	Yes	No	Yes	No
LapMentor [67–70]	Simbionix (www.simbionix.com)	Virtual reality	Yes	Yes	No	No
MIST-VR [6,71–73]	Mentice (www.mentice.com)	Virtual reality	Yes	No	No	No
LTS [57,58]	METI (www.meti.com)	Box	Yes	No	Yes	No
ProMIS [53–56]	Haptica (www.haptica.com)	Hybrid	Yes	No	Yes	No
LapEd	LapEd (www.LapEd.org)	Box	No	No	Yes	Yes
LapTrainer with Simuvision [74]	Simulab (www.simulab.com)	Box	No	No	Yes	Yes
SimEndo [75–78]	DeltaTech (www.simendo.eu)	Virtual reality	Yes	No	No	No

two-dimensional skills acquisition was demonstrated in a group of novice surgeons [79]. Contrary to popular belief and to studies in laparoscopic surgical training, video game experience among trainees correlated negatively with robotic knotting, while athletes and musicians were more adept at these skills [80]. Multiple studies have estimated the learning curve for the da Vinci–assisted laparoscopic radical prostatectomy to range from 20 to 70 cases [81]. Robotic surgical training is extremely expensive and can be difficult because of the high demand on equipment during the week for actual surgery, the high cost of purchasing a dedicated "training robot," and the space required to house the robot [82]. Mimic Technologies (Seattle, Washington), in collaboration with Intuitive Surgical, has released a beta version of the dV-trainer Movie 8: dV-trainer for robotic skills*). This is a virtual reality robotic simulator platform that provides a similar master console with finger cuff telemanipulators and binocular three-dimensional visual output. It incorporates multiple exercises for training in proper ergonomics, camera navigation, telemanipulator clutching, transfer skills, needle handling, needle driving, and suturing. This simulator uses a method known as *cross-sensory substitution*,

by which objects turn bright red if they are out of the "ergonomically ideal" position or if too much force is applied. The simulator tracking device also provides force-feedback, which may or may not have a role in the robotic skills training curriculum. Lendvay and colleagues [82] studied 27 randomized participants in an American Urological Association course for pediatric urologists to demonstrate acceptability and preliminary validity evidence that experience correlated with key performance metrics on the simulator. They are developing more accurate virtual tissue models specific to radical prostatectomy [83]. METI has just released a robotic surgery simulator (RSS) module for its SurgicalSIM platform [84].

When building any simulator, the requirement analysis follows very specific steps of development. First, it is important to determine what is intended to be accomplished and what learning domain the learning objective primarily falls into. As with any curriculum development, it is important to then define the specific learning objectives and what constitutes success and error within each domain. Next, the application must be justified and the metrics and feedback defined. The necessary sensory mode requirements, such as visual, auditory, olfactory, and tactile sensation must be delineated. It is then important to determine the best format for presentation of the simulation and whether this should be a completely immersive

* Videos for this article can be accessed by visiting www.urologic.theclinics.com. In the online table of contents for this issue, click on "add-ons."

environment or whether a two-dimensional computer screen or simple box will be sufficient. The fidelity and computer-processing requirements to accomplish these goals are then determined.

The biggest challenge of virtual reality high-fidelity simulation is modeling tissue behavior, not just gross appearance. In other words, simulation needs to mimic how the tissue responds when an instrument touches it, both visually and haptically. Finite element analysis/modeling represents the industry standard for re-creating realism, but this method is extremely time-consuming and cannot provide the user with a feeling of "real time." This becomes even more challenging when considering cutting and blunt dissection techniques. There are continuous mechanics equations of motion that involve space aspects, time aspects, collision detection, and collision response that all have to be taken into consideration. Such considerations are going into the collaborative American Urological Association–METI novel simulator designed to train transperitoneal laparoscopic nephrectomy.

Besides enhancing the realism of the simulated experience and expanding beyond basic-skills trainers toward more full "procedural" trainers, current design thrusts for simulation projects are focused on building integrated curriculum-driven trainers, not just simulators with cognitive rehearsal trainers on the front end. These integrated curriculum-driven trainers will have formative as well as summative feedback built in, creating "virtual mentorship." Rapid model conversion protocols will allow for patient-specific rehearsal and many groups are integrating training systems to provide for team-training opportunities. One of the other trends related to simulators is the movement to improve access for simulation beyond the confines of simulation centers.

Much like the forces influencing the development process, the progress of simulation and computer devices in minimally invasive surgery is being primarily driven by three forces: advances and trends in the clinical sciences, computer science/engineering, and education. In the clinical sciences, the trend of less and less "invasiveness" will obviously continue vis-à-vis Natural Orifice Transluminal Endoscopic Surgery (NOTES) and transcutaneous energy-directed ablative procedures, miniaturization and cavity-specific robotics, and femto-laser technology. In parallel, instrument design will, it is hoped, make procedures less technically challenging and reduce the steepness of the learning curve, just as the robot

has done for laparoscopic prostatectomy. Other modalities will likely integrate information, such as imaging and manipulative systems, and, via augmented reality, provide artificially intelligent intraoperative guidance [85]. All of these technologies also provide potential platforms for education and training. By reversing the master–slave concept, the integrated manipulative (robot) and visual system could take the training surgeon for a "ride" through a virtual procedure, with virtual mentorship and "intelligent tutoring." One could then predict automation of the procedure, whereby the information that the robot gathers is even more fully integrated. The resulting "black box" models created through this process would allow the robot to do certain maneuvers automatically, based on millions of "input" data points collected via memory from past procedures performed by master surgeons, until a "conflict in obvious judgment" occurs and the surgeon overtakes that particular step. This process would then contribute to the "black box" itself via hidden Markov models and other complex modeling techniques associated with artificial intelligence.

In the area of computer science/engineering, the trends of simulation and computer-assisted training will likely follow the path that video games have followed. First there was a transition from stand-alone "games" to game platforms. We are seeing this now as companies such as METI and Simbionix are steering away from single-procedure trainers toward platforms with pipelines of module development for purchase. As with gaming technology, the next phase of transition will be online, whereby a surgeon will be able to upload his or her patient's imaging dataset and then remotely rehearse the procedure on a "digital double." Also, we can expect significant advancements in the way virtual models look, interact, behave, and feel via advances in computer graphic software and hardware as well as computational mechanics and haptics. Such advancements will provide a more realistic environment in which the learner can practice and be evaluated. Advancements in training robots, multimodal sensory devices, and tracking solutions will also likely contribute to these improvements in simulated education.

Educational reform, though not a technological breakthrough, will probably have the largest impact on the future development of simulators and computer-assisted training devices. Governing bodies, such as the American College of Surgeons and the American Urological

Association, have taken steps toward the development and serious evaluation of simulators and computer-assisted devices for the purpose of residency training. The next step will be to evaluate these modalities for the more "high stakes" applications, such as credentialing and candidate screening. Research into what actually contributes to making a "good surgeon" is paramount and these devices will likely contribute to this research. Increasing emphasis is being placed on the cognitive domain and judgment of the surgeon whom simulators can now help train and assess. These devices are only as useful as the educational framework that supports them. There must be a clear understanding of the educational design, curriculum, metrics, and the very skills to be taught before embarking on a simulator development project. Through the development of standards and by following "backward design" concepts, the richness of simulation-based curriculum in urology is just beginning to be unleashed.

References

[1] Reznick RK, MacRae H. Teaching surgical skills—changes in the wind. N Engl J Med 2006;355(25): 2664–9.

[2] Das S. Susruta, the pioneer urologist of antiquity. J Urol 2001;65(5):1405–8.

[3] Kohn LT. The Institute of Medicine report on medical error: overview and implications for pharmacy. Am J Health Syst Pharm 2001;58(1):63–6.

[4] Merriam-Webster Online Dictionary Available at: http://www.m-w.com. Accessed February 12, 2008.

[5] Wilson KA, Burke CS, Priest HA, et al. Promoting health care safety through training high reliability teams. Qual Saf Health Care 2005;14(4):303–9.

[6] Moorthy K, Munz Y, Adams S, et al. A human factors analysis of technical and team skills among surgical trainees during procedural simulations in a simulated operating theatre. Ann Surg 2005; 242(5):631–9.

[7] Seymour NE, Gallagher AG, Roman SA, et al. Virtual reality training improves operating room performance: results of a randomized, double-blinded study. Ann Surg 2002;236(4):458–63 [discussion: 463–4].

[8] Norman GR. The adult learner: a mythical species. Acad Med 1999;74(8):886–9.

[9] Williams W. Effective teaching: gauging learning while teaching. J Higher Educ 1985;56(3):320–7.

[10] Davis D, O'Brien MA, Freemantle N, et al. Impact of formal continuing medical education: do conferences, workshops, rounds, and other traditional continuing education activities change physician behavior or health care outcomes? JAMA 1999; 282(9):867–74.

[11] Kolb D. Experiential learning: experience as the source of learning and development. Englewood (CO): Prentice-Hall Publishers; 1984.

[12] Gallagher AG, Ritter EM, Champion H, et al. Virtual reality simulation for the operating room: proficiency-based training as a paradigm shift in surgical skills training. Ann Surg 2005;241(2):364–72.

[13] Kahol K, Satava RM, Smith ML, et al. The effective short-term pretrial practice on surgical proficiency in simulated environments: a randomized trial of the preoperative warm up effect. (Personal Communication with Dr. Satava, submitted to J Am Coll Surg).

[14] Gallagher AG, Cates CU. Approval of virtual reality training for carotid stenting: what this means for procedural-based medicine. JAMA 2004; 292(24):3024–6.

[15] Rashid HH, Kowalewski T, Oppenheimer P, et al. The virtual reality transurethral prostatic resection trainer: evaluation of discriminate validity. J Urol 2007;177(6):2283–6.

[16] Freeman J, Cash C, Yonke A, et al. A longitudinal primary care program in an urban public medical school: three years of experience. Acad Med 1995; 70(Suppl 1):S64–8.

[17] Sachdeva AK, Pellegrini CA, Johnson KA. Support for simulation-based surgical education through American College of Surgeons–accredited education institutes. World J Surg 2008;32(2):196–207.

[18] Johnson KA, Sachdeva AK, Pellegrini CA. The critical role of accreditation in establishing the ACS Education Institutes to advance patient safety through simulation. J Gastrointest Surg 2008; 12(2):207–9.

[19] Sweet R, Hananel D, Lawrenz F. A new approach to validation, reliability and study design in technical skills training. Med Educ, submitted.

[20] Spencer F. Teaching and measuring surgical techniques: the technical evaluation of competence. Bull Am Coll Surg 1978;63:9–12.

[21] Bloom BS. Taxonomy of educational objectives. Handbook 1: the cognitive domain. New York: David McKay Co inc.; 1956.

[22] Peters JH, Fried GM, Swanstrom LL, et al. Development and validation of a comprehensive program of education and assessment of the basic fundamentals of laparoscopic surgery. Surgery 2004;135(1):21–7.

[23] Dall'Era M, Tran L, Sweet RM. An interactive computer-based simulator to train cognitive surgical skills. SanDiego (CA): Western Section AUA; 2004: Available at: http://www.redllamainc.com Accessed December 15, 2007.

[24] Moorthy K, Munz Y, Sarker SK, et al. Objective assessment of technical skills in surgery. BMJ 2003; 327(7422):1032–7.

[25] Reznick R, Regehr R, MacRae H, et al. Testing technical skill via an innovative "bench station" examination. Am J Surg 1997;173(3):226–30.

[26] Residency Competency Evaluation System. Available at: http://www.acgme.org/acWebsite/resEvalSystem/

reval_urology.asp. 2008, Accreditation Council for Graduate Medical Education. Accessed December 15, 2007.

[27] Yedidia MJ, Gillespie CC, Karchur E, et al. Effect of communications training on medical student performance. JAMA 2003;290(9):1157–65.

[28] Tubaro A. Initial experience of an objective structured clinical examination in evaluating urology residents. Curr Opin Urol 2001;11(1):110.

[29] Gettman MT, Karnes RJ, Arnold JJ, et al. Urology resident training with an unexpected patient death scenario: experiential learning with high fidelity simulation. J Urol 2008;180(1):283–6.

[30] Riley W, Davis S, Miller K, et al. High reliability healthcare: identifying and mitigating breeches in defensive barriers to reduce patient harm. In: UK Ergonomics Patient Safety Society. 2008. Cambridge.

[31] Tran L, D'allera M, Sweet RM. Validation study of a computer-based open surgical trainer: the Sim-Praxis simulation platform. Society for Simulation in Healthcare, in press.

[32] Matsumoto ED. Low-fidelity ureteroscopy models. J Endourol 2007;21(3):248–51.

[33] Brehmer M, Swartz R. Training on bench models improves dexterity in ureteroscopy. Eur Urol 2005; 48(3):458–63 [discussion: 463].

[34] Knoll T, Trojan L, Haecker A, et al. Validation of computer-based training in ureterorenoscopy. BJU Int 2005;95(9):1276–9.

[35] Ogan K, Jacomides L, Shulman MJ, et al. Virtual ureteroscopy predicts ureteroscopic proficiency of medical students on a cadaver. J Urol 2004;172(2): 667–71.

[36] Matsumoto ED, Pace KT, D'A Honey RJ. Virtual reality ureteroscopy simulator as a valid tool for assessing endourological skills. Int J Urol 2006; 13(7):896–901.

[37] Chou DS, Abdelshehid C, Clayman RV, et al. Comparison of results of virtual-reality simulator and training model for basic ureteroscopy training. J Endourol 2006;20(4):266–71.

[38] Bird VG, Fallon B, Winfield HN. Practice patterns in the treatment of large renal stones. J Endourol 2003;17(6):355–63.

[39] Watterson JD, Soon S, Jana K. Access related complications during percutaneous nephrolithotomy: urology versus radiology at a single academic institution. J Urol 2006;176(1):142–5.

[40] Hammond L, Ketchum J, Schwartz BF. A new approach to urology training: a laboratory model for percutaneous nephrolithotomy. J Urol 2004; 172(5 Pt 1):1950–2.

[41] Häcker A, Wendt-Nordahl G, Honeck P, et al. A biological model to teach percutaneous nephrolithotomy technique with ultrasound- and fluoroscopy-guided access. J Endourol 2007;21(5):545–50.

[42] Strohmaier WL, Giese A. Ex vivo training model for percutaneous renal surgery. Urol Res 2005;33(3): 191–3.

[43] Knudsen BE, Matsumoto ED, Chew BH, et al. A randomized, controlled, prospective study validating the acquisition of percutaneous renal collecting system access skills using a computer based hybrid virtual reality surgical simulator: phase I. J Urol 2006;176(5):2173–8.

[44] Gettman MT, Le CQ, Rangel LJ, et al. Analysis of a computer based simulator as an educational tool for cystoscopy: subjective and objective results. J Urol 2008;179(1):267–71.

[45] Sweet RM. Review of trainers for transurethral resection of the prostate skills. J Endourol 2007; 21(3):280–4.

[46] Wright JL, Hoffman HG, Sweet RM. Virtual reality as an adjunctive pain control during transurethral microwave thermotherapy. Urology 2005;66(6):1320. e1–1320e3.

[47] Sweet R, Kowalewski T, Oppenheimer P, et al. Face, content and construct validity of the University of Washington virtual reality transurethral prostate resection trainer. J Urol 2004;172(5 Pt 1):1953–7.

[48] Sweet R, Porter J, Oppenheimer P, et al. Simulation of bleeding in endoscopic procedures using virtual reality. J Endourol 2002;16(7):451–5.

[49] Oppenheimer P, Gupta A, Weghorst S, et al. The representation of blood flow in endourologic surgical simulations. Stud Health Technol Inform 2001; 81:365–71.

[50] Reich O, Noll M, Gratzke C, et al. High-level virtual reality simulator for endourologic procedures of lower urinary tract. Urology 2006;67(6):1144–8.

[51] Anastakis DJ, Regehr G, Reznick RK, et al. Assessment of technical skills transfer from the bench training model to the human model. Am J Surg 1999;177(2):167–70.

[52] Fried GM, Derossis AM, Bothwell J, et al. Comparison of laparoscopic performance in vivo with performance measured in a laparoscopic simulator. Surg Endosc 1999;13(11):1077–81 [discussion: 1082].

[53] Scott DJ, Bergen PC, Rege RV, et al. Laparoscopic training on bench models: better and more cost effective than operating room experience? J Am Coll Surg 2000;191(3):272–83.

[54] Van Sickle KR, McClusky DA, Gallagher AG, et al. Construct validation of the ProMIS simulator using a novel laparoscopic suturing task. Surg Endosc 2005;19(9):1227–31.

[55] McCluney AL, Vassiliou MC, Kaneva PA, et al. FLS simulator performance predicts intraoperative laparoscopic skill. Surg Endosc 2007;21(11): 1991–5.

[56] Botden SM, Buznik SN, Schijven MP, et al. Augmented versus virtual reality laparoscopic simulation: What is the difference? A comparison of the ProMIS augmented reality laparoscopic simulator versus LapSim virtual reality laparoscopic simulator. World J Surg 2007;31(4):764–72.

[57] Ritter EM, Kindelan TW, Michael C, et al. Concurrent validity of augmented reality metrics applied to

the fundamentals of laparoscopic surgery (FLS). Surg Endosc 2007;21(8):1441–5.

[58] Fichera A, Prachand V, Kives S, et al. Physical reality simulation for training of laparoscopists in the 21st century. A multispecialty, multi-institutional study. JSLS 2005;9(2):125–9.

[59] Hasson HM, Kumari NV, Eekhout J. Training simulator for developing laparoscopic skills. JSLS 2001; 5(3):255–65.

[60] Sørhus V, Eriksen EM, Grønningsaeter N, et al. A new platform for laparoscopic training and education. Stud Health Technol Inform 2005; 111:502–7.

[61] van Dongen KW, Tournoij E, van der Zee DC, et al. Construct validity of the LapSim: Can the LapSim virtual reality simulator distinguish between novices and experts? Surg Endosc 2007;21(8):1413–7.

[62] Hogle NJ, Briggs WM, Fowler DL. Documenting a learning curve and test-retest reliability of two tasks on a virtual reality training simulator in laparoscopic surgery. J Surg Educ 2007;64(6):424–30.

[63] Woodrum DT, Andreatta PB, Yellamanchilli RK, et al. Construct validity of the LapSim laparoscopic surgical simulator. Am J Surg 2006;191(1):28–32.

[64] Eriksen JR, Grantcharov T. Objective assessment of laparoscopic skills using a virtual reality stimulator. Surg Endosc 2005;19(9):1216–9.

[65] Duffy AJ, Hogle NJ, McCarthy H, et al. Construct validity for the LAPSIM laparoscopic surgical simulator. Surg Endosc 2005;19(3):401–5.

[66] Rodriguez-Covarrubias F, Martinez-Liévano L, Gabilondo Pliego B, et al. [Use of a virtual immersion computer simulator as a model for basic training in laparoscopic urology]. Actas Urol Esp 2006; 30(8):819–23 [in Spanish].

[67] Maass H, Chantier C, Trantakis C, et al. Fundamentals of force feedback and application to a surgery simulator. Comput Aided Surg 2003;8(6):283–91.

[68] McDougall EM, Corica FA, Boker JR, et al. Construct validity testing of a laparoscopic surgical simulator. J Am Coll Surg 2006;202(5):779–87.

[69] Ayodeji ID, Schijven M, Jakimowicz J, et al. Face validation of the Simbionix LAP Mentor virtual reality training module and its applicability in the surgical curriculum. Surg Endosc 2007;21(9):1641–9.

[70] Yamaguchi S, Konishi K, Yasunaga T, et al. Construct validity for eye-hand coordination skill on a virtual reality laparoscopic surgical simulator. Surg Endosc 2007;21(12):2253–7.

[71] Zhang A, Hünerbein M, Dai Y, et al. Construct validity testing of a laparoscopic surgery simulator (Lap Mentor): Evaluation of surgical skill with a virtual laparoscopic training simulator. Surg Endosc 2008;22(6):1440–4.

[72] Chaudhry A, Sutton C, Wood J, et al. Learning rate for laparoscopic surgical skills on MIST VR, a virtual reality simulator: quality of human-computer interface. Ann R Coll Surg Engl 1999;81(4): 281–6.

[73] Hackethal A, Immenroth M, Burger T. Evaluation of target scores and benchmarks for the traversal task scenario of the minimally invasive surgical trainer–virtual reality (MIST-VR) laparoscopy simulator. Surg Endosc 2006;20(4):645–50.

[74] Aggarwal R, Grantcharov T, Moorthy K, et al. A competency-based virtual reality training curriculum for the acquisition of laparoscopic psychomotor skill. Am J Surg 2006;191(1):128–33.

[75] Chung SY, Landsittel D, Chon CH, et al. Laparoscopic skills training using a webcam trainer. J Urol 2005;173(1):180–3.

[76] Verdaasdonk EG, Dankelman J, Lange JF, et al. Transfer validity of laparoscopic knot-tying training on a VR simulator to a realistic environment: a randomized controlled trial. Surg Endosc 2008;22(7): 1636–42.

[77] Verdaasdonk EG, Stassen LP, Monteny LJ, et al. Validation of a new basic virtual reality simulator for training of basic endoscopic skills: the SIMENDO. Surg Endosc 2006;20(3):511–8.

[78] Verdaasdonk EG, Stassen LP, Schijven MP, et al. Construct validity and assessment of the learning curve for the SIMENDO endoscopic simulator. Surg Endosc 2007;21(8):1406–12.

[79] Hubens G, Coveliers H, Balliu L, et al. A performance study comparing manual and robotically assisted laparoscopic surgery using the da Vinci system. Surg Endosc 2003;17(10):1595–9.

[80] Harper JD, Kaiser S, Edrahimi K, et al. Prior video game exposure does not enhance robotic surgical performance. J Endourol 2007;21(10):1207–10.

[81] Samadi D, Levinson A, Hakimi A, et al. From proficiency to expert, when does the learning curve for robotic-assisted prostatectomies plateau? The Columbia University experience. World J Urol 2007;25(1):105–10.

[82] Lendvay T, Casale P, Sweet RM, et al. Virtual reality simulation for robotic surgery. Surg Endosc, submitted.

[83] Rashid H, Bekley J, Vollenweider M, et al. Creating a patient specific interactive virtual reality model for robotic prostatectomy. J Endourol 2006; 20(Suppl 1):A326.

[84] Halvorsen FH, Elle OJ, Dalinin VV, et al. Virtual reality simulator training equals mechanical robotic training in improving robot-assisted basic suturing skills. Surg Endosc 2006;20(10):1565–9.

[85] Satava RM. Disruptive visions: a robot is not a machine. Surg Endosc 2004;18(4):617–20.

ELSEVIER
SAUNDERS

Urol Clin N Am 35 (2008) 533–542

UROLOGIC
CLINICS
of North America

Index

Note: Page numbers of article titles are in **boldface** type.

Moving?

Make sure your subscription moves with you!

To notify us of your new address, find your **Clinics Account Number** (located on your mailing label above your name), and contact customer service at:

E-mail: elspcs@elsevier.com

800-654-2452 (subscribers in the U.S. & Canada)
1-407-563-6020 (subscribers outside of the U.S. & Canada)

Fax number: 407-363-9661

Elsevier Periodicals Customer Service
6277 Sea Harbor Drive
Orlando, FL 32887-4800

*To ensure uninterrupted delivery of your subscription, please notify us at least 4 weeks in advance of move.